Understanding Medical Research
The Studies That Shaped Medicine

EDITED BY

John A. Goodfellow BM BCh, PhD
Honorary Clinical Academic Fellow
University of Glasgow
Glasgow, UK

WITH FOREWORD BY

Sir Liam Donaldson
Chief Medical Officer, 1998-2010
Department of Health
London, UK

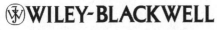

WILEY-BLACKWELL
A John Wiley & Sons, Ltd., Publication

Wiley-Blackwell is an imprint of John Wiley & Sons, formed by the merger of Wileys global Scientific, Technical and Medical business with Blackwell Publishing.

Registered office: John Wiley & Sons, Ltd, The Atrium, Southern Gate, Chichester, West Sussex, PO19 8SQ, UK

Editorial offices: 9600 Garsington Road, Oxford, OX4 2DQ, UK

The Atrium, Southern Gate, Chichester, West Sussex, PO19 8SQ, UK

111 River Street, Hoboken, NJ 07030-5774, USA

For details of our global editorial offices, for customer services and for information about how to apply for permission to reuse the copyright material in this book please see our website at www.wiley.com/wiley-blackwell.

Library of Congress Cataloging-in-Publication Data

Understanding medical research : the studies that shaped medicine / edited by
John A. Goodfellow ; with foreword by Sir Liam Donaldson.
       p. ; cm.
   Includes bibliographical references and index.
   ISBN 9780470654484 (pbk.)
   I. Goodfellow, John A.
   [DNLM: 1. Biomedical Research. 2. Peer Review, Research. W 20.5]
   LC classification not assigned
   610.72'4- -dc23

2011030825

A catalogue record for this book is available from the British Library.

Wiley also publishes its books in a variety of electronic formats. Some content that appears in print may not be available in electronic books.

Set in 9/11.5pt Minion by Thomson Digital, Noida, India
Printed and bound in Malaysia by Vivar Printing Sdn Bhd

1   2012

Understanding
Medical Research

To my wife Rosalyn

Contents

Contributors

Raza Alikhan
Consultant Haematologist
Haemophilia and Thrombosis Centre
University Hospital of Wales
Cardiff, UK

Nigel Arden
Professor of Rheumatology
Botnar Research Centre
Institute of Musculoskeletal Sciences
University of Oxford
Oxford, UK

Peter J. Barnes
Professor and Head of Respiratory Medicine
Airway Disease Section
National Heart and Lung Institute
Imperial College London
London, UK

Philip M.W. Bath
Professor of Stroke Medicine
Stroke Association
Division of Stroke
School of Clinical Sciences
University of Nottingham
Nottingham, UK

Colin Berry
Professor and Honorary Consultant
Physician and Cardiologist
BHF Glasgow Cardiovascular Research
Centre
University of Glasgow
Glasgow, UK

Alistair Burns
Professor of Old Age Psychiatry
Department of Old Age Psychiatry
School of Medicine
University of Manchester
Manchester, UK

Andrew K. Burroughs
Consultant Physician and Professor of
Hepatology
Royal Free Sheila Sherlock Liver Centre
Royal Free Hospital
London, UK

Andrew Bush
Professor of Paediatric Respirology
Imperial College London and Royal
Brompton Hospital
London, UK

Geraldine Cambridge
Principal Research Fellow and Honorary
Senior Lecturer in Rheumatology
Centre for Rheumatology
Division of Medicine
University College London
London, UK

Alasdair Coles
University Lecturer in Neuroimmunology
Department of Clinical Neurosciences
University of Cambridge
Cambridge, UK

Alastair Compston
Professor of Neurology
Department of Clinical Neurosciences
University of Cambridge
Cambridge, UK

Philip J. Cowen
Professor of Psychopharmacology
Department of Psychiatry
University of Oxford
Oxford, UK

Martin R. Cowie
Professor of Cardiology
National Heart and Lung Institute
Imperial College London
London, UK

Robert J.O. Davies
Professor of Respiratory Medicine
Respiratory Medicine Group
Experimental Medicine Division
University of Oxford
Oxford, UK

Sir Liam Donaldson
Chief Medical Officer for England and UK
Government Chief Medical Adviser
1998–2010
Department of Health
London, UK

Anahita Dua
Department of General Surgery
Medical College of Wisconsin
Milwaukee, Wisconsin, USA

Jonathan C.W. Edwards
Professor in Connective Tissue Medicine
Centre for Rheumatology
Division of Medicine
University College London
London, UK

Emad M. El-Omar
Professor of Gastroenterology
Gastrointestinal Group
Institute of Medical Sciences School of
Medicine & Dentistry Aberdeen University
Aberdeen, UK

Paul A. Ford
Senior Clinical Research Fellow
Airway Disease Section
National Heart and Lung Institute
Imperial College London
London, UK

John A. Goodfellow
Honorary Clinical Academic Fellow
Neuroimmunology Group
Division of Clinical Neuroscience
University of Glasgow
Glasgow, UK

Kaushik Guha
Clinical Research Fellow
National Heart and Lung Institute
Imperial College London
London, UK

Felix Greaves
Public Health Registrar and Clinical Research
Fellow
Department of Primary Care and Public
Health
Imperial College London
London, UK

Donald G. Grosset
Consultant Neurologist and Honorary Senior
Lecturer in Neurology
Greater Glasgow Movement Disorder Clinic
Institute of Neurological Sciences
Southern General Hospital
Glasgow, UK

Philip Home
Chair of Diabetes Medicine
Institute of Cellular Medicine
University of Newcastle upon Tyne
Newcastle, UK

Dame Eve C. Johnstone
Professor and Head of Division of Psychiatry
Centre for Clinical Brain Sciences
University Department of Psychiatry
University of Edinburgh
Edinburgh, UK

Mandy Johnstone
Clinical Lecturer in Psychiatry
Centre for Clinical Brain Sciences
University Department of Psychiatry
University of Edinburgh
Edinburgh, UK

Maria J. Leandro
Honorary Senior Lecturer
Centre for Rheumatology
Division of Medicine
University College London
London, UK

Tak H. Lee
Asthma UK Professor of Allergy and
Respiratory Medicine
Division of Asthma, Allergy and Lung Biology
Kings College London
London, UK

Wei Yao Lim
Academic Foundation Trainee
BHF Glasgow Cardiovascular Research
Centre
University of Glasgow
Glasgow, UK

Raashid Luqmani
Senior Lecturer in Rheumatology
Nuffield Department of Orthopaedics,
Rheumatology and Musculoskeletal Sciences
University of Oxford
Oxford, UK

Eleanor K. Mishra
Research Fellow
Oxford Centre for Respiratory Medicine
University of Oxford
Oxford, UK

Stanley Nattel
Associate Professor
Department of Medicine
Montreal Heart Institute
Université de Montreal
Canada

Edward J. Newman
Clinical Lecturer in Neurology
Greater Glasgow Movement Disorder Clinic
Institute of Neurological Sciences
Southern General Hospital
Glasgow, UK

Alexander S. Nicholls
Botnar Research Centre
Institute of Musculoskeletal Sciences
University of Oxford
Oxford, UK

Kunihiro Nishida
Assistant Professor
The Second Department
of Internal Medicine
University of Toyama
Toyama, Japan

Douglas Noble
Public Health Registrar and Honorary
Clinical Lecturer
Centre for Health Sciences
Barts and the London School of Medicine
and Dentistry
London, UK

James O'Beirne
Consultant Hepatologist
Royal Free Sheila Sherlock Liver Centre
Royal Free Hospital
London, UK

Jenny Papakrivopoulou
NIHR Clinical Lecturer in Nephrology
UCL Centre for Nephrology
Royal Free Hospital
London, UK

Charles Percy
Specialty Registrar in Haematology
Haemophilia and Thrombosis Centre
University Hospital of Wales
Cardiff, UK

Tica Pichulik
MRC Human Immunology Unit
Weatherall Institute of Molecular Medicine
University of Oxford
Oxford, UK

Qi Qian
Lecturer in Internal Medicine and
Nephrology
Division of Nephrology and Hypertension
Department of Internal Medicine
Mayo Clinic
Rochester, Minnesota, USA

Joanna Robson
Rheumatology Registrar
Nuffield Department of Orthopaedics,
Rheumatology and Musculoskeletal Sciences
University of Oxford
Oxford, UK

Fergus J. Rugg-Gunn
Consultant Neurologist
Department of Clinical and Experimental
Epilepsy
National Hospital for Neurology and
Neurosurgery
Queen Square
London, UK

Leonard Siew
Clinical Research Fellow
Department of Asthma, Allergy and
Respiratory Science
Kings College London
London, UK

Alison Simmons
Senior Clinical Lecturer
MRC Human Immunology Unit
Weatherall Institute of Molecular Medicine
University of Oxford
Oxford, UK

Dame Elizabeth Simpson
Emeritus Professor of Transplantation
Biology
Division of Immunology and Inflammation
Imperial College London
London, UK

Anushka Soni
Botnar Research Centre
Institute of Musculoskeletal Sciences
University of Oxford
Oxford, UK

Nikola Sprigg
Clinical Associate Professor
Division of Stroke
School of Clinical Sciences
University of Nottingham
Nottingham, UK

Ravi Suppiah
Rheumatology Clinical Fellow
Nuffield Department of Orthopaedics,
Rheumatology and Musculoskeletal Sciences
University of Oxford
Oxford, UK

Kevin Talbot
Professor of Motor Neuron Biology and
Honorary Consultant Neurologist
Oxford Motor Neuron Disease Centre and
Department of Clinical Neurology
University of Oxford
Oxford, UK

Gilbert R. Thompson
Emeritus Professor of Clinical Lipidology
Department of Medicine
Imperial College London
London, UK

Martin R. Turner
Lady Edith Wolfson Clinician Scientist and
Honorary Consultant Neurologist
Oxford Motor Neuron Disease Centre and
Department of Clinical Neurology
University of Oxford
Oxford, UK

Robert Unwin
Professor of Nephrology and Physiology
UCL Centre for Nephrology
Royal Free Hospital
London, UK

Sir David Weatherall
Regius Professor of Medicine Emeritus
Weatherall Institute of Molecular Medicine
University of Oxford
Oxford, UK
Chancellor
Keele University
Keele, UK

Mark W. Weatherall
Consultant Neurologist
Princess Margaret Migraine Clinic
Department of Clinical Neurology
Charing Cross Hospital
London, UK

Kirsten White
Botnar Research Centre
Institute of Musculoskeletal Sciences
University of Oxford
Oxford, UK

Gordon Wilcock
Professor of Clinical Geratology
Dementia Clinical Research Group
Experimental Medicine Division
University of Oxford
Oxford, UK

Hugh J. Willison
Professor of Neurology
Neuroimmunology Group
Division of Clinical Neuroscience
University of Glasgow
Glasgow, UK

John M. Wrightson
Clinical Research Fellow and Respiratory
Specialist Registrar
Oxford Centre for Respiratory Medicine
University of Oxford
Oxford, UK

Preface

Ars longa, vita brevis, occasio praeceps, experimentum periculosum, iudicium difficile.
[The art (of medicine) is long, life is short, opportunity fleeting, experiment treacherous, judgment difficult.]

Hippocrates

Understanding Medical Research is aimed at giving medical students and junior doctors a concise and authoritative overview of the landmark papers in medical research. Rather than summarising only recent developments, as review articles do, in each chapter the authors discuss ten or so papers that have contributed most to our understanding of the topic. It is distinct from *evidence-based medicine* in that it doesn't aim to summarise the 'best available' trial data; rather, it summarises the unique blend of science and pragmatism that has come together to form medical practice.

Such an enterprise is obviously a huge challenge to the authors, and I have allowed them some flexibility in how they approach this. For most a chronological approach is taken, but for some, such as the chapters on stroke, population health and patient safety, a slightly different approach is used. Regardless, the effect is the same: an authoritative summary of the key papers from people at the cutting edge of research.

The range of studies included is broad: from famous randomised clinical trials down to obscure case studies and biochemical reports. Likewise the range of journals from which the articles are selected is equally broad, although one or two recur again and again. These are the papers and journals that have changed our understanding of medicine, and every doctor should be familiar with them.

The reader should use this book as a starting point from which to enter the world of research. The chapters will give you a 'big-picture' overview of the topic. This will put you in an ideal place to then put into context current studies and clinical practice, and to formulate your own research questions.

JOHN A. GOODFELLOW

Foreword

Modern medicine is a discipline that over the last 150 years has developed in response to changing patterns of human disease, scientific understanding and technology. As such its origins, paradigm shifts and breakthroughs have at times come from human ingenuity, scientific scrutiny and serendipity. Much contemporary focus is rightly on determining best clinical practice through rigorous and tightly controlled clinical trials. However, this is only one part of the story of medicine in any given field. *Understanding Medical Research* is a book that seeks to give the reader a succinct and lively account of the colourful research that has made clinical practice what it is today.

For example, the 'shoe-leather epidemiology' of the great physician John Snow looks rather primitive in its methodology to the modern doctor: walking the streets of London to gather data by knocking on doors! This would not earn him a high-impact publication in today's journals, yet his painstaking observations allowed him to go beyond the 'miasma' theory of cholera and propose a waterborne pathogen, before even the germ theory of disease itself was widely accepted! Not to mention the countless lives he directly saved.

Not many of us have seen a case of familial hypercholesterolaemia; fewer still have read Goldstein and Brown's technical article on lipid metabolism in fibroblasts from patients with this disorder in a 1974 issue of the *Journal of Biological Chemistry*. However, we prescribe millions of statins on a daily basis and their Nobel Prize winning work began with this diligent piece of work. Other Nobel Prize winners have begun with more of a flair: the Australian gastroenterology registrar who, determined to convince rightly sceptical colleagues of his new theory on gastric ulcers, uses himself in an '*n* of one' trial by simply walking into his laboratory and swallowing a vial of *H. pylori*.

Of course, many of the most significant publications have been large, well-conducted trials. The Framingham study for example established a standard, perhaps never to be replicated, in conducting long-term observational studies on a large scale. So much of what we now believe about hypertension, ischaemic heart disease and much more comes directly from this mammoth enterprise. Or the trials in heart failure – CONSENSUS, RALES and many others – that now allow us to know with great confidence which drugs really work and save lives.

Understanding Medical Research is an attempt to put in one place these very different types of studies which have come together to shape modern medicine. I hope that in reading it you develop the same sense of enthusiasm and excitement about medicine with which the authors have written.

SIR LIAM DONALDSON

Acknowledgements

First and foremost I must thank each of the authors who have given their time, expertise and energy in making this textbook what it is. It isn't hard to get academics to talk about what they love, but nonetheless it is easy to underestimate the time needed to carefully and succinctly summarise a whole field of research, and to do so in the midst of busy academic and clinical commitments. Your efforts have been legion and will provide a generation of medical students and junior doctors with an introduction to the vast volumes of medical research.

My thanks to the whole team at Wiley-Blackwell in Oxford, particularly Elizabeth Johnston for giving the project a chance when it was just an idea in a medical student's head, and Karen Moore for her endless patience in putting the manuscript together.

Thanks to Sir Liam Donaldson for providing the Foreword.

A final thanks to a few fellow medics who encouraged me along the way: Jakub Scaber, Charles Williams and Wei Yao Lim.

1 Population Health

Douglas Noble[1], Felix Greaves[2] and Sir Liam Donaldson[3]

[1]Centre for Health Sciences, Barts and the London School of Medicine and Dentistry, London, UK
[2]Department of Primary Care and Public Health, Imperial College London, London, UK
[3]Chief Medical Officer, 1998–2010, Department of Health, London, UK

Introduction

There are many reasons why a paper could be selected as 'important' in public health. Some studies of the epidemiology of a disease have led to a clear understanding of their causation and opened up the scope for prevention. Iconic population studies of cancer, cardiovascular disease and industrial disease fall into this category. Other papers based on observational epidemiological studies of the pattern of disease by time, place or person have also made the case for public health action. Sometimes these have galvanised passion and commitment over long periods of time. Some studies of health inequalities will be seen in this way. Yet again, some contributions have laid the foundation of a new framework or approach to understanding public health problems or acting on them. Often they are associated with particular figures in history who have been the inspiration and guiding light for generations of public health practitioners. In selecting 'important' papers for this chapter, we have drawn from all these areas, recognising that in choosing these many other candidates for inclusion have been laid aside.

Shoe-Leather Epidemiology
Snow, London, 1855

> *Each epidemic of cholera in London has borne a strict relation to the nature of the water supply of its different districts, being modified only by poverty, and the crowding and want of cleanliness which always attend it.*

There are few doctors who can claim two places in medicine's hall of fame, but the Victorian physician John Snow (1813–1858) was one. Celebrated in the history of anaesthetics, he helped to develop the early scientific basis for deploying gases to sedate and relieve pain, then popularised their use by administering chloroform to Queen Victoria during childbirth.

Snow's contribution to public health was arguably even greater. Born in York, and apprenticed to a surgeon in Newcastle upon Tyne, Snow gravitated to London where he found himself in the midst of the great cholera outbreak of 1854. Cholera was one of

---

Understanding Medical Research: The Studies that Shaped Medicine, First Edition. Edited by John A. Goodfellow. © 2012 John Wiley & Sons, Ltd. Published 2012 by John Wiley & Sons, Ltd.

the major pandemic disease scourges of the 19th century. It took the lives of thousands in all walks of life, but particularly the poor who lived in filthy and overcrowded dwellings in the towns and cities of the industrial revolution. It struck fear and despair into the population. The prevailing and firmly held theory on its cause was that it arose in the form of an invisible and noxious gas seeping from rotting vegetation and decaying corpses.

Snow debunked this 'miasma' theory with a painstaking piece of public health detective work. He was perhaps the greatest exponent of so-called shoe-leather epidemiology. He quite literally walked the streets of London for weeks, gathering information, talking to people, recording deaths and mapping them. He concluded that the source of the outbreak was a water pump in Broad Street, Soho that had been contaminated by raw sewage. That explained the clustering of cholera deaths of residents in the street near the pump, but it did not explain cases occurring further afield (Figure 1.1). Snow had the answer. His enquiries showed him that a woman had her water sent from the pump because, over the years, she preferred the taste. He explained other exceptions. Snow petitioned the local parish, and the pump handle was removed and the epidemic waned. Some experts dispute whether it was declining anyway.

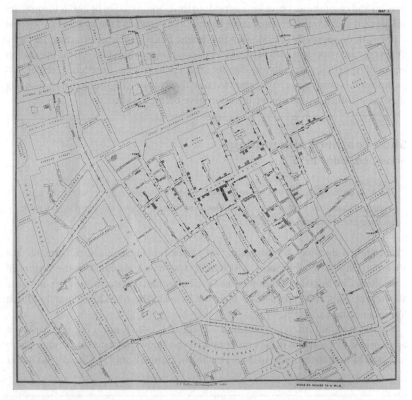

Figure 1.1 Mapping of cases around Broad Street pump. Reproduced with permission from Snow, London, 1855. © British Library Board.

In a less dramatic but equally important piece of work, Snow analysed the rates of attack from cholera in houses supplied by different London water companies. He found that two of these companies drew their supplies from the lower and most polluted parts of the Thames. Snow wrote up his findings in his celebrated monograph and postulated that a transmissible water-borne agent was the cause of cholera. His views were not accepted by establishment opinion at the time, and it would be many years before his conclusions were universally accepted, as the 'germ theory' of disease became established.

Smoking and Cancer: Association and Causality
Doll and Hill, British Medical Journal (1950)

It must be concluded that there is a real association between carcinoma of the lung and smoking.

The early part of the 20th century saw an explosion in the accuracy of collection of epidemiological information. Despite this increased reporting and enquiry, lung cancer incidence appeared to be dramatically increasing. Between 1922 and 1947 the yearly rate of cases causing death had risen from 612 to 9287 in England and Wales. This trend was being observed internationally. Doll and Hill hypothesised that the smoking of tobacco could be causal in the development of lung cancer.

Their first preliminary description in the *British Medical Journal* in 1950 reported on a case-control study in London hospitals. They compared patients with lung cancer versus inpatients with other diseases. Careful epidemiological study involved identifying suitable controls at the level of the hospital ward, within the same age group and of the same sex.

The most striking data revealed that both male and female smokers were more likely to have lung cancer compared with other diseases (males: 647/649 versus 622/649, $p < 0.05$; females: 41/60 versus 28/60, $p < 0.02$).

Further analysis of amount of smoking revealed that for males, increasing numbers of cigarettes per day equated with a higher likelihood of lung cancer (Figure 1.2).

There were many possible biases. The samples only represented London hospital patients and controls. The case-control method, whilst ideal for this type of study, has inherent weaknesses of recall bias, especially in cases where there is an increased likelihood of remembering possible causal factors when faced with severe terminal disease.

Despite these criticisms a compelling case for smoking being statistically associated with lung cancer had been made. Causality could not be proven from this study; Austin Bradford Hill himself was to develop a framework for implying causality, which would rest on far more than just statistical association. Yet the authors continued their quest to prove causality, publishing regularly on smoking and lung cancer from 1950 to 2004, including the famous study examining smoking habits and mortality in British doctors.

Doll and Hill not only went on to show conclusively the link between lung cancer and smoking, but also established smoking as a cause of premature death, as well as demonstrating causality with heart disease and other illnesses. Studies in the United States around the same time revealed the same findings.

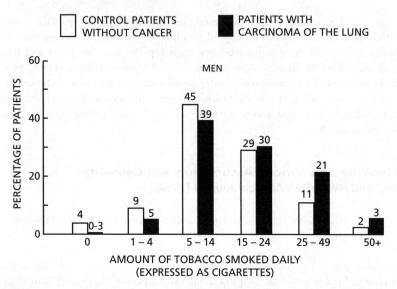

Figure 1.2 Increasing numbers of cigarettes per day equated with a higher likelihood of lung cancer. Reproduced with permission from Doll and Hill, *British Medical Journal* (1950), with permission from BMJ Publishing Group Ltd.

In the short term, Doll and Hill's paper had little influence on behaviour. Health education advice to the public was slow to emerge from the Ministry of Health as the powerful influence of the tobacco industry held sway. Their later longitudinal study of smoking amongst doctors, showing the now familiar smoking-related disease patterns, and the reduction of risk for quitters, ignited the war against tobacco. It is a war that is still being fought today around the world as the impact of tobacco on health is as great as any of the historical infectious disease pandemics. Doll and Hill's first study, however, remains the foundation stone of evidence from which the impetus for all subsequent public health progress was built.

The Inverse Care Law
Hart, Lancet (1971)

> *In areas with most sickness and death, general practitioners have more work, larger lists, less hospital support, and inherit more clinically ineffective traditions of consultation, than in the healthiest areas.*

Some papers in the history of public health have been influential less for the underpinning analysis than for the central idea that they communicate. It is no coincidence that the terminology used to describe the idea is often memorable in its own right. Julian Tudor-Hart practised for a whole professional lifetime as a general practitioner in one of the most deprived communities in Wales. Passionate about the links between poverty and poor health, angry about the opportunities for healthier lives denied to the populations he served and convinced of the benefits of a National

Health Service unfettered by the need to pay, he practised, researched and campaigned with equal passion.

He formulated the following principle: 'The availability of good medical care tends to vary inversely with the need for the population served'. Stated more simply, those who most need healthcare get less of it, whilst those who need less get more.

Hart based his assertion on a series of different sources of evidence. This included the observation that general practitioners saw more poor than wealthier patients, but with inadequate time to treat properly or keep themselves adequately skilled. The incentive was full waiting rooms, with each patient paying a low fee that resulted in a tidy profit. There were also quantitative studies that indicated the unfairness. In 1961 a study of 1370 patients and 552 doctors revealed that for the middle classes younger than 45 years old, general practitioner attendances were more than 50% less compared to working classes. However, over 75, the pattern was reversed. Hart infers that this leads to the conclusion that for all ages the middle classes received higher quality care.

The fabric of healthcare facilities also reflected the trend. In working-class areas 80% of practices were built before 1900, compared to 50% in middle-class areas.

The skill and time of doctors followed suit. In middle-class areas lists under 2000 were more common; four times as many general practitioners had a degree from Oxford or Cambridge; double the number had post-graduate qualifications; and five times as many had ready availability of physiotherapy. Hart argues this is because of the preponderance of higher social classes in medical school.

Hart showed himself a canny and brilliant advocate of his ideas. Years later he admitted that he had thought long and hard about what to call his principle. He thought of the 'inverse square law' which all adults would remember from their school mathematics classes. With one change of word he had the 'inverse care law', a term that has endured and continued to inspire idealists and pragmatists alike.

Framingham and the Heart
Dawber et al., American Journal of Public Health (1951)

> The study is focused on arteriosclerotic and hypertensive cardiovascular disease, because these are the most important of the cardiovascular diseases and the least is known about their epidemiology.

Epidemiologists often dream of 'population laboratories' – places which make sense in social and geographical terms, where the community is relatively stable, where data on health status are comprehensively collected and where partnership with the local community can be made with willing participants in generating evidence that will provide deep insights into disease causation and the scope for prevention. Framingham, Massachusetts, United States was such a place.

The Framingham heart study, established in 1948, studied cardiovascular disease over time. Naming one paper is problematic given that over 1000 studies have been published linked to this program. The study population initially included over 5000 participants of both sexes, ages 30–62, who had not experienced any symptoms of cardiovascular disease. Each of the participants initially underwent lifestyle interviews and detailed physical examinations. Participants returned every two years for continued follow-up, including medical histories, examination and laboratory investigations. In the 1970s the research extended the study to include over 5000 of the initial cohort's offspring and their partners. Over the last 20 years, it has continued to evolve and successive new groups of participants have been added, including the grandchildren of the first group.

The Framingham cohorts have allowed causality to be established between a range of risk factors and cardiovascular disease. These have included diabetes mellitus, hypercholesteroleamia, hypertension, lack of exercise, obesity and smoking. These core findings have transformed the understanding of cardiovascular disease the world over; few patients with symptoms suggestive of cardiovascular disease would fail to be screened for these core risk factors. They are comprehensive in establishing risk of disease and formative in determining individual patient management plans and population-level public health interventions. Findings have also included the link between cardiovascular disease and demographic factors, such as age and sex.

Ecological studies of this sort are complex to manage. They are susceptible to a well-described error, the ecological fallacy. This infers that the overall aggregated population statistics will apply to any one individual member of the population, which may not be true given the varying characteristics of every individual member of that population. Furthermore, the generalisability of the study to populations distinct from Caucasian Americans has been questioned. Yet, despite these epidemiological limitations, the principal findings have been reproduced in independent studies in many other population groups.

Much of the knowledge the world formed about the risks of cardiovascular disease initially came from the Framingham study. It set a new standard for the organisation and quality of methodologies needed to run effective large-scale longitudinal studies of natural populations.

The Evidence-Based Revolution
Cochrane, London, 1989

> It is surely a great criticism of our profession that we have not organised a critical summary, by specialty or subspecialty, adapted periodically, of all relevant randomised controlled trials

At a march before the Second World War to advocate the introduction of a national health service, participants were given placards which read 'All healthcare should be free'. One young marcher, Archie Cochrane, a medical student, amended his sign to read: 'All effective healthcare should be free'. Nearly 80 years later, that student's insight is astonishing. Health services and patients around the world continue to waste large sums of money on treatments that either do no good or actively harm people.

Cochrane was one of the generation of British doctors who fought fascism in the Spanish Civil War. He then came back to make his career in public health, for much of it carrying out seminal studies of lung disease with the population of the Welsh Valleys, many of them dominated by mining. He came to wider attention, though, through the publication of an extended essay which laid the foundation for the modern concept of evidence-based healthcare.

Cochrane's compelling thesis demanded that clinical practice be based on evidence of effectiveness and not reliant solely on tradition or subjective opinion. This was of profound public health significance effectively calling for a paradigm shift from gross and wasteful clinical variation to evidence-based treatments.

He argued for more than just evidence-based practice and policies. He recognised the age-old public health paradigm that demand always outstrips supply. In face of this truth of scarce resources, he upheld that intervention should always be based on evidence, not clinical preference or hearsay.

Critics warned that individual patients would be disadvantaged with treatments that may have been proven for a population of patients, but were not necessarily effective for individuals. Yet despite these objections, over the next 40 years evidence has become the cornerstone of modern clinical practice. Medical students are versed internationally with the critical appraisal demanded by Cochrane for medical intervention: 'What is the evidence for effectiveness?'

Cochrane advocated the use of randomised control trials as the highest form of medical evidence. Today the Cochrane name is immortalised in the Cochrane Library and Cochrane Collaboration. These resources are sustained by the tireless work of experts in all corners of the world who provide an accessible, readable database of world-class evidence for medical practice in multiple specialities.

The Black Report
Black Report, London (1980)

> *It will come as a disappointment to many that over long periods since the inception of the NHS there is generally little sign of health inequalities in Britain actually diminishing and in some cases, they may be increasing.*

Ever since the gathering of statistics on population health began, epidemiologists have used them to study the pattern of disease in the triad of time, place and person. For almost all diseases, causes of death, or known risk factors to health there is a gradient. The worst health is found amongst those in the lowest strata of society. This has been examined by social class (defined by occupation) or socioeconomic status as well as by comparing communities according to various population indices of deprivation.

The gap between the health of the worst and the least deprived has at different points of the United Kingdom's history been very wide. At times it has narrowed, but it has never closed. Globally the gap in health status between rich and poor communities is quite shocking.

The Black report did not coin the term 'health inequalities' to describe this phenomenon, but it did bring it to wider prominence and public attention.

Sir Douglas Andrew Kilgour Black was commissioned in 1977 by David Ennals, the Labour Government's Secretary of State for Health, to write a review on the state of health inequalities in the United Kingdom. A general election intervened, and the final report was received by an incoming Conservative government led by Margaret Thatcher.

Black's thesis stated that haphazard policy making leading to highly variable public services was important in causality, not just that the differences were accounted for by differences in social mobility, lifestyle, economic or educational factors.

Controversially he advocated radical societal changes, including limiting the advertising of tobacco, as well as changes to benefits.

The legacy of the Black Report has endured for three main reasons. Firstly, it was the first report since Victorian times to provide a comprehensive and compelling analysis of the key statistics linked to a proposed strategic programme of action. Secondly, it was led by a mainstream medical figure who could not be dismissed as a public health idealist or radical. Thirdly, the method of publication of the report (plain cover, limited print run, release over a bank holiday weekend) made it a *cause célèbre*.

Many reports and books have followed. Sadly, the problem of health inequalities in the United Kingdom and worldwide persists. However, the centrality of health inequality to government policy making and NHS strategy is impressive. It is a transformation that would not have been possible without the touchstone of the original Black Report.

The Prevention Paradox
Rose, British Medical Journal (1981)

> But, however much it [the public health intervention] may offer to the community as a whole, it offers little to each participating individual.

Geoffrey Rose described the concept, the prevention paradox: 'a measure that brings large benefits to the community offers little to each participating individual'.

Firstly, Rose deals with prevention at an individual level. Captured by the story of the man who arrives to see his doctor and is discovered to have high blood pressure, the man leaves a patient, confirmed by the endowing of pills. Rose confirms the perception that doctors do not traditionally interfere with men, only patients. Yet, in the above scenario this is not therapeutics; it is preventive medicine.

Secondly, intervention may have a high relative risk reduction, but if the population at risk is small in comparison to the whole population, absolute risk reduction will be less significant. Decision making, Rose argues, needs to be taken based on absolute figures. For example, if any one population were to simply target familial hypercholesterolemia (a condition with a high relative risk of cardiovascular disease), those individuals would benefit as they have a 50% higher mortality rate, but only 1% of all those at risk of death of cardiovascular disease would be targeted.

Rose refers to the Whitehall study (of the health of civil servants) and notes that those with marginally raised blood pressure were higher in number than those with very high blood pressure. More cases of stroke were observed in the marginally raised population. A strategy to target the high risk will not suffice as they are relatively few in numbers; to target the majority at risk of complications, a whole-population approach is required. Yet it is wasteful and of little benefit to any given individual with only a marginally raised blood pressure. Rose also gives the example of the first diphtheria programme in the United Kingdom. One child saved equated with 599 'wasted' vaccines. Likewise if male doctors adhered to seat belt laws their entire working life, 399/400 doctors for 40 years would have 'wasted' their time fastening their seat belt – it wouldn't have mattered whether they did or not.

Rose establishes this background as the basis for the prevention paradox – high benefits to the community overall has little impact on the individual person.

Rose's paradox has greatly influenced the practice of public health and in particular the design of interventions aimed at changing a population's behaviour. Many risk factors to health (e.g. blood pressure, cholesterol, obesity and physical inactivity) vary within the population. Sometimes if plotted graphically, they approximate a bell-shaped curve: the two tails representing the outliers (the best and the worst) with the majority falling on either side of the median. The challenge in prevention is to move the whole curve in the direction of the best, rather than target the small extreme ends. That is most effectively done by influencing the behaviour or risk factors of the many (the mass of people around the median of the distribution) and not the few (the outliers at the tails of the distribution).

The Principles of Screening
Wilson and Junger, Geneva, 1968

> *The central idea of early disease detection and treatment is essentially simple. However, the path to its successful achievement (on the one hand, bringing to treatment those with previously undetected disease, and, on the other, avoiding harm to those persons not in need of treatment) is far from simple though sometimes it may appear deceptively easy.*

Ask the person in the street, the politician, the journalist or even a doctor whether a society should concentrate effort on diagnosing disease early, and most would answer unequivocally 'Yes'. As a general principle it certainly holds true for individuals and in the assessment of patients. If symptoms and abnormal signs are recognised early, by and large the outcome of treatment is better. The problem comes when the same argument is applied to pro-actively offering a diagnostic test to a population whose members believe themselves to be healthy. Conceptually and ethically, this is different. It is no longer simply early diagnosis; it is presymptomatic or population screening.

This carries the implicit promise that people who are called forward with an offer of a test will benefit from earlier treatment. Unfortunately this is not always the case – a positive test result may simply reveal the knowledge of the presence of disease for the screened person earlier than for a patient who presents symptomatically. Both may live as long after treatment, but the screened person will appear to have lived longer than the symptomatic patient (so-called lead time bias) and the benefit of screening will be fallacious rather than real.

In the early 1960s, when cheap, quick tests to detect disease early were becoming more available, the pressure was to offer them to populations without a necessary sound basis. A discipline was brought to the screening bandwagon by a seminal set of scientific criteria to be applied before embarking on any population screening for a particular condition. This led to proper evaluation, sometimes including randomised controlled trials, before a decision to introduce a screening programme was made.

Wilson and Junger's criteria, published by the World Health Organisation in 1968, had ten conditions to be met before a screening programme should be initiated (Table 1.1).

Today in many countries extensive screening programmes have developed steered by Wilson and Junger's original criteria, and they have been developed further over time. Programmes of population screening in routine use include those for common cancers

Table 1.1 Wilson and Junger's Original Screening Criteria

The condition sought should be an important health problem.
There should be an accepted treatment for patients with recognized disease.
Facilities for diagnosis and treatment should be available.
There should be a recognizable latent or early symptomatic stage.
There should be a suitable test or examination.
The test should be acceptable to the population.
The natural history of the condition, including development from latent to declared disease, should be adequately understood.
There should be an agreed policy on whom to treat as patients.
The cost of case finding (including diagnosis and treatment of patients diagnosed) should be economically balanced in relation to possible expenditure on medical care as a whole.
Case finding should be a continuing process and not a 'once and for all' project.

Source: Wilson and Junger (1968).

such as breast, bowel and cervix, as well as rarer but devastating conditions such as fetal anomalies. This small but vital evaluation framework has stood the test of time and has prevented untold harm and wastage of resources on ineffective population screening programmes, whilst ensuring that money and effort have been targeted ethically on those that could save lives and prevent disease progression.

Determining Causation
Hill, Proceedings of the Royal Society of Medicine (1965)

> *Upon what basis . . . can we pass from observed association to a verdict of causation?*

Statistical association is at the heart of epidemiological study. Yet, simple association, be it statistically robust or not, does not prove causation.

The jump from statistical association to causation was becoming increasing prominent post-war, especially with the advent of computers that handled ever larger data sets. This gap in public health thinking was addressed by Hill some years after he and Richard Doll had embarked upon the famous smoking studies reviewed earlier in this chapter. There was an identified gap in practice in how to establish causation. Hill's paper outlined nine criteria for strengthening the case for causation. It is not dogmatic or prescriptive, but brought together many common elements required to uphold the case for assuming agent A caused effect B.

The nine criteria are as follows:

Strength of association: Mainly statistical, but of course in certain cases where numbers studied are so large and effect of an agent so likely even statistical tests do not add much evidence. Hill gives the 18th-century example of the vast increase of scrotal cancer in chimney sweeps. He also argues the importance of using relative risk when establishing aetiology, the commonest technique used in public health today.

Consistency of findings: Research findings replicated by separate study techniques, at different times, by new researchers in dissimilar places. This is particularly important for drawing causality about rare risks.

Specificity: The clarity of link between one agent and one effect. Whilst two or more agents may be responsible for causing disease, where one agent is identified the likelihood of causation is strengthened.

Temporality: This addresses the question: which is the chicken and which is the egg? This is an important factor especially in illnesses with very long incubation periods. Are those selected to work in a certain environment more susceptible to contracting a certain disease, or is that workplace the source of the vector of disease?

Biological gradient: Enabling a dose–response to be plotted. For example, increasing numbers of cigarettes smoked per day causes a concomitant increase in lung cancer.

Plausibility: Covering the biological sense of the mechanism. However, this criterion depends on current levels of knowledge.

Coherence: The apparent association should not be significantly contrary to the natural history of the disease in question.

Experiment: Does the removal of a supposed pathogen reduce the association of agent and disease? Hill suggests that this is where the strongest evidence of causality may lie.

Analogy: Making an inference to causality for similar agents. For example, it is a reasonable starting point to think that a drug closely related to thalidomide could cause foetal deformity.

These nine criteria have been variously used, tested, added to and modified. Over time they create a viable and lasting way of weighing statistical evidence of association with postulated causality. Clearly some, such as reversibility, have more credence, but all nine offer evidence of establishing the verdict of cause and this checklist has become a cornerstone of public health practice.

On the State of Public Health
Simon, London, 1858

> *The essential points which I deem it necessary to bring under your lordships' consideration ... the inequality with which deaths are distributed in different districts of the country.*

The post of Chief Medical Officer for England was established by the government of the day as part of its response to the great cholera epidemics that swept Victorian England. The post continues to present times and remains the main source of advice on medical and public health matters to the government. Although working for and within government, the Chief Medical Officer post is politically independent and public facing. One of the highest profile elements of the role is the production of an annual report on the nation's health. Over the years, post holders have used this opportunity differently. The best have highlighted a serious problem, championed the need for action and done so without fear or favour.

In 1858, the first Chief Medical Officer of the United Kingdom, Sir John Simon, wrote a report to the Privy Council on the state of the nation's health. His report was crucial in helping to set the direction for future public health laws and reforms. It also set clarity of focus in health communication that was a beacon to light the path of his successors.

Simon was a surgeon at St Thomas' Hospital, and he fought hard for the right to provide independent advice to the government. Appointed as the medical officer of health for London in 1848, he wrote a series of reports on issues including vaccination and sanitation. By working closely with the government, and contributing to the development of the Public Health Acts that went through parliament, he was able to secure the crucial function of an annual independent report on public health to the highest level of government.

Many of the issues he mentioned in his first report as Chief Medical Officer sound familiar today, even if the diseases involved do not. He described the epidemics sweeping England at the time, including an outbreak of cowpox in Wraybury and typhoid in Windsor. He also highlighted the problems of health inequalities between different parts of the country. This was a well-observed fact, given that the life expectancy of a young man in Liverpool was 26 years, compared to his peer in the leafy market town of Oakhampton, who could expect to live to 57.

This description of the health of a population, and in particular the independent nature of the report, is fundamental to the public health function. Working with government, but also maintaining distance and objectivity, Simon was well respected by his superiors and by influential newspapers of the day and consequently was able to push for real change.

Conclusion

Population health is a broad topic but one that has included some of the most influential and insightful studies and reports in the history of medicine. From the shoe-leather epidemiology of John Snow explaining cholera outbreaks; through the work of Doll and Hill establishing the link between smoking and lung cancer; the mammoth Framingham 'study'; to population screening, it is at once a discipline of immense practical benefit to millions and also one of academic rigour. Political and practical, academic and pragmatic, it represents the interface between society and healthcare and will continue to spearhead health policy for many generations.

Key Outstanding Questions
1. Can we improve health without increasing health inequalities?
2. What role will genetics play in the future of public health?
3. What future infectious disease threats remain unknown?

Key Research Centres
1. Johns Hopkins Bloomberg School of Public Health, Baltimore, United States
2. London School of Hygiene and Tropical Medicine, London, United Kingdom
3. The Cochrane Collaboration, Oxford, United Kingdom

References
Black Report (1980) *Department of Health and Social Security (1980) inequalities in health: report of a working group chaired by Sir Douglas Black*. DHSS, London
Cochrane, A.L. (1989) *Effectiveness and efficiency: random reflections of health services*. 2nd ed. Nuffield Provincial Hospitals Trust, London. http://www.cochrane.org/about-us/history/archie-cochrane

Dawber, T.R., *et al.* (1951) Epidemiological approaches to heart disease: the Framingham Study. *American Journal of Public Health*, **41**(3), 279–286. http://ajph.aphapublications.org/cgi/reprint/41/3/279?view=long&pmid=14819398

Doll, R., and Hill, A.B. (1950) Smoking and carcinoma of the lung: preliminary report. *British Medical Journal*, 739–748. http://www.ncbi.nlm.nih.gov/pmc/articles/PMC2038856/?tool=pubmed

Hart, J.T. (1971) The inverse care law. *Lancet*, **1**(7696), 405–412. http://www.thelancet.com/journals/lancet/article/PIIS0140-6736(71)92410-X/Abstract

Hill, A.B. (1965) The environment and disease: association or causation. *Proceedings of the Royal Society of Medicine*, **58**, 295–300. http://www.ncbi.nlm.nih.gov/pmc/articles/PMC1898525/?tool=pubmed

Rose, G. (1981) Strategy of prevention: lessons from cardiovascular disease. *British Medical Journal*, **282**(6279), 1847–1851. http://www.ncbi.nlm.nih.gov/pmc/articles/PMC1506445/?tool=pubmed

Simon, J. (1858) *On the state of public health in England*. Report of the Chief Medical Officer, London.

Snow, J. (1855) *On the mode of communication of cholera*. 2nd ed. John Churchill, London. http://johnsnow.matrix.msu.edu/work.php?id=15-78-52

Wilson, J.M.G., and Junger, G. (1968) *Principles and practice of screening for disease*. World Health Organization, Geneva. http://whqlibdoc.who.int/php/WHO_PHP_34.pdf

2 Patient Safety

Felix Greaves[1], Douglas Noble[2] and Sir Liam Donaldson[3]

[1]Public Health Registrar and Clinical Research Fellow, Department of Primary Care and Public Health, Imperial College, London, UK

[2]Public Health Registrar and Honorary Clinical Lecturer, Centre for Health Sciences, Barts and the London School of Medicine and Dentistry, UK

[3]Chief Medical Officer for England and UK Government Chief Medical Adviser 1998–2010

Introduction

Only in the last 20 years has patient safety emerged as a distinct academic discipline, and even then its progress has been hesitant and occasionally stumbling. In that time we have begun to understand the frequency of medical error, we have moved forward in our understanding of why care is unsafe and we have started to identify a small number of interventions that seem to make care safer. Despite these advances, the medical care of patients remains a high-risk activity and we have only just begun the process of making care safer.

Restricting a history of the patient safety movement to the peer-reviewed scientific press would neglect some of the more profound work. Whereas a story of the development of many fields of medicine would move from one learned journal to another, the nature of patient safety, often in opposition to the prevailing medical establishment, has used a wider variety of media.

A stream of ideas, captured in detailed experiments, tabloid exposes of individual stories, investigations into tragic accidents and moments of thought leadership, have all moved the field forward.

Florence Nightingale on Running a Hospital
Nightingale, London, 1863

Florence Nightingale was more than the caricatured 'lady of the lamp', floating down the corridors of the military hospital in Scutari during the Crimean War. She was also a writer, a policy reformer, a researcher and a statistician with an eye for a good graph.

Returning home after the Crimean war, she found herself a national heroine and set about writing a series of monographs. Several of them made a valuable contribution to thinking about patient safety (although it was not a recognised term then). In her most famous – *Notes on Nursing* – she describes her approach to improving healthcare standards by applying discipline, training and method to the practice of nursing. It laid the foundations of the profession we know today.

However, a lesser known work – *Notes on Hospitals* – contains many ideas that would become profoundly influential in reducing the risks from healthcare infection. In it she set out a comprehensive argument about how hospitals should be designed and run to minimise harm, match form with function and apply data collection and measurement to allow improvement of performance.

In the work she uses statistics and reasoning to argue that the many causes of preventable death are a result of the environment that the patient is nursed in, including space, ventilation and sanitation. She makes a strong call for the use of standardised data in hospitals and talks about the need for effective administration.

> With fixed data, arrived at on these principles, we can readily obtain the proportionate mortality, not only of the whole hospital, but of every ward of it.

She even included example tables for collecting hospital statistics so that they could be adopted and used locally to improve safety.

The report also discussed international best practice, reflecting on the way things are done in French hospitals amongst others and suggesting what could be learned from them. It talks about standardising procedure to make sure they are done correctly, even things as mundane as making the beds and scrubbing the floors. It even calls for regular annual reports on quality standards by hospitals.

Contemporary practice would recognise these concepts as benchmarking, standardisation and accountability. We struggle to do them well even now.

At times the report appears overly prescriptive, and some of the views expressed within it look strange to a modern worldview, particularly around gender roles and germ theory. But many aspects of it are relevant to the contemporary audience and to principles of evidence-based policy.

Her call to arms in the preface remains as valid now as it was then:

> It may seem a strange principle to enunciate as the very first requirement in a Hospital that it should do the sick no harm. It is quite necessary, nevertheless, to lay down such a principle, because the actual mortality in hospitals, especially in those of crowded cities, is very much higher than any calculation founded on the mortality of the same class of diseases among patients treated out of hospital would lead us to expect.

Codman and the End Results System
Codman, Boston, 1918

As is often the case with scientists who are ahead of their time, or who demonstrate unfortunate truths that go against the prevailing consensus, some pioneers of patient safety found themselves unpopular, marginalised and even ostracised. An early chapter of the story is that of a brave physician in Massachusetts in the early 20th century: Ernest Amory Codman.

Dr Codman was an orthopaedic surgeon who published formative work on the treatment of the shoulder and introduced ideas, such as anaesthetic charts, that remain commonplace today. These achievements would normally have marked him as a distinguished clinician and academic. However, he ended his career as an outcast of the medical establishment after he pushed his ideas on the improvement of healthcare too far.

At the start of the 20th century, he was working at Massachusetts General Hospital, systematically looking at what happened to his patients after he had operated on them. He became interested in what he termed an 'end results system'. In the modern language of healthcare, we recognise this idea as measuring patient outcomes:

> *Every hospital should follow every patient it treats long enough to determine whether or not the treatment had been successful and then to enquire, if not, why not?*

Amongst many papers on the subject, his work *A Study in Hospital Efficiency: The First Five Years* stands out as a piece that captured many of his progressive ideas. In it, he laid out his system of measuring the outcomes of patients leaving the hospital and a classification system for thinking about why errors occurred in their treatment. It also included a call to arms for the open and transparent publishing of hospital outcome data, to allow the ranking of different facilities and even individual clinicians. He argued that this information should be made public so that patients could make informed choices about their healthcare, and he was not afraid to lead by being critical of himself.

In a 5-year study, from 1911 to 1916, he described 337 patients who were treated in his hospital and he reported 123 errors.

Despite initial enthusiasm from his peers, in the rarefied academic environment of early 20th-century Boston Codman became seen as a trouble maker. Perhaps he was not helped by the directness of his attacks on prevailing standards of care, which led to allegations of arrogance. Eventually he removed himself from the established community, and set up his own hospital working to his own mechanisms.

Codman was a remarkable man. By family origin and schooling he was from the elite of Boston society. His challenges to the establishment were his undoing professionally, but in historical terms his ideas are still shaping healthcare today.

Understanding the Prevalence of Medical Error
Leape et al., New England Journal of Medicine (1991)

One of the main drivers of the patient safety movement that gathered force in the late 1990s was the publication of studies that had aimed to assess the scale of harm in healthcare. They demonstrated that medical error was much commoner than had previously been recognised.

The first of these was the Harvard Medical Malpractice Study. It was published by a team at Harvard led by Lucian Leape and Troyen Brennan in 1991 and looked at the medical records of more than 30,000 patients. Each record was reviewed by two physicians, and identified when harm had come to patients as a result of the care they received. Retrospective medical record review comes with inherent systematic biases. For example, results are dependent on what is committed to the written medical record, and it is well known that physicians are notorious under-reporters of medical errors.

Despite such hurdles, they identified that 1133 patients had disabling injuries caused by their medical treatments, amounting to 3.7% of all treated (a likely underestimation of actual harm, but still substantial). The conclusion of the study was that medical error was more common than was realised, and that a substantial proportion of it was preventable.

This initial study led the way to many similar studies around the world. The frequency of medical error in other geographical areas varied but not greatly. It led to the often-cited figure that roughly one in ten patients admitted to hospital in a developed country will experience some kind of error affecting their care.

The findings from these so-called prevalence studies were so striking that they led to patient safety programmes being established in many countries and raised a great deal of public concern about the safety of hospitals.

Models for Understanding Error
Reason, British Medical Journal (2000)

Understanding the scale of medical error is not sufficient to fix the problem. One of the biggest steps forward in understanding patient safety has been through the development of theoretical models. These models allow the problem of why we make mistakes to be thought about in a structured way. They also enable core ideas to be more easily understood by a wider audience.

Although several different models have been used to describe different aspects of safety and risk, the best example is that of the Swiss cheese model, as described by James Reason.

Professor Reason began his career as a researcher in psychology, who became interested in how and why we make mistakes. Much of his early work focussed on areas other than medicine, including high-risk industries such as the railways and aviation.

In a short piece in the *British Medical Journal*, now cited 5000 times, he argues that a systems approach to error is a better model for understanding error than a person-based approach.

He describes a person approach as centred on the errors of individuals, blaming them for their own weakness, forgetfulness and inattention. This contrasts with a systems approach, in which emphasis is placed on the conditions under which an individual works.

Although Reason states that 'Blaming individuals is emotionally more satisfying than targeting institutions', he argues that we need to understand the wider systemic factors that contribute. Once we have understood the many factors that contribute to errors, we can take more effective action to mitigate them.

Using Swiss cheese as a metaphor to describe the systems approach, he describes a series of defences which normally prevent errors from occurring. While these barriers would ideally be complete, he describes them as being more like slices of Swiss cheese: in reality containing many holes. At times, the holes in a series of these defensive layers line up and permit the trajectory of an accident opportunity to occur (Figure 2.1).

The holes in the defences, according to his theory, arise for two reasons: active failures and latent conditions. Nearly all adverse events involve a combination of these two sets of factors.

His thinking allowed mistakes and errors to be defined more clearly, and broken down into their constituent parts. More than that, his ideas were simple and understandable. It allowed people to see that the system was more often at fault rather than a single individual, and allowed professionals to be more accepting of the notion of a broader responsibility for error.

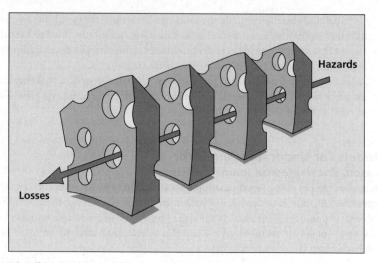

Figure 2.1 The Swiss cheese model of how defences, barriers and safeguards may be penetrated by an accident trajectory. Reproduced from Reason, *British Medical Journal* (2000), with permission from BMJ Publishing Group Ltd.

This systems model of thinking has been fundamental to our attempts to understand and reduce errors.

The Story of Wayne Jowett
Toft, Department of Health, London, 2001

The majority of tragic deaths due to medical error have been investigated and reported on in formats that do not reach an international (or sometimes even a national) audience. Most often those involved in the investigation are from professional bodies or healthcare organisations using time-honoured methods of enquiry. Alternatively major public enquiries into such incidents are legally based, lengthy and very expensive.

The Toft Report stands apart in the history of patient safety-related deaths. The lead investigator was an expert in safety in other sectors. He was not a healthcare insider. Moreover, he used an approach based on accident investigation in other sectors.

The death investigated resulted from a catastrophic mistake: the injection of the wrong therapeutic drug (vincristine) into a patient's spinal fluid. The error, whilst rare, had happened previously in other countries.

Among the failings demonstrated were the lack of induction and training for new staff, the poor labelling of the medications, the inappropriate storage of medications on the ward and their inappropriate release from pharmacy. The report concluded that there had been many opportunities for the error to have been prevented. Each was missed.

The patient's name and the harrowing story have been told to healthcare audiences around the world. It has all the ingredients of a classic accident. Toft's report was a revelation in exposing the systems causation of the death. He found 40 points on the pathway of care which contributed to the death.

It remains a landmark to enlighten those who do not see the purpose of systems thinking, those who sneer at comparisons between medicine and other industries and those who want a high-impact example to use in education and training in patient safety.

Setting the Agenda and Building Learning Organisations
Chief Medical Officer, Department of Health, London, 2000

As the scale of the problem had become better demonstrated by prevalence studies, individual stories had highlighted the effect of the epidemic of unsafe care and new ways of thinking had allowed us to move towards a systems-based approach, it became apparent that significant policy action was required.

The report *An Organization with a Memory*, produced by England's Chief Medical Officer supported by a team of expert advisers in 2000, was the UK government's attempt to deal with this situation. It complemented other policy setting reports such as *To Err Is Human*, by the Institute of Medicine in the United States the year before.

The report argued that the UK health system needed to learn from risk management in industry, particularly aviation, focusing less on human error and more on systemic factors.

> *The time is right for a fundamental re-thinking of the way that the NHS approaches the challenge of learning from adverse health care events. The NHS often fails to learn the lessons when things go wrong, and has an old-fashioned approach in this area compared to some other sectors. Yet the potential benefits of modernisation are tremendous – in terms of lives saved, harm prevented and resources freed up for the delivery of more and better care.*

It also made a compelling case about the scale of the problem with the UK health system, estimating that there are 850,000 adverse events a year, at a cost of £2 billion.

The UK report, however, went a step further than those in other nations by advocating the creation of a national reporting and learning system. Through this national system, incidents would be reported, trends in errors would be analysed and lessons learned would be implemented. It became the world's leading reporting system collecting and analysing millions of reports of medical error. It created the first National Patient Safety Agency in the world with a wide ranging remit for safety across the whole National Health Service.

This landmark report put patient safety right at the top of the United Kingdom's healthcare agenda and shaped the approach to making care safer in the decade ahead. It also set the pace for many other health systems around the world to learn and improve.

Technology and Patient Safety
Bates et al., Journal of the American Medical Association (1998)

Technology has often been held up as a potential panacea to prevent medical error, but as healthcare has become more complex, technology also presents further opportunities for mistakes to be made and care to be compromised. However in specific areas the use of technology has been demonstrated to have definite benefits to healthcare, and it was one of the first areas to establish itself as an intervention with an effective evidence base.

David Bates and colleagues at Brigham and Women's Hospital in Boston set the pace in proving the effectiveness of technology in reducing medical error. In a before-and-after comparison in a large tertiary care hospital, they investigated the effectiveness of a physician computer order entry system in reducing adverse drug events. The earlier Harvard medical practice study had identified adverse drug events as accounting for 19% of the serious errors that occurred, and represented the single largest category of error.

Using non-intercepted serious medication errors as their main outcome measure, they found that the introduction of a computerised physician order entry (CPOE) system led to a reduction from 10.7 events per 1000 patient days to 4.86 events per 1000 patient days, a fall of 55%.

The continued role of technology in reducing errors in healthcare, and in its converse action in improving healthcare quality by aiding diagnostic decisions and strengthening processes of care, has been demonstrated in many other areas. Computer simulations, for example, are now being used to improve the skill of surgeons before they operate on their patients. It appears likely that technology will be one of the tools that allow us to improve the safety of care in the future.

Hand Hygiene
Pittet et al., Lancet (2000)

The link between hand washing and disease transmission has been known since the work of Ignaz Semmelweis in 1847 in Budapest. Subsequent improvements in hospital hygiene and the introduction of aseptic practice transformed mortality and morbidity of healthcare during the 20th century. It was a matter of deep concern to publics and governments around the world to see at the end of that century, and into the 21st, the resurgence of healthcare infection and the rise in antimicrobially resistant organisms such as meticillin-resistant *Staphylococcus aureus* (MRSA). Even more alarming was the poor levels of hand hygiene particularly amongst doctors. Levels of compliance with hand hygiene protocols were below 20% in some developed countries.

During the mid- to late 1990s, Professor Didier Pittet and his team, based in Geneva, Switzerland, implemented a structured campaign to promote hand hygiene throughout their hospital. Before, during and after the campaign, they monitored hand washing behaviour, soap usage and clinical measures such as noscomial infection rates.

Over the period of the study, they were able to demonstrate increased hand washing (rising from 48% of the time to 66%) and a reduction in noscomial MRSA transmission (from 2.16 to 0.93 episodes per 10,000 patient-days; $p<0.001$). They also found that the amount of alcohol-based handrub solution used increased from 3.5 to more than 15 litres per 1000 patient days. Behaviour change is notoriously hard, but this study showed that it was possible at an organisational level.

This work is just one of many studies by the Geneva group that has provided a rigorous evidence base for the reinstitution of a practice that is as vital to modern healthcare as it was in Semmelweiss' time. It has also helped to stimulate numerous campaigns around the world to improve hand hygiene levels and set an example for numerous other hand hygiene campaigns.

This work also started to shift attitudes away from doctors seeing hand hygiene as an option if they had time, to a duty which if neglected could cost their patients their lives.

Standardising Care
Pronovost et al., New England Journal of Medicine (2006)
Amongst the many comparisons made between healthcare and other high-risk industries, one of the most striking is the acceptance in those other industries of the necessity to standardise process or procedures to reduce risk.

This has not been customary in medicine because it is at odds with the traditions and underlying philosophy of practice. Medicine evolved as a profession with autonomy in clinical decision making at its core. Certainly there has been great emphasis, since the second part of the 20th century, on best practice guidelines and other tools to encourage conformity to evidence-based practice, but ultimately it remains with the practitioners who choose whether to adopt them. The use of a standard procedure aims to remove the variability inherent in the practice of medicine.

Peter Pronovost succeeded in doing something very impressive in 108 intensive care units across the state of Michigan. The study team introduced a simple set of behavioural interventions to improve safety. These included the use of a checklist of things that must be done when inserting a central line, but also wider measures including daily goals sheet to improve clinician-to-clinician communication and a comprehensive unit-based programme to improve the safety culture.

Over an 18-month period, the intervention reduced the median rate of catheter (or central line-associated) blood stream infections from 2.7 per 1000 catheter days to 0.

Simple interventions like these have acted as a standard bearer to the patient safety movement. They have been easier to explain and roll out across large areas than other safety interventions. Resistance to the ideas has also been considerable at times, but it appears that in standardising high-risk procedures, and demonstrating a reduction in risk, the patient safety community has found something which has been a powerful tool in advancing its agenda.

Using Checklists
Haynes et al., New England Journal of Medicine (2009)
In 2006 the Chief Medical Officer for England and Chair of the World Health Organization's (WHO) Patient Safety Programme asked Atul Gawande, a Harvard surgeon and distinguished medical author, to lead a global challenge to make surgery safer.

The case for change was strong. Initial findings revealed that 234 million operations are performed across the world each year, more than the number of births per year. Although many of the dangers associated with surgery remain unknown, data from the developed world show a death rate of up to 0.8% and a major complication rate of up to 17%.

The key element of the World Health Organisation programme was the creation of a surgical safety checklist. This approach is rare in medical practice, yet the safety of aviation hinges on the routine use of checklists by every pilot and crew flying today.

The goal of Gawande and his team was not only to eliminate or reduce the incidence of operations on the wrong patient or the performance of the wrong procedure but also to ensure that a range of other essential measures were properly carried out (such as that antibiotics were given where necessary, thromboprophylaxis was in place and swab counts were correct).

To this end, a checklist was compiled to standardise pre-, intra- and post-operative elements of care in the form of a sign-in, time-out and sign-out checklist. The checklist was piloted in eight different countries representing each WHO region of the globe (Toronto, Canada; New Delhi, India; Amman, Jordan; Auckland, New Zealand; Manila, Philippines; Ifakara, Tanzania; London, United Kingdom; and Seattle, United States). The results were striking.

A prospective study collected data on approximately 4000 consecutive patients before and after introduction of the surgical checklist. Each had their death rates and complications of surgery analysed up to 30 days after their operation. Complications fell from 11% to 7% (P<0.001), and death rates from 1.5% to 0.8% (P = 0.003) before and after introduction of the checklist.

The use of a checklist has the additional advantage of bringing members of a team together to go through it, thus securing strong focus and coherence of teamwork. There will always be those who consider the use of a checklist simplistic and unnecessary. The number of such doubters is dwindling as more and more operations worldwide are taking place with a surgical checklist as routine.

Conclusions

A history of the patient safety movement is a difficult and fragmented story to tell. There has been no sequence of studies that has demonstrated a clear route of scientific progress. There are few seminal experiments that produced iconic images, traces of a graph or plots of a Western blot which definitely validated a hypothesis.

Its origins, sharing characteristics with a scientific discipline as well as a consumer movement, have been forged in the academic arena and also the environment of policy, lobbying and advocacy.

Patient safety has now moved into the mainstream of clinical thought. It is widely recognised as a discipline, and is elevated to a policy priority for the governments of many countries.

The papers described here show that the scientific community is starting to gain an understanding of some measures that can be taken to make care safer, but simple solutions have proved hard to find.

It is noticeable that several of the seminal works of patient safety have come from people working outside medicine. These people have been brave, or foolish, enough to challenge the existing hierarchies. Those from within the medical profession have sometimes felt the weight of peer opinion on their shoulders.

As the next generation of patient safety researchers set to work, they will do so with a strong base of ideas and enthusiasm. They will not need to fight the same battles against the establishment, or to gain recognition that many of their predecessors did. They will need to be creative, to borrow further ideas from other industries and to build experimental models that provide strong proof of effectiveness. The problem is real and pressing, and there is still much work to be done.

Key Outstanding Questions

1. What interventions work to improve patient safety?
2. Do reporting and learning systems act to improve patient safety?
3. How cost-effective are different methods of making care safer?

Key Research Centres

1. Center for Innovation in Quality Patient Care, Johns Hopkins University, Baltimore, USA
2. Center of Excellence for Patient Safety Research and Practice, Brigham and Women's Hospital and Harvard Medical School, Boston, USA
3. Infection Control Program at the University of Geneva Hospitals, Geneva, Switzerland

References

Bates, D.W., *et al.* (1998) Effect of computerized physician order entry and a team intervention on prevention of serious medication errors. *Journal of the American Medical Association*, **280**, 1311–1316. http://jama.ama-assn.org/content/280/15/1311.long

Chief Medical Officer (2000) *An organisation with a memory*. Department of Health, London. http://www.dh.gov.uk/en/Publicationsandstatistics/Publications/PublicationsPolicyAnd Guidance/DH_4065083

Codman, E. (1918) *A study in hospital efficiency: as demonstrated by the case report of the first five years of a private hospital*. Todd, Boston. http://www.archive.org/details/studyinhospitale00codm

Haynes, A.B., *et al.* (2009) A surgical safety checklist to reduce morbidity and mortality in a global population. *New England Journal of Medicine*, **360**, 491–499. http://www.nejm.org/doi/full/10.1056/NEJMsa0810119

Leape, L.L., *et al.* (1991) The nature of adverse events in hospitalized patients. Results of the Harvard Medical Practice Study II. *New England Journal of Medicine*, **324**, 377–384. http://www.nejm.org/doi/full/10.1056/NEJM199102073240605

Nightingale, F. (1863) *Notes on hospitals*. Longman, London. http://books.google.com/books?id=k_w5uPm0DcC&printsec=frontcover&source=gbs_ge_summary_r&cad=0#v=onepage&q&f=false

Pittet, D., *et al.* (2000) Effectiveness of a hospital-wide programme to improve compliance with hand hygiene. *Infection Control Programme. Lancet*, **356**, 1307–1312. http://www.thelancet.com/journals/lancet/article/PIIS0140-6736(00)02814-2/fulltext

Pronovost, P., *et al.* (2006) An intervention to decrease catheter-related bloodstream infections in the ICU. *New England Journal of Medicine*, **355**, 2725–2732. http://www.nejm.org/doi/full/10.1056/NEJMoa061115

Reason, J. (2000) Human error: models and management. *British Medical Journal*, **320**, 768–770. http://www.bmj.com/content/320/7237/768.long

Toft, B. (2001) *External inquiry into the adverse incident that occurred at Queen's Medical Centre, Nottingham*. Department of Health, London. http://www.who.int/patientsafety/news/Queens%20Medical%20Centre%20report%20(Toft).pdf

Additional References

1. Brennan, T.A., *et al.* (1991) Incidence of adverse events and negligence in hospitalized patients. Results of the Harvard Medical Practice Study I. *New England Journal of Medicine*, **324**, 370–376.
2. Friedman, R.C., *et al.* (1997) The intern and sleep loss. *New England Journal of Medicine*, **285**, 201–203.
3. Vincent, C G., *et al.* (2001) Adverse events in British hospitals: preliminary retrospective record review. *British Medical Journal*, **322**, 517–519.
4. Wilson, R.M., *et al.* (2005) The Quality in Australian Health Care Study. *Medical Journal of Australia*, **163**, 458–471.

3   Heart Failure

Martin R. Cowie and Kaushik Guha

National Heart and Lung Institute, Imperial College London, London, UK

Introduction

Heart failure is a syndrome characterised by fluid retention, fatigue and breathlessness. It is triggered by underlying cardiac dysfunction with haemodynamic, neurohormonal and immunological changes becoming more marked as the syndrome progresses. Any pathology that impairs the ability of the heart to function as an effective pump can lead to the syndrome of heart failure. Coronary artery disease is the main driver in the developed world, often with a history of hypertension or diabetes. Degenerative valve disease is becoming a more important aetiology as the population ages[1].

Heart failure care today bears little resemblance to practice in the 1980s. The treatment options for the failing heart, particularly with underlying systolic impairment of the left ventricle, have expanded impressively in the past two decades as a result of a large number of randomised studies. Consequently the prognosis has improved, with annual mortality of around 10% if the early high-risk period is survived. These studies have been driven by a better understanding of the underlying pathophysiology and the realisation that driving the failing heart harder is counterproductive except in the very short term. Much better outcomes can be achieved if the intense neurohormonal activation characteristic of the syndrome is gradually but progressively antagonised pharmacologically. Electrical therapies, with a range of implanted devices that improve the efficiency of cardiac pumping or treat life-threatening arrhythmia, have recently transformed the outlook for some patients. Monitoring the control of the syndrome is also becoming more sophisticated, particularly with increasingly expert patients and better access to home-based technologies.

In this chapter, we have chosen studies that have had a major effect on clinical practice in the past 20 years.

Disappointingly many people with heart failure do not receive the full benefits of the therapeutic advances outlined in these influential papers. Improving access to such advances will remain a challenge for all healthcare systems particularly with a rapidly ageing population and an increasing number of people living with heart failure.

The Landmark Trial of Renin-Angiotensin Inhibition
CONSENSUS Trial Group, New England Journal of Medicine (1987)

This randomised trial heralded the era of neurohormonal antagonism as an effective mechanism of improving the prognosis for heart failure. The angiotensin-converting enzyme (ACE) inhibitor enalapril was compared with placebo in patients with severe

---

Understanding Medical Research: The Studies that Shaped Medicine, First Edition. Edited by John A. Goodfellow. © 2012 John Wiley & Sons, Ltd. Published 2012 by John Wiley & Sons, Ltd.

heart failure. Enalapril reduces the conversion of angiotensin I to angiotensin II, a potent vasoconstrictor that also acts to stimulate release of aldosterone from the adrenal glands and thus increase fluid retention, myocardial fibrosis and potential arrhythmia.

In terms of today's clinical trials, this study was small with only 253 patients randomised before the data monitoring and safety board recommended the termination of the study on ethical grounds. This was because of the marked benefit in favour of enalapril, with the primary endpoint of death at 6 months being reduced 40% (from 44% to 26%; P = 0.001).

For the first time, a safe and effective therapy had been robustly proven to markedly improve the prognosis of severe heart failure. Since this trial there have been many others with ACE inhibitors: in asymptomatic left ventricular dysfunction, in mild to moderate heart failure and in heart failure in the context of acute myocardial infarction. ACE inhibitors are consequently recommended as first-line agents for all patients with heart failure due to left ventricular systolic dysfunction in all international guidelines. They are so effective that economic analyses suggest that they may be cost-saving for the healthcare system in this indication.

Under-dosing with ACE inhibitors (or indeed angiotensin-converting enzyme receptor blockers (ARBs)) remains a major problem for patients with heart failure. International guidelines suggest that patients should have the dose of these agents titrated up to the doses used in the randomised trials (e.g. enalapril 10 mg bd, ramipril 5 mg bd, candesartan 32 mg od and valsartan 160 mg bd), unless the patient experiences symptomatic hypotension or significant deterioration in renal function. Evidence exists that where doctors and patients adhere to such guidance, the outcome for patients is much better.

The Multidisciplinary Heart Failure Team
Rich et al., New England Journal of Medicine (1995)

The high readmission rate of patients after discharge from hospitalisation with decompensation was well recognised as a major problem in the 1990s. In addition to being very unsatisfactory from the patient's point of view, it was clearly consuming substantial healthcare resources. Year on year the number of admissions due to heart failure was climbing. Crisis management by hospital services was important, but improvement in monitoring of the condition, earlier detection of deterioration and better use of disease modifying therapies was clearly needed.

Michael Rich and colleagues were the first group to robustly assess the impact of a nurse-led post-discharge programme on the outcome for patients with heart failure. A group of 282 elderly patients hospitalised with heart failure were randomised to standard care or a programme consisting of comprehensive education of the patient and family, a prescribed diet, social-service consultation, planning for early discharge, review of medication, and intensive follow-up including home visits and telephone contact. The primary endpoint was that of survival to 90 days without readmission. This was achieved in 91 of 142 patients in the treatment group as compared with only 75 of the 140 patients in the control group (a 20% increase, albeit not reaching statistical significance with a p value of 0.09). However, the important secondary endpoints, including the total number of readmissions and readmissions due to heart failure, were reduced significantly by 44% and 56% respectively. Because of the large reduction in the number of admissions, the intensive programme was cost-saving compared with usual care.

Although small in size, the study led to a marked change in practice. No longer were heart failure patients just treated for decompensation and then discharged to routine follow-up. Instead comprehensive disease management programmes were set up, and the discipline of heart failure nursing was born. Today most developed countries have good examples of strong multidisciplinary heart failure management programmes, working across secondary and primary care, with evidence of an important impact on readmission rates.

Other randomised trials of such programmes have been published subsequently, with meta-analysis confirming the beneficial impact on hospital readmission rates and mortality.

An About-Turn in Medical Thinking: Beta-Blockers Are Good for Heart Failure
Packer et al., New England Journal of Medicine (1996)

For 30 years after the discovery of beta-blockers, all doctors were taught that such drugs should be avoided at all costs in patients with heart failure. The acute negative inotropic and chronotropic effects could lead to decompensation of the syndrome. However, astute clinical observation coupled with small studies had led to the hypothesis that careful introduction and subsequent up-titration of dosage of beta-blockers might improve the outcome in heart failure.

The first large randomised trial to support this 'Beta-blockers are good for heart failure' hypothesis was published in 1996. The US Carvedilol Heart Failure Study Group randomised 1094 patients with mild, moderate or severe heart failure, with left ventricular ejection fractions of 0.35 or less, to placebo (398 patients) or carvedilol (696 patients), in addition to standard therapy with digoxin, diuretics and an ACE inhibitor. The target dose for carvedilol was 25 mg bd, with an initial starting dose of 6.25 mg bd.

The effect of the beta-blocker was so impressive that the Data and Safety Monitoring Board recommended early termination of the study: overall mortality was reduced by 65% (P < 0.001). In addition, there was a 27% reduction in the risk of hospitalisation for cardiovascular reasons, and a 38% reduction in the combined endpoint of hospitalisation or death. Interestingly, worsening heart failure was less common in the group randomised to carvedilol compared with those randomised to placebo.

Since publication of this study, this effect has been confirmed in other large randomised studies using metoprolol, bisoprolol and nebivolol. Carvedilol was shown to be more effective than metoprolol in a head-to-head comparison in a large randomised trial. International guidelines recommend beta-blockers be prescribed in all patients with heart failure due to left ventricular systolic dysfunction, provided there is no absolute contraindication (e.g. asthma or severe hypotension). The drug is introduced at low dose and titrated up as tolerated to the doses used as targets in the randomised trials. Sadly, many patients with heart failure are still not considered for beta-blocker therapy due to excessive caution in the treating physicians.

B-Type Natriuretic Peptide in Helping to Identify Heart Failure
Cowie et al., Lancet (1997)

Heart failure is often not a straightforward diagnosis. The symptoms are nonspecific, and clinical signs may be difficult for a non-expert to pick up and not always present.

Many studies have shown that only about a third of patients in whom a primary care physician suspects heart failure have this diagnosis confirmed on full cardiological assessment. Access to cardiac imaging, such as echocardiography, may help improve this but often the physician may not be confident to interpret the results of the imaging.

Natriuretic peptides are a family of polypeptides, with both the atria and ventricles excreting these (atrial natriuretic peptide and B-type natriuretic peptide (BNP), respectively) in response to increased cardiac strain.

The first proper assessment of the clinical utility of B-type natriuretic peptide in helping a primary care physician to diagnose heart failure was performed in Hillingdon, West London and published by the author of this chapter. All patients with a suspected diagnosis of new heart failure from a network of 81 general practitioners were assessed in a rapid access clinic. A panel of three cardiologists reviewed the clinical history, examination findings, electrocardiograms, blood results (not including BNP), chest radiographs and echocardiograms, and decided whether heart failure was present or not. This 'gold standard' diagnosis was then compared with the plasma BNP measurement. The receiver operating characteristics curve is shown in Figure 3.1, with an area under the curve of 0.96 (where 0.5 means no discriminatory ability, and 1.0 is perfect discrimination between heart failure and not heart failure). In other words, the BNP test on its own was in virtually all cases as good as the expert panel at picking up heart failure in this referred population.

The data from this study, and many subsequently, have proven the utility of measuring plasma BNP concentration (or NT-proBNP) as a diagnostic test in the diagnostic work-up of patients with suspected heart failure in both the acute and chronic setting. International guidelines now recommend access to this test for diagnostic purposes[2]. The peptide is also a useful marker of prognosis, but the evidence for its role in monitoring and titrating therapy remains less clear.

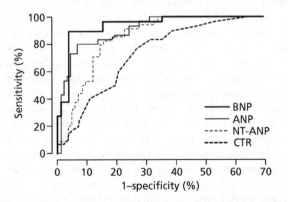

Figure 3.1 Receiver operating characteristics curve for natriuretic peptides and cardiothoracic ratio (CTR) in patients referred from primary care with a suspected diagnosis of heart failure. Area under the curves: BNP (0.96), ANP (0.93), NT-ANP (0.89) and CTR (0.79). Reprinted from Cowie *et al.*, *The Lancet*, Copyright (1997), with permission from Elsevier.

The Digoxin Trial in Heart Failure Study
The Digitalis Investigation Group, New England Journal of Medicine (1997)

Digoxin has been used in a variety of forms for the treatment of heart failure and an irregular pulse since at least the time of the description of the medicinal uses of digitalis (an extract from the foxglove plant) by William Withering in 1785. Along with diuretics it was the mainstay of treatment of heart failure well into the latter part of the 20th century.

Digoxin increases cardiac contractility by increasing intracellular calcium concentrations via the sodium/potassium co-transporter on the cell surface. It was thought to be useful for patients with heart failure because of its intrinsic inotropic properties. It is also vagotonic and thereby increases atrioventricular block in patients with atrial fibrillation. However, it has a narrow therapeutic index and digoxin toxicity was well recognised in clinical practice.

The Digitalis Investigation Group (DIG) trial investigators wished to evaluate the safety and efficacy of digoxin in a formal randomised controlled trial. They randomised 6800 patients with heart failure and an ejection fraction of 0.45 or less to digoxin or placebo in addition to standard treatment with diuretics and ACE inhibitors. All patients were in sinus rhythm at the time of randomisation.

Digoxin did not reduce overall mortality, but it reduced the overall rate of hospitalisation by 6% and the rate of hospitalisation for heart failure by 28%. Suspected digoxin toxicity led to hospitalisation in 2% of the digoxin group and 0.9% in the placebo group.

This study has led to a gradual reduction in the usage of digoxin in patients with heart failure except where persistent atrial fibrillation is present. In UK practice it is generally confined to those who are in atrial fibrillation or those in sinus rhythm who remain very symptomatic despite optimal drug therapy with diuretics, ACE inhibitors (or ARBs), beta-blockers and spironolactone.

The Randomized Aldactone Evaluation (RALES) Study
Pitt et al., New England Journal of Medicine (1999)

ACE inhibitors were a major breakthrough in improving the prognosis of heart failure. However, the prognosis remained disappointing and the search was on for additional agents that might help. It was known that aldosterone levels were high in heart failure, particularly in those with a poor prognosis. ACE inhibitors did decrease the circulating concentrations of aldosterone, but over time the levels tended to creep back up again, a phenomenon termed 'aldosterone escape'.

The Randomized Aldactone Evaluation Study (RALES) was published in 1999 and demonstrated the large additional benefit from directly antagonising the effects of aldosterone in patients with severe heart failure and left ventricular systolic dysfunction. 1663 patients were randomised to either best medical therapy or best medical therapy along with the aldosterone antagonist spironolactone at a target dose of 25 mg once per day.

The trial was terminated early because of overwhelming evidence of benefit to those randomised to spironolactone. There was a highly significant 30% reduction in the relative risk of death from both progressive heart failure and sudden death. There was also a 35% relative risk reduction for heart failure hospitalisations and an improvement in symptoms. Gynaecomastia or breast pain was reported in 10% of men on spirono-lactone compared with only 1% on placebo, but only ten men needed to stop therapy because of this.

It is important to monitor serum creatinine and potassium concentrations in patients with heart failure particularly if there are on neurohormonal antagonists such as aldosterone. Rather indiscriminate use of spironolactone in patients after the publication of the RALES study was shown to be associated with increased rates of life-threatening hyperkalaemia. International heart failure guidelines give clear instructions as to the frequency of monitoring required and the need to temporarily reduce or occasionally stop this medication if renal function deteriorates or serum potassium is too high.

The benefit of aldosterone antagonism in patients with heart failure after myocardial infarction has been subsequently demonstrated in a randomised trial using the more selective aldosterone antagonist, eplerenone[3]. Randomised trials are ongoing in milder chronic heart failure and in heart failure with normal ejection fraction.

Flogging a Dying Horse: The Sad Tale of Intravenous Inotropes
Cuffe et al., Journal of the American Medical Association (2002)

Despite the clinically obvious short-term haemodynamic benefits of intravenous inotropic therapy, it was not clear whether routine use of such therapy was beneficial even in the medium term for patients with acute decompensation of heart failure. The first large randomised trial to examine this was Outcomes of a Prospective Trial of Intravenous Milrinone for Exacerbations of Chronic Heart Failure (OPTIME-CHF).

951 patients admitted with exacerbations of systolic heart failure but not requiring inotropic therapy for low blood pressure or critical organ hypoperfusion were randomised to receive a 48-hour infusion of either milrinone or saline placebo. The primary endpoint was the cumulative days of hospitalisation within 60 days following randomisation.

There was no difference in the primary endpoint between the two arms of the study, but sustained hypotension requiring intervention and new atrial arrhythmias occurred more frequently in the milrinone arm. There was no difference in in-hospital mortality, mortality at 60 days or the composite endpoint of death or readmission by 60 days.

This trial stopped the fashion current at that time to use intravenous inotropes as a routine treatment in patients with acute decompensation of chronic heart failure. Of course, inotropes are still used for a small minority of patients who require resuscitation from marked hypotension and low organ perfusion, but such therapy is used for as short a time as possible.

A Paradigm Shift: The Development of Cardiac Resynchronisation Therapy: CARE HF
Cleland et al., New England Journal of Medicine (2005)

Despite improvements in the drug therapy of chronic heart failure, many patients with heart failure remain symptomatic and have a poor life expectancy. It had been recognised for some time that many such patients had dysynchronous contraction of the left ventricle with regional delay in contraction. This is particularly marked in those with a broad bundle branch block on the surface electrocardiogram.

Small, short-term studies of an electrical technology that 'resynchronised' ventricular contraction in such patients by pacing both the right ventricle through its apex and the left ventricle via a tributary of the coronary sinus had suggested there were benefits on patient symptoms, neurohormonal activation and left ventricular function. Data on the effect of such therapy on clinical outcomes were lacking.

This changed with the publication of the Cardiac Resynchronisation Heart Failure (CARE-HF) study in 2005. 813 patients with moderate to severe symptoms despite optimal medical therapy and left ventricular dysynchrony were randomised to medical therapy alone or cardiac resynchronisation with an atrio-biventricular pacemaker. The primary endpoint was the time to death from any cause or an unplanned hospitalisation for a major cardiovascular event. The principal secondary endpoint was all-cause mortality.

Much to many physicians' surprise, CARE-HF reported a highly significant 37% reduction in the primary endpoint, and a similarly significant 36% reduction in all-cause mortality over an average follow-up of 30 months. Measures of ventricular function also improved, as did patient symptoms.

It appears that cardiac resynchronisation therapy (CRT) reduces the risk of death from progressive heart failure and from sudden cardiac death, presumably related to an anti-arrhythmic effect of improving cardiac function without increasing myocardial oxygen requirements (unlike the situation with intravenous inotropes).

CRT is now recommended in all international guidelines for patients with systolic left ventricular dysfunction, bundle branch block, and moderate-to-severe symptoms despite optimal drug therapy. It is likely in the future that patients with milder symptoms will be included in such recommendations as a result of ongoing studies.

Preventing Sudden Death by an Implantable Cardioverter Defibrillator
Bardy et al., New England Journal of Medicine (2005)

Patients with heart failure generally die from either progressive pump failure or sudden, presumed arrhythmic, death. Patients with milder symptoms are more likely to die suddenly than from progressive heart failure. Medical therapy with neurohormonal antagonists reduces the risk of sudden as well as progressive heart failure death, but the possibility was raised that an implantable cardioverter defibrillator might further reduce this risk.

The Sudden Cardiac Death in Heart Failure Trial (SCD-HeFT) investigators set out to test the hypothesis that a simple single-chamber implantable cardioverter defibrillator (ICD) would reduce all-cause mortality when compared with optimal medical therapy alone. They also wished to examine whether treatment with amiodarone in addition to optimal medical therapy alone would reduce this risk, and how much this differed from the effect of a defibrillator.

The results were published in 2005 after an average follow-up of almost 4 years. 847 patients with mild to moderate heart failure (NYHA Class II or III) and a left ventricular ejection fraction of 0.35 or less had been randomised to optimal medical therapy plus placebo medication, 845 patients to optimal medical therapy plus oral amiodarone and 829 patients to a simple single-lead ICD (without amiodarone, but with optimal medical therapy). Patients could be included if the heart failure was of ischaemic origin or dilated cardiomyopathy. 29% of the patients had died in the placebo group, 28% in the amiodarone group and 22% in the ICD group – a 23% relative risk reduction for this group (P = 0.007). The benefit appeared to take 2 years to become apparent, and increased with time, with some evidence that greater benefit was found in those with milder symptoms (NYHA Class II).

Currently international guidelines recommend that patients should be considered for an ICD provided they are not symptomatic at rest (NYHA Class IV), have a reasonable life expectancy and have an ejection fraction of 0.35 or less, whatever the aetiology of heart failure. Many such patients do not receive such therapy due to referral problems or lack of capacity to implant such technologies.

Amiodarone is now not used routinely in patients with heart failure and low ejection fraction even if they have markers of higher risk of sudden death. An ICD is the treatment of choice for such patients, in addition to optimal medical therapy. Amiodarone is still used for other indications, such as an attempt to maintain sinus rhythm in those with paroxysmal atrial fibrillation and heart failure, or to reduce the frequency of ICD discharges in patients with frequent serious ventricular arrhythmia.

ICD technology can be combined with a CRT platform, to provide appropriate patients with maximum protection from the risk of sudden death. Such a combination is considerably more expensive than straightforward CRT, but most recent analyses suggest it is cost-effective.

Telemonitoring: An Important Technological Advance in Monitoring Heart Failure
Cleland et al., Journal of the American College of Cardiology (2005)

It is generally accepted that to optimise the outcome for patients living with chronic heart failure, monitoring of the condition is necessary. The traditional model was to arrange periodic clinical review in either primary or secondary care. Patients often decompensated over a period of time without this being noticed, necessitating emergency admission to hospital for control to be re-established. Such an approach was inefficient, inconvenient, expensive and potentially harmful to the long-term outcome of the patient.

More intensive post-discharge care is now the norm for patients who come to the attention of a heart failure service, although sadly not to the many who are cared for by generalists or purely in primary care. Such monitoring is usually nurse-led and involves a combination of telephone contact, clinic reviews and occasionally home visits.

A variety of systems have been developed that enable physiological measurements to be made in the patient's home or implanted device. Such information can be transmitted to a health care professional remotely, who can review the data and decide whether to contact the patient for further information about their symptoms or to arrange a clinical review in primary or secondary care. Such timely attention might enable earlier detection of decompensation and help reduce the need for subsequent emergency hospitalisation. This approach is termed 'telemonitoring' and is one example of how eHealth is transforming the healthcare environment.

The Trans-European Network – Home Care Management Study (TENS-HMS) trial was one of the first large multicentre, pan-European trials designed to evaluate the effect of telemonitoring on the outcome of patients with heart failure.

426 patients with a recent admission to hospital with heart failure and a left ventricular ejection fraction of less than 0.40 were assigned randomly to home telemonitoring, nurse

telephone support alone or usual care in a 2:2:1 ratio. Those who were allocated to home telemonitoring self-monitored weight, blood pressure, heart rate and rhythm with automated devices linked to a cardiology centre. In the nurse telephone support group, patients could contact the nurses if they had a concern about their heart failure (such as an increase in weight).

There was a trend to a reduction in the number of days dead or hospitalised at 240 days (the primary endpoint) in both the nurse telephone support group and home tele-monitoring compared with usual care. Mortality was higher ($P = 0.032$) in the usual care group (45% 1-year mortality) compared with the other two groups (27% nurse telephone support and 29% home telemonitoring). The duration of admissions was shortest in the home telemonitoring group.

Combined with meta-analysis of other studies of telemonitoring, there is increasing evidence that such systems reduce mortality compared with usual care, and although not decreasing overall admissions to hospital they do reduce the proportion of such admissions that are due to heart failure and are unplanned. The increased convenience of the monitoring, and reduction in the need for 'routine' clinic visits, is perhaps most important for the frail elderly and for those living remotely from healthcare settings.

More sophisticated monitoring of a range of physiological items, such as transthoracic impedance, heart rate variability, atrial arrhythmia and patient activity, is currently possible for patients with implanted devices. Making sense of the data stream, and ensuring interventions are triggered appropriately, is a challenge that needs to be robustly assessed in the near future. Several trials are underway.

Undoubtedly heart failure services will increasingly adopt a menu-based approach to the chronic management of the patients under their care, with a range of possible models being employed including traditional clinic review, self-monitoring supplemented by contact with healthcare professionals either in person or by telephone, telemonitoring and even hospital-at-home services. Such an individually tailored approach is likely to maximise the efficiency of services and support the patient to obtain optimal benefit from all the therapies now available[4].

Key Outstanding Questions
1. How best can nonsystolic heart failure be diagnosed? Will measurement of plasma natriuretic peptide concentration have a role?
2. What therapies can improve survival and quality of life in patients with nonsystolic heart failure?
3. Will heart replacement with mechanical pumps become a feasible and cost-effective option in the foreseeable future?
4. Considering that many promising new drugs have failed at the large randomised controlled trial stage, how can the outcome of acute heart failure be improved?

Key Laboratories and Clinics
1. National Heart & Lung Institute, Imperial College London, in partnership with Royal Brompton and Harefield NHS Foundation Trust, United Kingdom
2. University of Hull, Yorkshire, United Kingdom
3. University Medical Centre Groningen, Groningen, the Netherlands
4. Cleveland Clinic, Cleveland, United States

5. Duke University Medical Center, Durham, United States
6. Monash University and Alfred Hospital Health Centre, Melbourne, Australia

References

Bardy, G.H., *et al.* (2005) Amiodarone or an implantable cardioverting defibrillator for congestive heart failure (Sudden Cardiac Death in Heart Failure Trial SCD-HeFT). *New England Journal of Medicine*, **352**, 225–237. http://www.nejm.org/doi/full/10.1056/NEJMoa043399

Cleland, J.G.F., *et al.* (2005) The effect of cardiac resynchronisation on morbidity and mortality of heart failure (Cardiac Resynchronisation Therapy in Heart Failure CARE-HF). *New England Journal of Medicine*, **352**, 1539–1549. http://www.nejm.org/doi/full/10.1056/NEJMoa050496

Cleland, J.G.F., *et al.* (2005) Non invasive home telemonitoring for patients with heart failure at high risk or recurrent admission and death. (The Trans-European Network – Home Management System Study). *Journal of the American College of Cardiology*, **45**, 1654–1664. http://content.onlinejacc.org/cgi/content/full/45/10/1654

CONSENSUS Trial Group (1987) Effects of Enalapril on mortality in severe congestive heart failure. Results of the Cooperative North Scandinavian Enalapril Survival Study (CONSENSUS). *New England Journal of Medicine*, **316**(23), 1429–1435. http://www.ncbi.nlm.nih.gov/pubmed/2883575

Cowie, M.R., *et al.* (1997) Value of the natriuretic peptides in assessment of patients with possible new heart failure in primary care. *Lancet*, **350**, 1349–1352. http://www.thelancet.com/journals/lancet/article/PIIS0140-6736(97)06031-5/fulltext

Cuffe, M.S., *et al.* (2002) Short-term intravenous milrinone for acute exacerbations of chronic heart failure: a randomized controlled trial. *Journal of the American Medical Association*, **287**(12); 1541–1547. http://jama.ama-assn.org/content/287/12/1541.long

The Digitalis Investigation Group (1997) The effect of digoxin on mortality and morbidity in patients with heart failure. *New England Journal of Medicine*, **336**, 525–533. http://www.nejm.org/doi/full/10.1056/NEJM199702203360801

Packer, M., *et al.* (1996) The effect of carvedilol on morbidity and mortality in patients with chronic heart failure. *New England Journal of Medicine*, **334**, 1349–1355. http://www.nejm.org/doi/full/10.1056/NEJM199605233342101

Pitt, B., *et al.* (1999) The effect of spironolactone on morbidity and mortality in patients with severe heart failure. *New England Journal of Medicine*, **341**(10), 709–717. http://www.nejm.org/doi/full/10.1056/NEJM199909023411001

Rich, M.W., *et al.* (1995) A multidisciplinary intervention to prevent the readmission of elderly patients with congestive heart failure. *New England Journal of Medicine*, **333**(18), 1190–1195. http://www.nejm.org/doi/full/10.1056/NEJM199511023331806

Additional References

1. Mosterd, A. and Hoes, A.W. (2007) Clinical epidemiology of heart failure. *Heart*, **93**, 1137–1146.
2. The Task Force for the Diagnosis and Treatment of Acute and Chronic Heart Failure 2008 of the European Society of Cardiology (2008) ESC Guidelines for the diagnosis and treatment of acute and chronic heart failure. *European Heart Journal*, **29**, 388–442.
3. Pitt, B., *et al.* (2003) Eplerenone, a selective aldosterone blocker, in patients with left ventricular dysfunction after myocardial infarction. *New England Journal of Medicine*, **348**, 1309–1321.
4. Riley, J.P. and Cowie, M.R. (2009) Telemonitoring in heart failure. *Heart*, **95**, 1964–1968.

4 Acute Coronary Syndrome (NSTEMI)

Wei Yao Lim and Colin Berry

BHF Glasgow Cardiovascular Research Centre, University of Glasgow, Glasgow, UK

Introduction

Acute coronary syndrome (ACS) constitutes a spectrum of disorders ranging from unstable angina to transmural myocardial infarction (MI). ACS is driven by a common underlying pathophysiology that usually involves the formation of thrombus on an inflamed and complicated coronary artery plaque. The resulting perfusion imbalance evolves from myocardial ischaemia (unstable angina) to myocardial infarction where there is evidence of myocardial cell death.

Clinically, the diagnosis of MI requires biochemical evidence of myocyte necrosis derived from the measurements of cardiac enzymes (mainly troponin) coupled with at least one of the following features:

– Typical history of cardiac sounding chest pain
– New electrocardiogram (ECG) changes indicating ischaemia: ST-T changes, new onset left bundle brunch block and the development of pathological Q-waves
– Evidence from imaging demonstrating new loss of myocardial viability or new abnormal regional wall features

For management purposes, MI is further divided into two categories based on ECG changes: (1) ST-elevation MI (STEMI) and (2) non-ST elevation MI (NSTEMI). Patients presenting with STEMI require urgent reperfusion therapy often in the form of primary percutaneous coronary intervention. This has resulted in most cases of STEMI now being triaged to hospitals (regional or tertiary) which provide primary angioplasty.

NSTEMI, on the other hand, is often seen and managed by general medical staff, and for this reason the focus of this chapter is to highlight the ten studies that have shaped our current management of this common presentation.

Troponin: The Basis of Diagnosis
Hamm et al., New England Journal of Medicine (1992)

A consensus document by the European Society of Cardiology (ESC) and the American College of Cardiology (ACC) published in 2000 caused a paradigm shift in our definition of MI. It emphasised the usage of cardiac biomarkers and recommended the use of troponin in routine clinical practice.

Troponin is a protein that regulates the interaction of actin and myosin in striated muscles, and leakage of troponin into the blood is an indication of myocardial damage. Although troponin measurement is now routine, the original work on troponin was

Understanding Medical Research: The Studies that Shaped Medicine, First Edition. Edited by John A. Goodfellow. © 2012 John Wiley & Sons, Ltd. Published 2012 by John Wiley & Sons, Ltd.

rejected for publication by *Circulation* and *Clinical Chemistry* because CKMB was considered the cardiac marker of choice back in the 1980s.

Hamm and colleagues set out to investigate whether troponin T would have any prognostic value in patients with unstable angina. 'Unstable angina' described patients suffering from cardiac sounding chest pain, without ECG changes and normal creatine kinase (CK) levels. Patients were further divided into two groups: (3) accelerated or subacute angina ($n = 25$) and (4) angina at rest ($n = 84$).

Troponin T (≥ 0.20) CK and CKMB were taken in all patients every 8 hours for 2 days, and the outcome of interest was in-hospital MI and death. All patients were given a standard medical regime and investigators were blinded to the patients' troponin status. None of the 25 patients with accelerated or subactue angina had a positive troponin, and none died. For the other 84 patients with angina at rest, troponin was detected in 33 patients (39%) whilst CKMB was present in only three patients. Ten of the 33 patients went on to develop MI (defined by ECG changes ± raised CK), of which five died during hospitalisation. Only one patient with a negative troponin developed MI and died. The authors concluded that troponin T was more sensitive than CKMB and had a role in determining the prognosis of patients with 'unstable angina'.

This study not only managed to demonstrate the superiority of troponin compared to CKMB but also gave rise to the idea that troponin-positive patients who did not fit the criteria for MI were suffering from 'minor myocardial necrosis'. This, together with subsequent studies on the cardiac specificity of troponin, paved the way for troponin to be recognised as an important marker and eventually led to the change in the definition of MI centred on the role of troponin.

Today troponin testing is part of routine clinical practice and a positive troponin is defined as a value greater than the 99th centile for a local reference population. The use of troponin as a sensitive cardiac-specific marker allows us to diagnose myocardial necrosis in those patients who we would previously label as unstable angina thereby triggering more appropriate management. High-sensitivity troponin assays (e.g. ARCHITECT *STAT*, Abbott Diagnostics) which have a detection limit of around 1 pg/mL are emerging as a much more sensitive test for detection of myocardial injury. A key outstanding question is whether management based on these new assays will lead to improved clinical outcomes compared with standard care.

Aspirin: The Cornerstone of MI Management
ISIS-2, Lancet (1988)

There is now extensive evidence on the beneficial effects of aspirin in the acute management and secondary prevention of patients with MI. We now turn to one of the most famous cardiology studies, the Second International Study of Infarct Survival (ISIS-2), one of the first papers that demonstrated the mortality benefit of aspirin in patients with acute MI.

This was a 2×2 factorial study assessing the role of IV streptokinase and aspirin either alone or in combination in patients with acute MI and successfully highlighted the efficacy of both these agents. However, as this section is on the role of aspirin, we will focus on the results pertaining to aspirin alone.

17,187 patients presenting 24 hours within the onset of symptoms of suspected MI were recruited into this double-blind randomised control trial. 8587 were allocated to aspirin. MI was diagnosed clinically and ECG changes at entry were not a requirement. Prior to this study, there was only one small randomised trial which administered a single dose of aspirin in acute MI with no further treatment. Patients in ISIS-2 were given a dose of 162.5 mg of aspirin immediately at presentation and continued for one month. The primary outcome measure was 5-week vascular-mortality.

When compared to placebo, aspirin had a 23% odd reduction in 5-week mortality. This would translate to preventing 25 deaths and 10–15 nonfatal reinfarctions or strokes if aspirin was started in 1000 patients.

It is worth noting that the diagnosis of MI was made clinically, and ECG changes and enzyme measurements were not essential. From the ECGs, 54% of patients in this trial would today be diagnosed as having a STEMI and possibly 35% of patients an NSTEMI. Nevertheless, ISIS-2 beautifully demonstrated the efficacy of aspirin in both STEMI and NSTEMI patients when given acutely.

Today aspirin has become one of the most widely used anti-platelets, and ISIS-2 was the landmark trial that provided the first piece of solid evidence of its efficacy. Patients with both STEMI and NSTEMI are now given aspirin acutely and continued indefinitely as well. Meta-analyses have proven the long-term benefits in secondary prevention.

The Additive Effect of Clopidogrel: A Case for Dual Anti-Platelet Therapy
CURE Trial Investigators, New England Journal of Medicine (2001)
Dual antiplatelet therapy with aspirin and clopidogrel is now recommended in acute NSTEMI patients. Clopidogrel inhibits adenosine diphosphate-induced platelet aggregation acting on a different pathway than the thromboxane-mediated pathway of aspirin. Other evidence-based alternatives to clopidogrel include prasugrel and ticagrelor.

The Clopidogrel in Unstable Angina to prevent Recurrent Events (CURE) trial is considered the landmark paper that established the first evidence of clopidogrel on top of aspirin in patients with acute coronary syndrome without ST-segment elevation.

This double-blind randomised controlled trial recruited patients on the basis of their symptoms and ECG findings. Patients were either given clopidogrel, with a loading dose of 300 mg followed by 75 mg per day for 3 to 12 months (mean 9 months), or an equivalent placebo. Patients were followed up at 1 month, 3 months and every subsequent third month until the end of the study date. The primary outcome assessment was a composite endpoint of cardiovascular death, nonfatal MI and nonfatal stroke.

It successfully showed a 2.1% absolute risk reduction and a 20% relative risk reduction in the primary composite endpoint and a 14% reduction in refractory ischaemia. The clopidogrel group also demonstrated a 34% higher incidence of major bleeding, defined as a disabling bleed, intraocular bleed causing loss of vision or bleeding resulting in transfusion of at least two units. For this reason, it was worth taking a closer look to see if the long-term benefits of clopidogrel were sustainable.

A further analysis of the CURE study population by Yusuf and colleagues demonstrated benefits of clopidogrel emerging within 24 hours and sustained beyond 30 days[2]. However, the data also suggested most of the benefit was derived within the first

3 months. Hence, it is now recommended that clopidogrel is given to patients with NSTEMI for 3 months.

Following this successful demonstration of combination therapy in the acute treatment of acute coronary syndrome, a subsequent study (CHARISMA)[3] set out to determine if dual anti-platelets in the form of aspirin and clopidogrel are appropriate for primary prevention. Unfortunately this combination did not show an overall benefit in reducing MI, stroke and cardiovascular causes of death and is not recommended as a choice of primary prevention in high-risk patients.

Today, the evidence is robust for the usage of aspirin and clopidogrel in all NSTEMI patients, STEMI patients and patients who have undergone percutaneous coronary intervention (PCI) and stent insertion. It is important to note, however, that the duration of treatment is dependent on the diagnosis and intervention undertaken. A future key outstanding question is how new anti-platelet drugs, such as prasugrel and ticagrelor, will impact the secondary prevention of cardiovascular disease, especially in selected non-ST elevation ACS subgroups such as those treated by PCI.

The New Kid on the Block: Fondaparinux
Yusuf et al., New England Journal of Medicine (2006)

Anticoagulation with low molecular weight heparin has been standard practice in the management of NSTEMI and is supported by evidence that it is modestly superior to unfractionated heparin in reducing death or MI. The trade-off is that it increases the risk of bleeding, translating into higher mortality.

The Fifth Organization to Assess Strategies in Acute Ischaemic Syndrome (OASIS-5) trial is to date the largest double-blind randomised control trial on ACS involving 20,078 patients. It compared the efficacy and safety of fondaparinux with enoxaparin in high-risk patients with unstable angina or NSTEMI.

Fondaparinux is a synthetic pentasaccharide that exerts its anticoagulation effect by inhibiting factor Xa. Patients were randomised to either fondaparinux (2.5 mg sc once daily) or enoxaparin (1 mg/kg sc twice daily) for 2–8 days. The primary efficacy outcome was a composite of death, MI and refractory ischaemia at day 9. The primary safety outcome was major bleeding at day 9. The secondary endpoint looked at each of the above components separately at day 30 and 6 months.

This non-inferiority trial demonstrated that fondaparinux was as effective as enoxaparin in preventing the primary outcome with a hazard ratio of 1.01 (95% CI 0.90–1.13). Fondaparinux had a 47% reduction of major bleeding at day 9 compared to enoxaparin. This marked decrease in bleeding rate contributed to an overall improved outcome of patients at day 30 and 6 months. The fondaparinux arm had a 17% reduction in 30-day mortality which was sustained at 6 months with a 13% relative risk reduction of MI, refractory ischaemia, major bleeding and death.

These encouraging results have helped to propel fondaparinux into clinical practice making it a more attractive agent of anticoagulation compared to enoxaparin. However, there are several issues that have been raised regarding usage of fondaparinux in NSTEMI. Firstly, some critics have pointed out that the efficacy of fondaparinux over enoxaparin might be due to the suboptimal usage of enoxaparin rather than the superiority of fondaparinux. This is because the study had a higher threshold than routine clinical practice in reducing the dosage of enoxaparin in patients with renal impairment. The authors have countered this by stating that fondaparinux was used in accordance to its licensing approval and that the reduction in bleeding risk was seen in all subgroups.

In OASIS-5, fondaparinux was associated with an increased risk of catheter thrombosis in patients undergoing PCI. These concerns were confirmed by the subsequent OASIS-6 study.

Current recommendations by the Scottish Intercollegiate Guideline Network (SIGN93, 2007) include fondaparinux for treatment of NSTEMI patients. A future question is the potential impact of fondaparinux in the cath lab management of patients with non-ST elevation myocardial infarction in ordinary clinical practice.

Percutaneous Coronary Intervention: Who Should Get It?
Fox et al., Lancet (2002)

Immediate revascularisation with PCI has formed the mainstay of treatment in patients presenting with STEMI. The management of NSTEMI usually involves the initiation of medical therapy, and patients would either undergo PCI as an inpatient or be investigated at a later stage.

Current guidelines recommend the use of risk stratification scores (GRACE, TIMI, PURSUIT and FRISC) to allow us to decide which patients would benefit from early interventions. In a clinical setting, patients classified as medium to high risk are offered an inpatient angiogram with or without PCI as part of an early invasive approach.

There are four large RCTs that have compared a conservative versus early invasive approach. Although the RITA-3 trial was not the largest among the four trials, it is selected as the key study because it comes equipped with 5-year follow-up data. This prospective, randomised control trial recruited 1810 patients, randomising 895 to early intervention and 915 to conservative management. The co-primary endpoints were a combined rate of death, nonfatal MI or refractory angina at 4 months and combined rate of death or nonfatal MI at 1 year. The trial was published in two parts; the first part was in 2002, and data from its 5-year follow-up were published in 2005[4].

The intervention was to perform an angiogram as soon as possible after randomisation and ideally within 72 hours. Depending on the findings, patients went on to have PCI or coronary artery bypass grafting or were treated medically.

At 4 months, RITA-3 demonstrated a 34% relative risk reduction (95% CI 15–59%) in its combined primary endpoint in the intervention group. Reduction in angina was the main driving force behind these results as there was no significant reduction in mortality and MI at 4 and 12 months in the intervention group.

The 5-year follow-up data are what caused the paradigm shift in practice. It successfully demonstrated a sustained benefit in the combined endpoint of MI or death in the intervention group. Although there was no initial benefit in MI and death, the 5 year follow-up data showed a relative risk reduction in all-cause death or MI by 24% and a 26% relative risk reduction in cardiovascular death and MI in patients who underwent an early invasive approach.

The RITA-3 trial recruited patients who were deemed to be at moderate risk; this, coupled with failure of the ICTUS trial[5] to demonstrate a benefit of early intervention in low-risk patients, has thus shaped our practice in adopting an early invasive approach for patients deemed moderate and high risk. A question for future research is how to best manage multivessel coronary disease in non-ST elevation MI patients at the time of initial angiography: treat all stenoses significant in the operator's judgment (e.g. as evaluated angiographically or by a coronary pressure wire study) or defer for non-invasive stress testing?

The Role of GPIIb/IIIa Inhibitors
EPIC investigators, New England Journal of Medicine (1994)

Glycoprotein IIb/IIIa (GP IIb/IIIa) receptors are involved in the final common pathway of platelet aggregation making agents blocking these receptors an attractive pharmacological target in ACS. National guidelines recommend its use in intermediate and high-risk patients, particularly if they are scheduled for PCI.

The Evaluation of 7E3 in Preventing Ischemic Complications (EPIC) study was the first large-scale randomised control trial using GPIIb/IIIa inhibitors in ACS. Abciximab was given in three regimes: (5) bolus and infusion of placebo, (6) bolus of abciximab and infusion of placebo and (7) bolus and infusion of abiciximab. It selected only high-risk patients who were due to undergo coronary angioplasty or directional atherectomy. 'High risk' was defined as severe unstable angina, evolving acute MI or high-risk coronary morphologic characteristics.

The primary endpoint was a composite of the following after 30 days: death from any cause, nonfatal MI, coronary artery bypass grafting (CABG) or repeat PCI for acute ischemia, coronary endovascular stent (in an era where stenting was not common) and placement of intra-aortic balloon pump to relieve refractory ischemia. Abciximab (bolus + infusion) demonstrated a convincing 35% relative risk reduction in the primary endpoint ($p = 0.008$) when compared to placebo. Its efficacy was primarily seen in reducing the rate of nonfatal MI and the need for emergency PCI or CABG. However, therapy with abciximab was associated with 14% incidence of bleeding compared to a 7% in the placebo group.

Further clinical trials like CAPTURE[6], EPILOG[7] and EPISTENT[8] cemented the use of GPIIb/IIIa inhibitors in patients with ACS undergoing PCI. The next phase of clinical trials involving PRISM[9], PARAGON[10], PURSUIT[11] and GUSTO-IV ACS[12] looked at whether this class of drug was beneficial in patients who were not scheduled for early PCI.

A meta-analysis of these trials showed GPIIb/IIIa inhibitors having a 9% relative risk reduction for death or MI at 30 days. This event reduction was most meaningful in high-risk patients. It confirmed a higher bleeding risk in the intervention group but stressed that stroke and intracranial bleeding were not increased. It did not answer the question on whether GPIIb/IIIa inhibitors would reduce complications if no PCI was performed because up to 14% of patients had undergone PCI within 5 days of randomisation.

We should be cautious in assuming a class effect for these drugs, as PARAGON, which randomised patients to lamifiban, had no clear benefit over placebo; and abciximab (48-hour infusion group,) used in patients not scheduled for PCI in the GUSTO-IV ACS study, was associated with a 15% increased risk of cardiac events.

The evidence points towards a benefit in GPIIb/IIIa inhibitors in high-risk patients. Interestingly patients who meet the criteria for a GPIIb/IIIa agent would also 'qualify' for angiography meaning these two treatment modalities go hand in hand. Current NICE recommendations are to use either eptifibatide or tirofiban in intermediate to high-risk patients scheduled for angiography within 96 hours. Abciximab is recommended as an adjunct to PCI in intermediate to high-risk patients who have not received another GPIIb/IIIa agent. Now that new arguably more potent anti-platelet drugs such as ticagrelor and prasugrel have emerged, are GpIIbIIIa inhibitors still as effective in non-ST elevation ACS patients who are treated with ticagrelor or prasugrel rather than clopidogrel?

Use of ACE Inhibitors Post Myocardial Infarction: Dawn of a New HOPE
The Heart Outcomes Prevention Evaluation Study Investigators, Yusuf et al., New England Journal of Medicine (2000)

Angiotensin-converting enzyme inhibitors (ACE-I) are an important evidence-based treatment for left ventricular dysfunction and heart failure.

The Heart Outcomes Prevention Evaluation (HOPE) study was a double-blind randomised control trial that recruited 9927 patients not known to have heart failure or impaired left ventricular (LV) dysfunction but deemed to be of high cardiovascular risk (known vascular disease (coronary artery disease, stroke, peripheral vascular disease) or diabetes plus either hypertension, dyslipidaemia, smoking or microalbuminuria).

The study drug was ramipril and showed remarkable results having a 16% relative risk reduction in all-cause mortality and a 26% relative risk reduction in cardiovascular mortality. Ramipril was also found to reduce the risk of future MI, strokes and heart failure. All of these benefits were independent of its blood pressure lowering effect.

Although HOPE did not include patients in the post-MI period, its selection of high-risk patients with normal LV function challenged the exclusive use of ACE-I in patients with establish heart failure. The EUROPA[13] study 3 years later recruited 13,655 patients with stable coronary artery disease regardless of their risk profile. Perindopril conferred a 20% relative risk reduction in the combined primary endpoint of cardiovascular death, cardiac arrest and MI.

Together, both EUROPA and HOPE have shown that ACE-inhibition prevents death in patients with coronary artery disease. This has resulted in the current guidelines to commence all patients on long term ACE-I treatment after an NSTEMI event. The potential benefits of ACE inhibitors (and angiotensin receptor blockers) have been extensively investigated in ACS patients.

Beta-Blockers: When to Give Them?
Chen et al., Lancet (2005)

Beta-blockers are now routinely given to all patients post MI, and their benefits have been consistently demonstrated by large meta-analysis. Unfortunately, there are no large randomised control trials describing the use of beta-blockers in NSTEMI and most of our understanding is extrapolated from STEMI trials.

Despite general consensus on their long-term benefits, it was not until 2005 that robust evidence emerged on whether beta-blockers would be beneficial if given in the acute setting. The ISIS-1 study suggested that IV atenolol was associated with a 15% relative risk reduction in cardiovascular mortality if given immediately. However, it was associated with a wide confidence interval and the study was also criticised for being unblinded with no placebo control.

The COMMIT/CCS study randomised 45,852 patients with STEMI to placebo or metoprolol 15 mg IV followed by oral metoprolol 200 mg OD until discharge or up to 4 weeks in hospital. The co-primary outcomes were a composite of death, reinfarction or cardiac arrest and all-cause mortality.

The study failed to demonstrate a significant effect on both primary endpoints and had a 30% relative risk increase in cardiogenic shock in the intervention group. There was an absolute risk reduction of reinfarction by 0.5% and an absolute risk reduction of 0.5% in ventricular fibrillation that might have accounted for the benefits noted by early trials. The benefits of beta-blockers became apparent in stable patients after day 1, but beta-blockers were found to be harmful in unstable patients with hypotension or in Killip class III.

Largely from this trial, beta-blockers are now started in patients in the acute setting if they are not bradycardic or hypotensive or demonstrate features of instability. In unstable patients these are withheld initially but given the convincing evidence on long-term effects, all patients presenting with an NSTEMI should be on a beta-blocker indefinitely if tolerated regardless of their LV function.

Should All Post-MI Patients Get Statins?
Scandinavian Simvastatin Survival Study Group, Lancet (1994)

A large body of evidence supports the use of statins in primary and secondary prevention. The Scandinavian Simvastatin Survival Study (4S) study provided the first robust evidence of the efficacy of statins in patients with established coronary heart disease.

This double-blind trial randomised 4444 patients to either placebo or simvastatin. Patients with angina or previous MI and serum cholesterol of 5.5–8.0 mmol/L were recruited and had a median follow-up period of 5.4 years.

The primary endpoint was all-cause mortality. The secondary endpoint included coronary deaths, nonfatal acute MI, resuscitated cardiac arrest and silent MI. Simvastatin demonstrated a 30% relative risk reduction in all deaths. The relative risk of patients in the simvastatin group meeting the secondary endpoint was 0.66 (95% CI 0.59–0.75). Four tertiary endpoints were also examined: (1) any coronary event – simvastatin showed a 27% relative risk reduction; (2) death or any arteriosclerotic event – relative risk reduction of 26%; (3) a 37% relative risk reduction of incidence of myocardial revascularisation procedures in the simvastatin group and (4) simvastatin did not demonstrate a reduction in hospital admissions with non-MI coronary heart disease events.

The 4S study was pivotal in proving that statins were safe and effective in improving survival for patients with coronary heart disease. However, on its own, it does not reflect current practice. 4S excluded patients presenting with an MI in the preceding 6 months, and it only recruited patients with a cholesterol level between 5.5 and 8.0 mmol/L.

The first piece of evidence on the efficacy of statins in the early post-infarction period was derived from the MIRACL study where atrovastatin was given to patients with unstable angina or non-Q wave acute MI within 24 to 96 hours of hospital admission. MIRACL[14] showed a significant reduction of the primary endpoint (death, nonfatal MI, cardiac arrest or recurrent symptomatic ischemia) after 16 weeks of follow-up (RR 0.84; 95% CI 0.7–1.0). The study also did not set a lower limit for cholesterol.

By 2006, atrovastatin had managed to become the bestselling drug for 5 consecutive years. This was made possible by the robust evidence derived from various trials which in the context of ACS was spearheaded by the 4S study. Statins not only work by lowering cholesterol, but also stabilise athereosclerotic plaques and modulate inflammation. Current clinical practice is that statins should be started on all patients with ACS regardless of their cholesterol level.

Aldosterone Antagonists
Pitt et al., New England Journal of Medicine (2003)

MI is one of the main causes of LV systolic dysfunction. For over two decades the pharmacological management of LV systolic dysfunction has targeted neurohumoral pathways including both angiotensin II and aldosterone to prevent adverse remodeling of the heart. There is now robust evidence to support the use of ACE-I routinely in patients post MI regardless of their LV function suggesting that early prevention of this remodeling effect would confer future benefit.

The EPHESUS study involved 6632 patients who were randomly assigned to either eplenerone or placebo in addition to optimal medical therapy and with a mean-follow of up of 16 months. Patients with acute MI between 3 to 14 days were eligible if they had clinical features of heart failure and an LV systolic function of <40%. The primary endpoint investigated was time to all-cause mortality or time to first cardiovascular hospitalisation or death. It demonstrated a 15% relative risk reduction of all-cause mortality and a 13% relative risk reduction in cardiovascular hospitalisation and 13% reduction in death in the group receiving eplenerone at 16 months.

Current guidelines recommend the use of eplenerone in post-MI patients with LV systolic function < 40% and NYHA class III/IV heart failure based on the population in EPHESUS.

However, with the recent publication of the EMPHASIS-HF study, these guidelines might change. EMPHASIS-HF[15] examined the effect of eplenerone in patients with mild heart failure and demonstrated a 24% relative risk reduction in both all-cause mortality and cardiovascular death at 21 months making eplenerone now applicable to a wider population of patients. A currently unanswered question is the potential benefit of aldosterone receptor antagonism in patients with non-ST elevation ACS.

Conclusion

Patients with an acute NSTEMI may now be offered a number of different drugs which have cardioprotective effects acutely and in the longer term. The evidence base to support the use of drugs such as aspirin, beta-blockers, ACE inhibitors and eplerenone has been developed in clinical trials over the past 30 years. Coronary heart disease remains the commonest cause of death in the developed world and, along with primary prevention, drug treatments and nonpharmacological interventions (such as with exercise) have pivotal importance to reduce the public health burden of ACS.

Key Outstanding Questions

1. Will management based on the new high-sensitivity troponin assays lead to improved clinical outcomes compared with standard care?
2. What is the best management approach for multivessel coronary disease in non-ST elevation ACS patients at the time of initial angiography: treat all stenoses in the operator's judgment to be significant (e.g. as evaluated angiographically or by a coronary pressure wire study) or defer for non-invasive stress testing?
3. How will new anti-platelet drugs, such as prasugrel and ticagrelor, impact the secondary prevention of cardiovascular disease, especially in selected non-ST elevation ACS subgroups such as those treated by PCI?
4. What is the potential benefit of aldosterone receptor antagonism with eplerenone in patients with non-ST elevation ACS?
5. A final area of uncertainty is the timing of coronary artery bypass surgery in patients with recent non-ST elevation ACS; should this occur early after admission or following a recovery period at least 30 days later?

Key Research Centres

There are multiple major research centres around the world involved in research into non-ST elevation ACS. The research is broad ranging from a focus on epidemiology to the development of novel drugs.

References

Chen, Z., *et al.* (2005) Early intravenous then oral metoprolol in 45, 582 patients with acute myocardial infarction: randomized placebo-controlled trial. *Lancet,* **366**, 1622–1632. http://www.ncbi.nlm.nih.gov/pubmed/16271643

The CURE Trial Investigators (2001) Effects of clopidogrel in addition to aspirin in patients with acute coronary syndromes without ST-segment elevation. *New England Journal of Medicine,* **345**, 494–502. http://circ.ahajournals.org/cgi/content/full/106/13/1622

The EPIC Investigators (1994) Use of monoclonal antibody directed against the platelet glycoprotein IIb/IIIa receptor in high risk coronary angioplasty. *New England Journal of Medicine,* **330**(14), 956–961. http://www.ncbi.nlm.nih.gov/pubmed/8121459

Fox, K.A., *et al.* (2002) Interventional versus conservative treatment for patients with unstable angina or non-ST-elevation myocardial infarction: the British Heart Foundation RITA 3 randomised trial. Randomised Intervention Trial of unstable Angina. *Lancet,* **360**(9335), 743–751. http://www.ncbi.nlm.nih.gov/pubmed/12241831

Hamm, C.W., *et al.* (1992) The prognostic value of serum troponin T in unstable angina. *New England Journal of Medicine,* **327**(3), 146–150. http://www.ncbi.nlm.nih.gov/pubmed/1290492

ISIS-2 Collaborators (1988) Randomised trial of intravenous streptokinase, oral aspirin, both, or neither among 17, 187 cases of suspected acute myocardial infarction: ISIS-2. *Lancet,* **2**(8607), 349. http://www.ncbi.nlm.nih.gov/pubmed/2899772

Pitt, B., *et al.* (2003) Eplenerone, a selective aldosterone blocker, in patients with left ventricular dysfunction after myocardial infarction. *New England Journal of Medicine,* **348**, 1309–1321. http://www.ncbi.nlm.nih.gov/pubmed/12668699

Scandinavian Simvastatin Survival Study Group (1994) Randomised trial of cholesterol lowering in 4444 patients with coronary heart disease: the Scandinavian Simvastatin Survival Study (4S). *Lancet,* **344**, 1383–1389. http://www.ncbi.nlm.nih.gov/pubmed/7968073

Yusuf, S., *et al.* (2000) Effects of an angiotensin-converting-enzyme inhibitor, ramipril, on cardiovascular events in high-risk patients. The Heart Outcomes Prevention Evaluation Study Investigators. *New England Journal of Medicine*, **342**(3), 145–153. http://www.ncbi.nlm.nih.gov/pubmed/10639539

Yusuf, S., *et al.* (2006) Comparison of Fondaparinux and Enoxaparin in acute coronary syndromes: the OASIS-5 investigators. *New England Journal of Medicine*, **354**, 1464–1476. http://www.ncbi.nlm.nih.gov/pubmed/16537663

Additional References

1. Antithrombotic Trialists' (ATT) Collaboration (2009) Aspirin in the primary and secondary prevention of vascular disease: collaborative meta-analysis of individual participant data from randomised trials. *Lancet*, **373**, 1849–1860.
2. Yusuf, S., *et al.* (2003) Early and late effects of clopidogrel in patients with acute coronary syndromes. *Circulation*, **107**(7), 966–972.
3. CHARISMA trial investigators (2004) Clopidogrel added to aspiring versus aspirin alone in secondary prevention and high-risk primary prevention: rationale and design of the Clopidogrel for High Atherothrombotic Risk and Ischaemic Stabilization, Management and Avoidance trial. *American Heart Journal*, **148**(2), 263–268.
4. Fox, K.A., *et al.* (2005) 5-year outcome of an interventional strategy in non-ST-elevation acute coronary syndrome: the British Heart Foundation RITA 3 randomised trial. *Lancet*, **336**(9489), 914–920.
5. De Winter, T., *et al.* (2005) Early invasive selectively invasive management for acute coronary syndrome. *New England Journal of Medicine*, **353**, 1059–1104.
6. The CAPTURE Investigators (1997) Randomised placebo-controlled trial of abiciximab before and during coronary intervention in refractory unstable angina: the CAPTURE study. *Lancet*, **349**, 1429–35.
7. The EPILOG Investigators (1997) Platelet glycoprotein IIb/IIIa receptor blockade and low-dose heparin during percutaneous coronary revascularization. *New England Journal of Medicine*, **336**, 1689–1696.
8. The EPISTENT Investigators (1998) Randomised placebo–controlled and balloon-angioplasty-controlled trial to assess safety of coronary stenting with use of platelet glycoprotein IIb/IIIa blockade. *Lancet*, **352**, 87–92.
9. The PRISM Study Investigators (1998) A comparison of aspirin plus tirofiban with aspirin plus heparin for unstable angina. *New England Journal of Medicine*, **338**, 1489–1505.
10. The PARAGON Investigators (1998) International, randomized, controlled trial of lamifiban (a platelet glycoprotein IIb/IIIa inhibitor), heparin, or both in unstable angina. Platelet IIb/IIIa antagonism for the reduction of acute coronary syndrome events in a global organization network. *Circulation*, **97**, 2386–2395.
11. The PURSUIT Trial Investigators (1998) Inhibition of platelet glycoprotein IIb/IIIa with eptifibatide in patients with acute coronary syndromes. *New England Journal of Medicine*, **339**, 436–443.
12. The GUSTO-IV ACS Investigators (2001) Effect of glycoprotein IIb/IIIa receptor blocker abciximab on outcome in patients with acute coronary syndromes without early coronary revascularization: the GUSTO IV-ACS randomized trial. *Lancet*, **357**, 1915–1924.
13. Fox, K.M. (2003) Efficacy of perindopril in reduction of cardiovascular events among patients with stable coronary artery disease: randomized, double-blind, placebo-controlled, multicentre trial (the EUROPA study). *Lancet*, **362**(9386), 782–788.

14. Schwartz, G.G., *et al.* (2001) Effects of atrovastatin on early recurrent ischemic events in acute coronary syndrome: the MIRACL study: a randomized controlled trial. *Journal of the American Medical Association*, **285**(13), 1711–1718.

15. Zannad, F., *et al.* (2011) Eplerenone in patients with systolic heart failure and mild symptoms. *New England Journal of Medicine*, **364**, 11–21.

5 Lipids, Dyslipidaemia and Cardiovascular Disease

Gilbert R. Thompson

Department of Medicine, Imperial College London, London, UK

Introduction

Atherosclerosis is characterised by the accumulation of cholesterol in the arterial wall, leading to inflammation and localised narrowing of affected vessels. This process is accelerated and accentuated in subjects with dyslipidaemia and manifests itself clinically as coronary heart disease and stroke.

During the 19th century, Virchow proposed that atherosclerosis was initiated by mechanical injury, which caused constituents of the blood to be deposited within the arterial wall and evoke a localised inflammatory response. Evidence of a specific role for lipids in this process came in 1910 when the Nobel Prize winning German chemist Windaus discovered large quantities of cholesterol in atheromatous aortas. Subsequently two Russian Army doctors, Anitchkov and Chalatov, showed that atherosclerosis could be induced experimentally by feeding cholesterol to rabbits. In the 1950s the American physicist Gofman demonstrated an association between coronary artery disease and raised levels of the cholesterol carried in plasma by low-density, but not high-density, lipoproteins. Oliver and Boyd, working in Edinburgh, utilised paper electrophoresis to separate α and β lipoproteins and showed that the α:β ratio was decreased in men with coronary disease, confirming Gofman's results. Despite their importance, these findings were greeted with apathy or scepticism by cardiologists on both sides of the Atlantic.

Widespread recognition of the clinical relevance of lipids came in 1967 when Fredrickson and his colleagues at the US National Institutes of Health published a five-part article in the *New England Journal of Medicine* describing a novel classification of dyslipidaemia. This publication stimulated a decade of productive research in the 1970s, resulting in major advances in knowledge concerning lipoprotein metabolism and the pathogenesis of atherosclerosis. The ten papers exemplifying the most important advances made during and since that time are reported here in chronological order.

The Beginnings of Clinical Lipidology: Fredrickson's Classification of Lipoprotein Phenotypes
Fredrickson et al., New England Journal of Medicine (1967)

Knowledge of lipid disorders was rudimentary or non-existent among clinicians half a century ago. That all changed in 1967 following the publication of this five-part *magnum opus*, which aimed to provide physicians with the information needed to manage

---

Understanding Medical Research: The Studies that Shaped Medicine, First Edition. Edited by John A. Goodfellow. © 2012 John Wiley & Sons, Ltd. Published 2012 by John Wiley & Sons, Ltd.

dyslipidaemia in a rational manner. To this end, Fredrickson and colleagues introduced the idea of classifying the various disorders in terms of lipoproteins rather than lipids. The existence of distinct classes of lipoprotein particles differing in their lipid composition was already well established, and these authors pointed out that abnormal levels of plasma cholesterol and/or triglyceride simply reflected changes in the concentrations of the lipoproteins which transported them.

Lipoproteins can be separated according to their density on ultracentrifugation into very low-density lipoprotein (VLDL), low-density lipoprotein (LDL) and high-density lipoprotein (HDL), or by differences in their electrophoretic mobility into the corresponding preβ, β and α lipoproteins. Because of its greater convenience, Fredrickson and colleagues adopted the latter approach. Drawing upon the unique collection of patients referred to the National Institutes of Health (NIH) in Bethesda, they described five distinct lipoprotein phenotypes, each of which reflected genetically determined or acquired forms of hyperlipoproteinaemia, the numbering of the phenotypes being based upon the electrophoretic mobility of the lipoprotein present in excess. Inherited forms of hypolipoproteinaemia were characterised by decreases in α lipoprotein (Tangier disease) or β lipoprotein (aβlipoproteinaemia and hypoβlipoproteinaemia).

As acknowledged by the authors, the typing system was a temporary expedient and, as knowledge of the underlying metabolic defects increased, it gradually became redundant. However, at the time it served a vital purpose in drawing attention to the role of specific lipoproteins in predisposing to atherosclerosis, which was especially severe and premature in type II patients with an inherited increase in LDL.

Fredrickson, Levy and Lees concluded their article by commenting, 'The plasma is often the only window from which one can see the state of intracellular metabolism. The view is limited and all ingenuity is needed to gain the sharpest perspective'. The insights into lipoprotein metabolism gained from the ingenuity of those pioneers inspired a whole generation of researchers and marked the inauguration of lipidology as a clinically relevant entity.

Dietary Saturated Fat and Cardiovascular Disease: The Seven Countries Study
Coronary Heart Disease in Seven Countries, Circulation Suppl. (1970)

An entire supplement to *Circulation* was devoted to 20 articles describing the design and 5-year results of the Seven Countries Study. The latter was the brain child of Ancel Keys who pioneered research into the role of dietary fats in cardiovascular disease.

Ancel Keys, who died recently aged 100, was a physiologist at the University of Minnesota with a strong interest in the epidemiology of coronary heart disease (CHD). In 1947 he initiated the first prospective study of this disorder in a group of local businessmen and found a correlation between a raised serum cholesterol and coronary mortality and morbidity. Surveys had suggested that differences in diet were responsible for geographical differences in the prevalence of CHD between countries such as South Africa and the United States. To pursue this question further, Keys undertook feasibility studies in countries with the lowest and highest recorded rates of CHD, namely Japan and Finland, which became the Seven Countries Study in 1957.

The seven countries involved were Finland, Greece, Italy, Japan, the Netherlands, the United States and Yugoslavia. All men aged 40–59 in defined areas of each country were examined at 5-yearly intervals over a period of at least 10 years. This involved investigating a total of 12,270 men using standardised methods, each examination including a questionnaire, blood and urine analysis, and electrocardiograms at rest and after exercise. Dietary intake was assessed by random surveys which involved weighing all food consumed over 1 week and chemical analysis of replicate meals. All deaths and major illnesses were recorded.

The results confirmed that the age standardised prevalence of CHD at entry was much higher in Finland and the United States than in most other countries. Over the next 5 years, the incidence in men free of CHD at entry followed a similar pattern, being highest in Finland and the United States and lowest in Japan and Greece. Differences in the incidence of CHD correlated with differences in the frequency of hypercholesterolaemia and in the percentage of calories provided by saturated fat in each country. For example, as illustrated in Figure 5.1, 56% of Finnish men had a serum cholesterol of >250 mg/dl (6.5 mmol/l) and 20% of their calories were provided by dietary saturated fat compared with 7% and 3% respectively in Japan, with comparable differences in the incidence of CHD between the two countries.

In the light of these findings Keys lobbied for, and subsequently achieved, major dietary changes in the United States, Finland and most other Western nations, resulting in a reduction in saturated fat consumption and its partial replacement with polyunsaturated fat. After he retired, he went to live in southern Italy and helped to popularise the benefits of the olive oil-based Mediterranean diet, now a cornerstone of healthy lifestyle strategies to prevent CHD.

Risk Factors for Coronary Heart Disease: The Framingham Study
Kannel et al., Annals of Internal Medicine (1971)

The word Framingham has become synonymous with 'risk factors', inherited or acquired traits that increase the likelihood that the bearer will develop CHD. Framingham, a small town near Boston, Massachusetts, gave its name to the prospective study which started there in 1948 and has been going on ever since. The main objective was to examine a representative sample of adults for characteristics that might predispose them to CHD and then follow them up for 20 years to determine which developed the disorder.

The study population was relatively small, consisting of slightly more than 2000 men and just under 3000 women aged 30–62. Anyone with evidence of pre-existing CHD at the first examination was excluded, and the remainder were re-examined every 2 years. Serum cholesterol was measured on each occasion, and LDL and VLDL were measured at the first two examinations. Other measurements performed routinely were blood pressure, body weight, blood glucose, uric acid and ascertainment of smoking status. The occurrence of coronary events was based on electrocardiogram (ECG) and enzyme changes and, if fatal, autopsy evidence. 80% were followed up for 14 years plus an additional 8% who died during that time.

During the follow-up period, 323 men and 169 women developed CHD, the incidence being threefold greater in those with serum cholesterol and LDL and VLDL concentrations in the top versus the bottom quartile. Except for VLDL in postmenopausal women, measurement of lipoprotein fractions was not more predictive than serum cholesterol alone. The discovery that an increase in VLDL was a risk

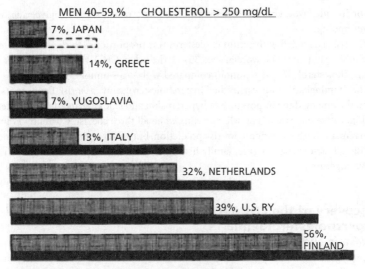

MEN 40–59,% CHOLESTEROL > 250 mg/dL

7%, JAPAN

14%, GREECE

7%, YUGOSLAVIA

13%, ITALY

32%, NETHERLANDS

39%, U.S. RY

56%, FINLAND

NARROW, SOLID BARS SHOW CHD INCIDENCE RATE

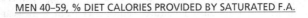

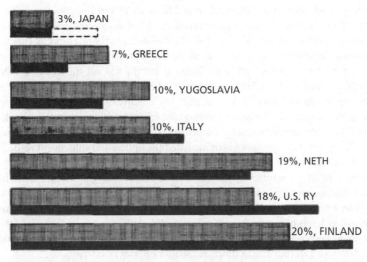

MEN 40–59, % DIET CALORIES PROVIDED BY SATURATED F.A.

3%, JAPAN

7%, GREECE

10%, YUGOSLAVIA

10%, ITALY

19%, NETH

18%, U.S. RY

20%, FINLAND

NARROW, SOLID BARS SHOW CHD INCIDENCE RATE

Figure 5.1 Percentage of men with serum cholesterol >250 mg/dl (6.5 mmol/l) (upper panel) and percentage of calories provided by saturated fat (lower panel). The lower, solid bars show the incidence of coronary heart disease in each country, the rate in Finland being 2% per year. Reproduced with permission from Coronary Heart Disease in Seven Countries, *Circulation*, 1970.

factor in older women, which manifests itself as a raised serum triglyceride, was a novel finding.

The risk associated with serum cholesterol was proportional to the latter's concentration so that in men and women aged 35–44, the risk of CHD was fivefold greater if the serum cholesterol was >6.8 mmol/l compared with < 5.7 mmol/l.

The Framingham study established hypercholesterolaemia as a risk factor in its own right, documented the importance of hypertension and smoking and demonstrated the multiplicative increase in risk which occurs when all three coexist. Currently Framingham remains the gold standard for risk prediction, but newer approaches, which include additional factors such as race, family history and C-reactive protein, may eventually prove superior.

Discovery of the LDL Receptor and the Cause of Familial Hypercholesterolaemia
Goldstein and Brown, Journal of Biological Chemistry (1974)

Homozygous familial hypercholesterolaemia (FH) is a very rare disorder, affecting one in a million people. A patient with this condition fascinated Joseph Goldstein when he was a clinical associate to Fredrickson at the NIH and led to his forming a Nobel Prize winning partnership with Michael Brown to study its cause. Working together in Dallas, they studied cholesterol synthesis in cultured fibroblasts from a 12-year-old FH homozygote whose serum cholesterol ranged between 18 and 26 mmol/l and who had sustained a myocardial infarct a year previously[1]. They discovered that the activity of hydroxymethylglutaryl coenzyme A (HMG CoA) reductase, the rate limiting enzyme on the cholesterol synthesis pathway, was 60–80 times greater in her fibroblasts than in control fibroblasts and that, unlike the latter, its activity was not suppressed by adding LDL to the culture medium. Fibroblasts from FH heterozygotes exhibited a partial defect in the regulation of HMG CoA reductase, but Goldstein and Brown considered it unlikely that a defect in the gene encoding that enzyme could explain their results.

In 1974 they demonstrated that ^{125}I-labelled LDL was bound to normal fibroblasts by a high-affinity, saturable process which mediated the uptake and subsequent proteolytic degradation of LDL and resulted in the suppression of HMG CoA reductase activity and therefore cholesterol synthesis. Fibroblasts from FH homozygotes lacked these high-affinity binding sites, failed to degrade LDL and failed to suppress their HMG CoA reductase activity when exposed to LDL. Fibroblasts from FH heterozygotes showed intermediate levels of high-affinity binding of LDL. At higher concentrations LDL was taken up by both normal and FH fibroblasts by a low-affinity process which resulted in degradation of LDL but not in down-regulation of HMG CoA reductase.

Goldstein and Brown concluded that high-affinity binding of LDL normally results in endocytosis and lysosomal degradation of LDL and that cholesterol is released during this process, leading to inhibition of HMG CoA reductase. They therefore proposed that FH was caused by an abnormality of a gene whose product was the LDL receptor. Their observations explain how inhibition of HMG CoA reductase by statins lowers LDL cholesterol by stimulating expression of hepatic LDL receptors and thereby increasing LDL catabolism. The discovery of the LDL receptor was a groundbreaking discovery which resulted in Goldstein and Brown being awarded the Nobel Prize for Physiology or Medicine in 1985.

Recognition of the Protective Role of HDL against Cardiovascular Disease
Miller and Miller, Lancet (1975)

HDL levels tend to be lower in situations associated with an increased risk of CHD, such as being male rather than female, and studies had shown that patients with CHD had lower HDL:LDL ratios than control subjects. However, it was not until Norman and George Miller published their paper in 1975 that the protective effects of HDL really grabbed the scientific headlines.

Analysing published data from Finland, the Millers showed that HDL cholesterol levels were significantly lower in eight normocholesterolaemic patients with CHD than in 14 controls with similar levels of VLDL and LDL cholesterol. They also demonstrated an inverse correlation between HDL cholesterol concentration and the mass of cholesterol present in both the rapidly and slowly exchangeable pools of tissue cholesterol. Since the latter included arterial wall cholesterol, these authors proposed that having a low HDL cholesterol level promotes the development of atherosclerosis by impairing the clearance of cholesterol from the arterial wall.

Miller and Miller noted that accumulation of tissue cholesterol is a feature of Tangier disease, in which HDL is absent, and that HDL cholesterol is the preferred substrate of lecithin cholesterol acyltransferase (LCAT) which, together with cholesterol ester transfer protein (CETP), is involved in the movement of cholesterol from plasma to the liver, otherwise known as reverse cholesterol transport. They therefore concluded that strategies designed to raise HDL cholesterol would have a favourable effect on atherosclerosis. Thus far, however, the evidence for this has been decidedly limited, depending mainly on the somewhat equivocal results of trials using fibrates. The most recent attempt at answering this question ended in disaster when the CETP inhibitor torcetrapib was shown to double the concentration of HDL cholesterol in the ILLUMINATE trial but at the cost of increasing total mortality by almost 60%.

Considering its paucity of original data, Miller and Miller's paper had an astonishing impact, being the second most frequently cited of the ten papers in this chapter. It undoubtedly established the inverse correlation between HDL cholesterol and risk of CHD, a relationship which was soon confirmed in other studies, including the Framingham Study.

The Discovery of Compactin: The First Statin
Endo et. al., Journal of Antibiotics (1976)

In 1971 Akira Endo, a Japanese microbiologist working for Sankyo, started searching for microbial metabolites which would inhibit HMG CoA reductase. His belief that this would provide a novel means of lowering plasma cholesterol was vindicated when, after testing more than 6000 microbial strains, he and his colleagues isolated a potent inhibitor from *Penicillium citrinum* which lowered serum cholesterol in experimental animals. Initially known as ML-236B, this compound was later called compactin and became the first HMG CoA reductase inhibitor to be used in humans.

Using the cultured fibroblast system devised by Goldstein and Brown, Endo and colleagues showed that compactin was a potent inhibitor of cholesterol synthesis *in vitro* in cells from both normal subjects and patients with FH. *In vivo* studies showed that compactin lowered serum cholesterol levels in dogs and monkeys but not in rats.

The first clinical studies were carried out in FH homozygotes in 1980 and subsequently it was shown that co-administration of compactin and cholestyramine lowered LDL cholesterol to an unprecedented extent in heterozygotes. However, at that stage Sankyo abruptly suspended their clinical trial programme for undisclosed reasons and compactin was never licensed.

Endo had collaborated with the US drug company Merck several years earlier by providing them with samples of compactin. In 1980 workers at Merck discovered a second HMG CoA reductase inhibitor, mevinolin, which they isolated from *Aspergillus terreus* and which was later renamed lovastatin[2]. Endo isolated this compound simultaneously but independently from a different mould, naming it monocolin K[3]. Merck proceeded with the clinical development of lovastatin, and in 1987 it became the first HMG CoA reductase inhibitor to be licensed for use in humans. Other statins soon followed including pravastatin (which was derived from compactin), simvastatin, fluvastatin, atorvastatin and rosuvastatin, the latest and most potent of these compounds.

During the 1990s a series of clinical trials established unequivocally that lowering LDL cholesterol with statins resulted in significant decreases in cardiovascular and total mortality without any increase in noncardiovascular mortality and with few serious side effects. As a result, these drugs are now used routinely to treat and prevent cardiovascular disease throughout the world. They have revolutionised the practice of cardiology, and it has been estimated that one third of adults in the United States and United Kingdom would benefit from taking them.

Endo's discovery of the hypocholesterolaemic properties of *Penicillium citrinum* was undoubtedly a first in the prevention and cure of atherosclerotic cardiovascular disease, akin to the Nobel Prize winning discovery half a century earlier of the antibiotic properties of *Penicillium notatum*.

ApoE Polymorphism and Type III Hyperlipoproteinaemia
Utermann et al., Nature (1977)

The clinical and laboratory features of type III hyperlipoproteinaemia, namely palmar striae, a broad β band on electrophoresis and increased risk of vascular disease, were described by Fredrickson and colleagues in 1967. The cause was unknown, but those authors speculated that the disorder represented the homozygous expression of a mutant gene that resulted in an abnormal lipoprotein with the density of VLDL but the electrophoretic mobility of LDL, giving rise to the term 'dysbetalipoproteinaemia'. Subsequently it was shown that the abnormal lipoprotein represented the accumulation of partially degraded chylomicrons and VLDL particles, nowadays termed 'remnants'.

In 1975 Utermann and colleagues reported that VLDL from normal subjects contained three arginine-rich polypeptides which they termed apoE-I, II and III, the third of these polypeptides being absent from the remnant particles of type III patients. They hypothesised that a recessively inherited deficiency of this isoform of apoE was the cause of the disorder[4].

Further light was thrown on the matter in 1977 by Utermann's paper in *Nature*. They showed that apoE polymorphism was determined by two alleles which they termed apoE[n] and apoE[d]: patients with type III hyperlipoproteinaemia were homozygous for apoE[d]. But so too were 1% of the German population, although only a small minority of these were hyperlipidaemic. The authors suggested that additional genetic factors had to coexist with apoE^d homozygosity to produce the full-blown type III phenotype. They also described a third apoE variant that occurred in 27% of the samples analysed, which they termed apo E-IV (+).

Later investigators published an alternative nomenclature for apoE isoforms. To resolve the confusion, the various groups involved got together and agreed on a common nomenclature reflecting the existence of three major alleles for apoE, giving rise to six commonly occurring apoE phenotypes. Under this system all type III patients were homozygous for ε2 (i.e. they had an E2/E2 phenotype). Subsequent research at the Gladstone Institute showed that apoE2 differs from apoE3 and apoE4 by the substitution of cysteine for arginine at amino acid 158. This causes a change in the conformation of apoE2 which inhibits its ability to act as a ligand for the LDL receptor, which normally mediates the uptake of VLDL remnants containing apoE3 and apoE4, and explains the accumulation of remnant particles in type III hyperlipoproteinaemia.

This has had wide ranging consequences. It has not only revealed the cause of type III hyperlipoproteinaemia but also showed that apoE phenotype influenced serum cholesterol and triglyceride levels in the population at large. Inherited differences in the frequency of the three common alleles also help to explain racial differences in lipid levels and predisposition to cardiovascular disease. Lastly, it has been established that inheritance of the ε4 allele increases the risk of early-onset Alzheimer's disease, especially in homozygous carriers.

Role of the Scavenger Receptor in Atherosclerosis
Goldstein et al., Proceedings of the National Academy of Sciences of the USA (1979)

Having shown that FH was due to an inherited lack of LDL receptors, Goldstein and colleagues were intrigued by the presence of cholesterol ester-filled macrophages (foam cells) in the atherosclerotic lesions of FH homozygotes, since it implied that macrophages took up LDL cholesterol by an LDL receptor-independent pathway. They investigated this paradox using mouse peritoneal macrophages and showed that the latter took up and degraded acetyl LDL 20 times faster than native LDL despite accumulating large amounts of cholesterol. They demonstrated that this process reflected the presence of a high-affinity binding site which recognised acetylated but not native LDL. At the same time, Brown and colleagues[5] showed that uptake and degradation of acetylated LDL markedly stimulated cholesterol esterification in mouse peritoneal macrophages and greatly increased their cholesterol ester content. This reflected the activity of acylcholesterol acyltransferase (ACAT) within macrophages, which re-esterified cholesterol linoleate (the main form in which cholesterol occurs in LDL) to cholesterol oleate, the main form in which it accumulates in foam cells.

Goldstein and Brown suggested that some chemical or physical modification of LDL occurred in human plasma or tissue fluid which made it a suitable ligand for what they termed the scavenger pathway for LDL in FH. Subsequently it became clear that this pathway plays a key role in atherogenesis in general, not just in FH, and that oxidised LDL is probably its main substrate.

The discovery of the scavenger receptor by Goldstein was a crucial step in the development of the inflammatory-response-to-injury theory of atherosclerosis originally proposed by Virchow, a concept which has been advanced further by Libby[6] and others during the past decade. Although definitive proof of a causal role for oxidized LDL is lacking, there is ample evidence of its presence in atherosclerotic lesions.

Atheromatous Plaque Fissuring and Fatal Coronary Events
Davies and Thomas, New England Journal of Medicine (1984)

The importance of plaque rupture or fissuring as the mechanism underlying sudden death from coronary heart disease was decisively established in this paper by Davies and Thomas. These authors undertook post-mortem coronary arteriography in a consecutive series of 100 patients who had died from cardiac ischaemia within 6 hours of onset and in control subjects dying from noncoronary causes. This involved injecting the coronary arteries with a barium/gelatine suspension, dissecting the vessels intact and sectioning them every 3 mm. The presence of thrombus and plaque fissuring and the extent of stenosis in each section were then painstakingly recorded in a blinded manner.

A total of 115 intraluminal thrombi were found in 74 of the coronary cases, 44 of whom had major acute thrombi occluding >50% of the vessel lumen. Forty-two of the 44 major thrombi and 103 of all the 115 thrombi had a coexisting intra-intimal thrombus resulting from plaque fissuring. Of the 26 cases without a luminal thrombus, 21 had an intra-intimal thrombus, 19 of which were associated with plaque fissuring. The authors noted that there was a preponderance of lesions in the right coronary artery, which supplies the conducting system of the heart. In a minority of instances, 14 out of 44 major thrombi occurred in pre-existing lesions with <50% diameter stenosis, all of these being associated with massive fissuring of lipid-rich plaques. Only 5% of the cases had no coronary lesions compared with 90% of controls. These findings established that plaque fissuring was far more common than had been recognised and suggested that it played a major role in effecting the progression of coronary atherosclerosis. Subsequent studies by Davies and colleagues[7] showed that the likelihood of a plaque developing a fissure is influenced by its cellular content and mechanical properties.

4S: The Trial That Proved the Lipid Hypothesis
Pedersen et al., Lancet (1994)

The publication in 1994 of the results of the Scandinavian Simvastatin Survival Study (4S) provided the first clear evidence that lowering cholesterol reduced both cardiovascular events and total mortality. In this epic trial, 4444 predominantly male patients from Denmark, Finland, Iceland, Norway and Sweden, aged 35–70 with angina or previous myocardial infarction and serum cholesterol averaging 6.8 mmol/l on diet, were randomised to receive simvastatin or placebo. During the study, simvastatin reduced total cholesterol by 25% and LDL cholesterol by 35% and increased HDL cholesterol by 8%.

The median duration of treatment was 5.4 years after which the trial was stopped because of a highly significant 30% reduction in total mortality. This was entirely due to a 42% reduction in coronary mortality, and there was no increase in noncardiovascular causes of death such as cancer or trauma. Unexpectedly simvastatin also reduced the occurrence of cerebrovascular events. The mean level of LDL cholesterol in subjects on simvastatin was similar to that seen in earlier trials where the effects of statins had been assessed by coronary angiography. Taken together the findings showed that a 30–35% reduction in LDL cholesterol resulted in decreased progression of coronary lesions and fewer clinical events.

The beneficial effects of statins were confirmed by the Cholesterol Treatment Trialists' Collaboration meta-analysis[8] of the data from over 90,000 individuals who participated in 14 statin trials published between 1994 and 2004. The results showed decreases of 12% and 19% in total and coronary mortality, respectively, for each 1 mmol/l (29%) reduction in LDL cholesterol. Overall the risk of a major vascular event, including strokes, was reduced by one fifth, and no significant changes in noncardiovascular mortality were observed.

Some authors have suggested that the cardiovascular benefits of statins are exerted via their so-called pleiotropic effects, which reflect inhibition of the synthesis of products of HMG CoA reductase other than cholesterol itself. Alternative means of lowering LDL cholesterol upregulate the HMG CoA reductase pathway and so cannot exert the pleiotropic effects attributed to statins. However, meta-analyses show that the reductions in coronary events seen in statin and nonstatin trials were similar and consistent with a one-to-one relationship between LDL cholesterol lowering and coronary heart disease reduction. Thus the effects of statins in reducing coronary events seem to be explicable entirely on the basis of their cholesterol lowering properties, a conclusion supported by the results of recent trials of more potent statins, which show that the greater the decrease in LDL, the greater the reduction in cardiovascular events.

Summary and Conclusions

It has been said that 'Without cholesterol there can be no atherosclerosis',[9] and it is clear that our current understanding of this disorder greatly benefitted from the advances in lipid research which occurred over the past 40 years. These reflect a broad spectrum of research activity encompassing clinical, epidemiological, biochemical, cell biological, pharmacological and pathological studies of the role of lipids in vascular disease. Consequently the causal role of LDL cholesterol in atherosclerosis is now an established fact, confirmed by studies showing that lowering LDL cholesterol arrests or reverses the pathological process and reduces the frequency of clinical events.

The discovery of statins is on a par with that of penicillin and has dramatically improved the management of dyslipidaemia and prevention of coronary heart disease. The finding that familial hypercholesterolaemia was caused by mutations of the LDL receptor gene heralded an increasingly strong genetic emphasis on research in this field, which not only has enhanced understanding of the causes of atherosclerosis but also may engender novel forms of therapy such as the use of anti-sense oligonucleotides to apoB mRNA to inhibit synthesis of LDL and Lp(a) or, when directed against proprotein convertase subtilisin/kexin type 9 (*PCSK9*), to enhance LDL catabolism[10].

Key Outstanding Questions

1. If raising HDL cholesterol is protective against vascular disease, is pharmacological inhibition of CETP a safe and effective means of achieving this objective?
2. In view of the evidence that oxidised LDL is atherogenic, why have trials of anti-oxidants had such a negative outcome?

3. Do statins which cross the blood–brain barrier favourably influence cognitive decline and/or Alzheimer's disease?
4. Are plant sterols when consumed as functional foods pro- or anti-atherogenic?
5. Should measurement of inflammatory markers such as hs-CRP be included in the prediction of cardiovascular risk?

Key Research Centres

1. Department of Molecular Genetics, University of Texas Southwestern Medical Center, Dallas, United States
2. Medical Research Council Clinical Sciences Centre and Imperial College London, London, United Kingdom
3. Department of Vascular Medicine, Academic Medical Center, University of Amsterdam, the Netherlands
4. Gladstone Institute of Neurological Disease, San Francisco, United States
5. Center for Cardiovascular Disease Prevention, Brigham and Women's Hospital and Harvard Medical School, Boston, United States

References

Coronary heart disease in seven countries (1970) *Circulation*, **41** (Suppl. 1), I–1-198. http://circ.ahajournals.org/content/vol41/issue4S1

Davies, M.J. and Thomas, A. (1984) Thrombosis and acute coronary artery lesions in sudden cardiac ischemic death. *New England Journal of Medicine*, **310**, 1137–1140. http://www.ncbi.nlm.nih.gov/pubmed/6709008 ML-236A, ML-236B, and ML-236C, new inhibitors of cholesterologenesis produced by Penicillium Citrinum. *Journal of Antibiotics*, **29**, 1346–1348. http://www.journalarchive.jst.go.jp/english/jnlabstract_en.php?cdjournal=antibiotics1968&cdvol=29&noissue=12&startpage=1346

Fredrickson, D.S., *et al.* (1967) Fat transport in lipoproteins: an integrated approach to mechanisms and disorders. *New England Journal of Medicine*, **276**, 34–42, 94–103, 148–156, 215–225, 273–281. http://www.nejm.org/doi/full/10.1056/New England Journal of Medicine196701052760107

Goldstein, J.L., *et al.* (1979) Binding site on macrophages that mediates uptake and degradation of acetylated low density lipoprotein, producing massive cholesterol deposition. *Proceedings of the National Academy of Sciences of the USA*, **76**, 333–337. http://www.ncbi.nlm.nih.gov/pmc/articles/PMC382933/?tool=pubmed

Goldstein, J.L. and Brown, M.S. (1974) Binding and degradation of low density lipoproteins by cultured human fibroblasts. *Journal of Biological Chemistry*, **249**, 5153–5162. http://www.jbc.org/content/249/16/5153.long

Kannel, W.B., *et al.* (1971) Serum cholesterol, lipoproteins and risk of coronary heart disease – Framingham Study. *Annals of Internal Medicine*, **74**, 1–8. http://www.annals.org/content/74/1/1.Abstract

Miller, G.J. and Miller, N.E. (1975) Plasma-high-density-lipoprotein concentration and development of ischaemic heart disease. *Lancet*, **1**, 16–19. http://www.thelancet.com/journals/lancet/article/PIIS0140-6736(75)92376-4/Abstract

Pedersen, T.R., *et al.* (1994) Randomised trial of cholesterol lowering in 4444 patients with coronary heart disease: the Scandinavian Simvastatin Survival Study (4S). *Lancet*, **344**, 1383–1389. http://www.ncbi.nlm.nih.gov/pubmed/7968073

Utermann, G., et al. (1977) Polymorphism of apolipoprotein-E and occurrence of dysbeta-lipoproteinemia in man. *Nature*, **269**, 604–607. http://www.nature.com/nature/journal/v269/n5629/abs/269604a0.html

Additional References

1. Goldstein, J.L. and Brown, M.S. (1973) Familial hypercholesterolemia: identification of a defect in the regulation of 3-hydroxy-3-methylglutaryl coenzyme A reductase activity associated with overproduction of cholesterol. *Proceedings of the National Academy of Sciences of the USA*, **70**, 2804–2808.

2. Alberts, A.W., et al. (1980) Mevinolin: a highly potent competitive inhibitor of hydro-xymethylglutaryl-coenzyme A reductase and a cholesterol-lowering agent. *Proceedings of the National Academy of Sciences of the USA*, **77**, 3957–3961.

3. Endo, A. and Monacolin, K. (1979) A new hypocholesterolemic agent produced by a *Monascus* species. *Journal of Antibiotics*, **32**, 852–854.

4. Utermann, G., et al. (1975) Familial hyperlipoproteinemia type III: deficiency of a specific apolipoprotein (apoE-III) in the very-low-density lipoproteins. *FEBS Letters*, **56**, 352–355.

5. Brown, M.S., et al. (1979) Reversible accumulation of cholesteryl esters in macrophages incubated with acetylated lipoproteins. *Journal of Cellular Biology*, **82**, 597–613.

6. Libby, P. (2002) Inflammation in atherosclerosis. *Nature*, **420**, 868–874.

7. Davies, M.J., et al. (1993) Risk of thrombosis in human atherosclerotic plaques: role of extracellular lipid, macrophages, and smooth muscle cell content. *British Heart Journal*, **69**, 377–381.

8. Baigent, C., *et al.* (2005) Efficacy and safety of cholesterol-lowering treatment: prospective meta-analysis of data from 90, 056 participants in 14 randomised trials of statins. *Lancet*, **366**, 1267–2378.

9. Anitchkov, N.N. (1915) New data on pathology and etiology of atherosclerosis. *Russian Physician*, **8**, 184–186 (in Russian).

10. Stein, E.A. (2009) Other therapies for reducing low-density lipoprotein cholesterol: medications in development. *Endocrinology Metabolism Clinics of North America*, **38**, 99–119.

6 Atrial Fibrillation

Kunihiro Nishida[1] and Stanley Nattel[2]

[1]The Second Department of Internal Medicine, University of Toyama, Toyama City, Japan
[2]Department of Medicine, Montreal Heart Institute, Université de Montreal, Canada

Introduction

Atrial fibrillation (AF) is characterised by rapid and irregular atrial activation, intermittently passing the AV node and causing irregular ventricular contraction. The electrocardiogram (ECG) demonstrates loss of P waves, irregular or flat baseline and irregular QRS rhythm. Atrial rate is so rapid that uniform atrial excitation does not occur.

Ventricular heart rate may be too fast or too slow depending on the conductivity of the AV node. Fast and irregular ventricular contraction may cause palpitations, and excessively low or high ventricular heart rate may lead to heart failure.

Thromboembolic stroke is one of the most serious complications of AF. Rapid atrial activation prevents effective relaxation and contraction and causes blood stasis in atria which promotes clot formation, particularly in the left atrial appendage. These clots are able to propagate to the brain and other organs, such as kidneys, mesenteric circulation and extremities, potentially leading to infarction.

Here, we will review the historical evolution of our understanding of AF in order to provide insights into the mechanisms underlying this common and clinically significant cardiac arrhythmia.

Basic Mechanisms: The Multiple-Wavelet Hypothesis
Moe et al., American Heart Journal (1964)

In 1964, Moe and colleagues developed a computer model of impulse propagation in a non-uniform two-dimensional system and elegantly simulated atrial activation during AF in order to demonstrate the mechanism of AF perpetuation. Based on observations from their experimental animal AF models, they proposed the multiple-wavelet hypothesis, which claimed that AF is maintained by irregular wanderings of many small excitation waves (Figure 6.1).

Their computer model made a number of simple assumptions. The atrial tissue consisted of a definite number of discrete units, which were arranged as a one-unit thick flat sheet. When a unit fired, it transmitted constant amplitude of excitation to all its neighbours and after some delay these neighbours would fire or not, depending on their state of excitability. The refractory period of each unit was defined by the preceding cycle length and a time constant, which varied from unit to unit and created heterogeneity in excitability.

Their model exhibited self-sustained atrial activity and resembled animal models of experimental AF in many aspects. The atrial activity was turbulent, but not rhythmic

Understanding Medical Research: The Studies that Shaped Medicine, First Edition. Edited by John A. Goodfellow. © 2012 John Wiley & Sons, Ltd. Published 2012 by John Wiley & Sons, Ltd.

and regular. The activity was not the result of fixed impulse generators of circuits, but was sustained by irregular drifting eddies or wave fronts, which varied in position, number and size at every moment.

In the multiple-wavelet hypothesis, the likelihood of AF persistence is determined by the number of wavelets present. If there are a large number of wavelets, there is little chance that all elements will fall into phase simultaneously. However, if there are only a small number of wavelets they may fuse and permit restoration of a sinus rhythm. The average number of the wavelets, in turn, depends on the atrial mass, the duration of the refractory period and the conduction velocity. A larger tissue supports a larger number of wavelets. A brief refractory period allows a larger number of coexisting wavelets. If the refractory period were sufficiently long, the entire atrial mass would soon be left in a refractory state. Conduction velocity also affects the number of wavelets so that if every impulse propagated rapidly to the most remote extremity, fractionation and disorganization of atrial behaviour would not occur.

In their computer model, reduction of the area and prolongation of the refractory period were shown to alter the self-sustained activity in the direction of termination, in agreement with the multiple-wavelet hypothesis.

Basic Mechanisms: Wavelength
Rensma et al., Circulation Research (1988)

Rensma and colleagues directly confirmed the effect of refractory period and conduction velocity on the occurrence of atrial arrhythmias by using an *in vivo* canine model. The investigators chronically stimulated conscious dogs with recording multi-electrodes implanted on the surface of both atria, and examined the electrophysiological measurements under various conditions.

Conduction velocity was calculated after various rates of constant basic stimuli (S1) and the first premature stimuli (S2). The refractory period was also measured by applying another premature stimulus (S2 or S3). The shortest possible atrial activation interval (shortest A1–A2 or A2–A3) measured by the recording electrode closest to the stimulation site was considered as the functional refractory period. The wavelength was defined as the distance travelled by the impulse during its functional refractory period and was calculated as the product of the conduction velocity and refractory period. Data were obtained from four distinct atrial sites.

Shortening of the pacing interval resulted in a gradual and progressive decrease in refractory period, conduction velocity and wavelength. For example, the refractory period, conduction velocity and wavelength measured in Bachmann's bundle were 114 msec, 127 cm/sec and 14.5 cm respectively during a 350 msec interval of slow basic stimuli. Those values decreased to 80 msec, 82 cm/s and 6.6 cm after a 110 msec interval of premature stimuli. The influences of the autonomic nervous system and several cardiac drugs were also studied.

Acetylcholine substantially reduced the refractory period without affecting conduction velocity, and resulted in a shortening of the wavelength. Parasympathetic blockade by atropine produced the opposite effect, resulting in an increase in the refractory period and the wavelength.

Cardiac drugs, such as propafenone, quinidine and d-sotalol, significantly prolonged atrial refractoriness. However, the effects on conduction velocity were markedly different.

Propafenone depressed conduction velocity so that the effect of the refractory prolongation was completely neutralized. Consequently it did not change the wavelength. Although quinidine mildly decreased the conduction velocity, it never exceeded the drug's prolonging effect of the refractory period. As a result, quinidine prolonged the wave length. D-sotalol exhibited no significant effect on conduction. Therefore the drug's action on the wavelength was solely determined by its effect on the refractory period, both of which were prolonged by 40% during normal rhythm and by 45% after the earliest premature stimuli.

Atrial arrhythmias were frequently induced by single premature stimuli. Three types of atrial arrhythmias were distinguished: (1) rapid repetitive response (RRR), defined as a series of no more than five spontaneous premature beats with a cycle length shorter than 150 msec; (2) atrial flutter (AFL), a regular rapid rhythm of more than five beats with monomorphic electrograms and a cycle length between 90 and 150 msec; and (3) AF, an irregular and extremely rapid rhythm with polymorphic electrograms. In total, 549 episodes of atrial arrhythmias were induced in 19 dogs (RRR, n = 223; AFL, n = 118; AF, n = 208).

Both the refractory period and conduction velocity were poor predictors of arrhythmia events. Although a relatively higher incidence of AF occurred at shorter refractory periods, prolongation of the refractory period did not prevent its induction. The predictive power of the conduction velocity was also low. However, the combination of both properties (i.e. wavelength) was a more reliable index for predicting the induction of the different arrhythmias correctly. Although the different arrhythmias were still not completely separated by wavelength, the degree of overlap was far less compared with the refractory period and conduction velocity.

Basic Mechanisms: Pulmonary Veins
Haïssaguerre et al., New England Journal of Medicine (1998)

The multiple-wavelet hypothesis and the concept of wavelength explained the mechanism of AF maintenance in the atrial tissue very well. However, the mechanism of its spontaneous onset remained unknown. Haïssaguerre and Clémenty discovered that focal arrhythmic substrate (focal firing within pulmonary veins) played a very important role in initiating AF, and elegantly demonstrated that the modification of the focal substrate produced a large therapeutic effect.

They studied 45 patients with frequent paroxysmal AF episodes. These were patients exhibiting frequent isolated atrial ectopic beats (>700 beats per 24 hours) and AF episodes (344 ± 326 minutes per 24 hours), which were refractory to drug therapy. Several multi-electrode catheters were introduced percutaneously into the atria, and the earliest electrical activity preceding the spontaneous initiation of AF and associated atrial ectopic beats were recorded. The timing of the atrial activity was assessed relative to the intra-atrial reference electrograms or the onset of the surface ECG P waves.

A total of 69 ectopic foci were identified in the 45 patients, among which 65 foci (94%) in 41 patients were found in the pulmonary veins. The depolarization was marked by a localized sharp spike, which preceded the onset of the ectopic P wave by 106 ± 24 msec. The spike occurred earliest deep in the vein and later progressively towards the ostium, resulting in distal-to-proximal activation.

Spontaneous initiation of AF was recorded in 36 patients. In most of those cases, AF was initiated by a short burst of two or more repetitive focal discharges within the pulmonary veins, which showed irregular cycle lengths, ranging from 110 to 270 msec, with a mean of 175 ± 30 msec (340 per minute).

Radiofrequency catheter ablation was performed at the site with the earliest ectopic activity, and the accuracy of the mapping was confirmed by the abrupt disappearance of triggering atrial ectopic beats. Successful ablation of ectopic foci in the hospital setting was achieved in 38 patients. AF was eliminated completely in 28 patients (62%) without any anti-arrhythmic agent during a mean follow-up period of 8 ± 6 months.

Basic Mechanisms: Mother Rotor
Mandapati et al., Circulation (2000)

This paper elegantly demonstrated that the focal arrhythmic mechanism plays an important role not only in the initiation of AF but also in AF maintenance.

The investigators employed an 'optical mapping' strategy. Isolated sheep hearts were perfused with a voltage-sensitive dye, which emitted fluorescent light when the membrane potential of the myocytes was depolarized. The fluorescence signal was recorded using a charge coupled device (CCD) camera. AF was induced by rapid pacing in the presence of acetylcholine, and the right and left atria were optically mapped simultaneously.

The frequency spectrogram of optical signals was analysed in each recording site using a fast Fourier transform algorithm. The frequency with the highest spectrum peak was identified as the dominant frequency of each recording site.

The left atrium exhibited a higher average of dominant frequency as compared with the right atrium suggesting the driving source resided in the left atrium while passive activation occurred in the right atrium. The highest dominant frequency was most often (80%) localised to the posterior left atrium near the ostium of pulmonary veins. Spatial and temporal periodicity was also seen in the left atrium, indicating regular stable activity. A single site with periodic activity and the highest dominant frequency was identified in five of the seven experiments.

Optical mapping identified small re-entrant activities (rotors) occurring frequently in the left atrium at the sites with the highest dominant frequency. Their rotating frequencies closely matched the highest dominant frequency value of the entire atria. High-resolution video imaging demonstrated that such sources corresponded to vortex-like re-entry around minuscule cores, suggesting 'spiral re-entry' (functional re-entry in the form of spiral waves rotating around a very small core; Figure 6.1) as the most likely underlying mechanism of AF in their model.

This study demonstrated that the sustained activity of a single or a small number of stable re-entry sources ('mother rotors') localised primarily in the left atria is at least partially responsible for AF maintenance (Figure 6.1).

Atrial Remodelling: Atrial Tachycardia-Induced Remodelling
Wijffels et al., Circulation (1995)

It had been recognised that paroxysmal AF often progresses to chronic AF and that the success rate of pharmaceutical or electrical defibrillation gradually decreases when AF

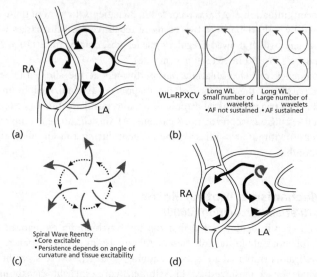

Figure 6.1 Mechanisms of AF. (a) Schema of atrial fibrillation maintained by multiple wavelets. (b) Wavelength and AF maintenance. RA, right atrium; LA, left atrium; WL, wavelength; RP, refractory period; CV, conduction velocity. (c) Spiral wave re-entry. (d) Schema of atrial fibrillation maintained by a mother rotor. Adapted by permission from Macmillan Publishers Ltd: *Nature* 2002, **415**, 219–226.

persists over a long period of time. These observations suggested that AF itself may cause progressive changes to the atria and perpetuate the condition.

In this study, Wijffels and colleagues demonstrated experimentally that AF alters atrial electrophysiology to enhance AF vulnerability and persistence. The investigators implanted goats with multiple pacing and recording electrodes sutured to the epicardium of both atria. Then the animals were connected to a fibrillation pacemaker which artificially maintained AF. Atrial electrogram was recorded and analysed continuously, and a 1-second burst stimulation was delivered automatically as soon as sinus rhythm was detected. This promptly induced AF and AF was maintained continuously by giving burst stimulation immediately after the AF converted to sinus rhythm.

Episodes of the pacing-induced AF were very short lasting (6 ± 3 seconds) in the control condition. However artificial maintenance of AF progressively increased over the duration of AF and AF became sustained (>24 hours) after 7 days in 10 of the 11 goats. During the first 24 hours of artificial AF maintenance, the median interval of atrial activation shortened from 145 ± 18 to 108 ± 8 ms. The atrial effective refractory period (ERP) shortened by 35% from 146 ± 19 to 95 ± 20 ms, and rate adaptation of the ERP (shortening of ERP during rapid rate) was impaired. All electrophysiological changes were found to be reversible within one week; sinus rhythm could be fully restored. The authors coined the term 'atrial remodelling' to describe those phenomena.

Following the discovery of the atrial electrical remodelling in this paper, our laboratory has been extensively exploring the underlying mechanisms using similar canine models of AF. The atrial rate increases to 400–600 beats/min during AF roughly tenfold more than the sinus rhythm. Rapid atrial activation causes frequent Ca^{2+} influx and cellular Ca^{2+} overloading, which threatens cell viability. Those changes also promote a decrease in L-type Ca^{2+} current (I_{CaL}) in an attempt to restore intracellular Ca^{2+} at the expense of arrhythmogenic changes in action potential duration. Short-term mechanisms involve voltage-dependent and intracellular Ca^{2+}-concentration-dependent inactivation of I_{CaL}. Over the longer term, I_{CaL} is reduced via the down-regulation of the mRNA and protein expression of its channel pore forming $\alpha 1$ subunit. Similar changes are produced by any form of sufficiently rapid atrial rate and are known as 'atrial tachycardia-induced remodelling'.

Atrial Remodelling: Congestive Heart Failure-Related Atrial Remodelling
Li et al., Circulation (1999)

Wijffels and colleagues demonstrated the remodelling mechanisms by which 'AF begets AF', but fell short of characterising the substrates that initially promote AF before the remodelling occurs. Li and Nattel and colleagues emphasised the importance of another type of atrial remodelling using a canine model of congestive heart failure induced by rapid ventricular pacing. This emphasized structural remodelling of the atrial architecture, particularly that of enhanced fibrosis.

Dogs were implanted with a pacemaker which stimulated the ventricle to high rates. After 5 weeks of rapid ventricular pacing, the dogs developed significant congestive heart failure (CHF), which was confirmed by clinical signs (such as lethargy, dyspnoea and oedema) and hemodynamic measurements. During electrophysiological study under anaesthesia, burst pacing-induced AF was able to be sustained for only a short duration (8 ± 4 seconds) in normal control dogs but was markedly prolonged to 535 ± 82 seconds in CHF dogs after 5 weeks of rapid ventricular pacing.

In contrast to atrial tachycardia-induced remodelling, CHF did not alter the atrial refractory period or global atrial conduction velocity, leaving wavelength unchanged. Focal conduction abnormality was precisely evaluated by analysing 'phase delay', the difference in activation time between each neighbouring electrode pair; CHF was found to significantly increase the spatial heterogeneity of phase delay by creating focal areas of slow conduction. Histology revealed increased atrial fibrous tissue content within and between muscle bundles (interstitial fibrosis) in CHF dogs, which interfered with local conduction, increased spatial conduction heterogeneity and stabilised re-entrant circuits.

This study provided the first detailed insights into the functional and structural changes underlying the ability to sustain AF in an animal model of CHF. These results have been important in elucidating the potentially different electrical and structural substrates of AF in different settings and when considering the mechanisms and potential treatments of AF.

Drug Therapy: Anticoagulation Therapy
Petersen et al., Lancet (1989)

AF is complicated by a high risk of thromboembolic strokes. The thromboembolic risk is reduced by the administration of oral anticoagulant drugs at the cost of an increased risk of bleeding complications.

This study was a randomised trial designed to compare the effects of warfarin, aspirin and placebo on the incidence of thromboembolic complications in patients with chronic nonrheumatic AF. A total of 1007 patients with chronic nonrheumatic AF were enrolled in the study. 335 received warfarin, 336 aspirin and 336 placebo. Because warfarin requires frequent blood tests and dose changes, it was given openly while aspirin and placebo were given in a double-blind fashion. Patients were followed up for 2 years or until the termination of the trial. The primary endpoint was a thromboembolic complication, such as stroke and transient ischemic attack, and the secondary endpoint was death.

Five patients on warfarin had strokes; four were disabling cerebral infarctions and one was a fatal intracerebral haemorrhage. Of the four infarcts, only one occurred during sufficient anticoagulation. Two occurred during discontinuation of the warfarin therapy, which occurred for evaluation of haematuria and before elective operation, and one suffered a stroke on the day of randomisation before treatment was started. In contrast, 20 and 21 thromboembolic complications occurred in the aspirin and placebo groups respectively. The yearly incidence of thromboembolic complications was 2.0% on warfarin and 5.5% on aspirin and placebo. The difference in frequency of events in the three groups was statistically significant; warfarin significantly lowered the incidence of thromboembolic complications, while aspirin did not.

Cerebrovascular and cardiovascular mortality was also lowered by warfarin administration. Only three vascular deaths occurred in the warfarin group, whereas 12 occurred in the aspirin group and 15 in the placebo group. However, 21 patients on warfarin were withdrawn from the study because of nonfatal bleeding complications, as opposed to only two on aspirin and none on placebo.

The results lead to the conclusion that anticoagulation therapy with warfarin should be recommended to prevent thromboembolic complications in patients with chronic nonrheumatic AF. Today antithrombotic therapy is tailored to the individual's risk factors. Warfarin therapy is considered for AF patients who have one or more risk factors for stroke, including but not limited to congestive heart failure, hypertension, aging, diabetes mellitus and previous stroke.

Drug Therapy: Rhythm Control versus Rate Control
Wyse et al. and AFFIRM Investigators, NEJM (2002)

Currently there are two strategies to treat AF: one is treatment with antiarrhythmic drugs to maintain sinus rhythm ('rhythm control'), and the other is the use of rate-controlling drugs while allowing AF to persist ('rate control'). The Atrial Fibrillation Follow-up Investigation of Rhythm Management (AFFIRM) study is the largest randomised, multicentre study in which these two treatment strategies have been compared.

A total of 4060 patients were enrolled. Enrolees were at least 65 years old or had at least one risk factor for stroke in addition to AF. Overall mortality was evaluated as the primary endpoint.

In the rhythm control group, the following drugs were acceptable for use: amiodarone, disopyramide, flecainide, moricizine, procainamide, propafenone, quinidine, sotalol, dofetilide and combinations of these drugs. More than two thirds of patients started therapy with amiodarone or sotalol. Almost two thirds of the patients had undergone at least one trial of amiodarone by the end of the study. The prevalence of sinus rhythm in the rhythm control group at follow-up was 82.4%, 73.3% and 62.6% at 1, 3 and 5 years, respectively.

In the rate control group, β-blockers, Ca^{2+}-channel blockers, digoxin and combinations of these drugs were used. Continuous anticoagulation was mandated by the protocol for the rate control group. However, in the rhythm control group continuous anticoagulation was encouraged but could be stopped if sinus rhythm was apparently maintained with antiarrhythmic drug therapy.

During the mean follow-up period of 3.5 years, there were 356 deaths in the rhythm control group and 310 deaths in the rate control group, and mortality at 5 years was 24% and 21%, respectively. More deaths occurred in the rhythm control group than in the rate control group, but the difference in mortality between the two groups was not considered statistically significant.

Although the difference in mortality was not statistically significant between the two groups, patients were hospitalised more frequently in the rhythm control group than in the rate control group, specifically 1374 patients (80%) in the rhythm control group versus 1220 patients (73%) in the rate control group, $p < 0.001$. Adverse drug effects, such as QT prolongation, torsade de pointes, bradycardiac arrest and pulmonary events, were also significantly more common in the rhythm control group.

Ischemic strokes occurred in 77 and 80 patients in the rate control and rhythm control groups, respectively, for an annual rate of approximately 1% in each group. In both groups, the majority of strokes occurred after interruption of warfarin therapy or when the effect of warfarin was subtherapeutic.

These results indicated that the rhythm control strategy does not offer a survival advantage over the rate control strategy, and that the rate control strategy has potential advantages, such as a lower risk of adverse drug effects. The use of anticoagulant drugs is recommended in both approaches and should be continued in those high-risk stroke patients, even if they are in sinus rhythm.

Subsequently published sub-analysis of the AFFIRM study revealed that the presence of sinus rhythm was associated with a lower risk of death, as was warfarin usage. However, currently available antiarrhythmic drugs were not associated with improved survival, which indicated that any beneficial antiarrhythmic effects of antiarrhythmic drugs were offset by their adverse effects.

Drug Therapy: Upstream Therapy
Li et al., Circulation (2001)

The AFFIRM study showed that while being in sinus rhythm showed a benefit for the survival of AF patients, treatment with conventional antiarrhythmic drug therapy did not. An effective method for maintaining sinus rhythm with fewer adverse effects is therefore a major therapeutic goal. A potential new approach is to target the underlying substrate of AF.

CHF and other heart diseases induce atrial structural remodelling which creates a substrate for AF; however, the precise underlying mechanisms and their signal transduction pathways have remained largely unsolved. Li and Nattel and colleagues demonstrated in this study the beneficial effects of angiotensin-converting enzyme (ACE) inhibition on arrhythmogenic atrial remodelling and the mechanistic involvement of mitogen-activated protein kinase (MAPK) changes in a canine model of rapid ventricular pacing-induced CHF.

Dogs were subjected to rapid ventricular pacing (220 to 240 bpm) in the presence or absence of oral administration of the ACE inhibitor enalapril. Five weeks of pacing induced CHF, which produced local atrial conduction slowing, interstitial fibrosis and prolonged atrial burst pacing-induced AF.

Left atrial tissues were obtained after various duration of pacing period, and angiotensin II concentrations and MAPK expression were examined in those tissues. Atrial angiotensin II concentration and phosphorylated ERK were found to have increased within 1 day, and they peaked at 1 week. Other MAPKs, including JNK and p38, and their phosphorylated forms increased on the first day and thereafter decreased.

Enalapril significantly reduced pacing-induced changes in atrial angiotensin II and phosphorylated ERK. The enalapril-treated dogs demonstrated significantly improved hemodynamics compared with placebo-treated animals. Enalapril also significantly attenuated the effects of rapid ventricular pacing on atrial conduction, atrial fibrosis and mean AF duration.

Rapid pacing dogs treated with the vasodilator hydralazine/isosorbide exhibited left ventricular diastolic and atrial pressures similar to those of enalapril-treated dogs, but lower than those of rapid pacing-only dogs. Despite this hemodynamic improvement, hydralazine/isosorbide did not affect rapid pacing-induced atrial fibrosis or AF promotion.

The effectiveness of ACE inhibition showed that interrupting signalling pathways is able to prevent development of the AF substrate, a process that might potentially be used to develop a new therapeutic approach.

Genetics
Chen et al., Science (2003)

Genetic research is one of the hottest topics in atrial fibrillation and arrhythmia. Chen and colleagues first identified a causative gene mutation in a family with hereditary AF in this 2003 *Science* paper. The authors studied a four-generation family with autosomal dominant persistent AF and identified a gain-of-function mutation in the KCNQ1 gene. Whole-genome linkage analysis was used to screen 14 affected and 25 unaffected family members.

Linkage analysis mapped the AF locus to chromosome 11p15.5 between D11S1363 and D11S1346. In a gene data bank search, KCNQ1, which encodes the pore-forming α subunit of the cardiac IKs channel (KCNQ1/KCNE1) and the KCNQ1/KCNE2 and the KCNQ1/KCNE3 potassium channels, was identified as a candidate gene. Sequence of the KCNQ1 coding region was analysed and a missense mutation S140G was revealed in all of the affected family members, but not in the unaffected individuals of the AF family or in 188 healthy control individuals.

To assess the S140G mutant KCNQ1 channel protein function, the S140G mutant protein was expressed in cultured COS-7 cells and analysed by a whole-cell patch clamping technique. Expression of the S140G mutant alone did not produce a substantial current. When S140G mutant KCNQ1 was co-expressed with KCNE1, the current density was increased by a factor of three compared with wild-type KCNQ1/KCNE1.

Co-expression of mutant KCNQ1 and KCNE2 induced a sixfold increase in current density compared with wild-type KCNQ1/KCNE2.

Thus the S140G mutation was likely to increase repolarisation potassium currents and initiate and maintain AF by reducing the action potential duration and effective refractory period in atrial myocytes. This contrasts with the dominant negative or loss-of-function effects of the KCNQ1 mutations previously identified in patients with long QT syndrome.

Several other loci, such as 21q22, 17q, 7q35–36, 5p13, 6q14–16 and 10q22, have been mapped for monogenetic AF thus far. Some of these loci encode subunits of potassium channels and are associated with a gain-of-function mutation involving repolarisation of potassium currents while the others are not yet identified. Ongoing genetic studies will improve our understanding of the mechanisms of AF and may allow for the development of novel therapeutic approaches in not only hereditary arrhythmia but also other clinical settings.

Conclusions

The mechanistic understanding of AF began with the multiple-wavelet hypothesis and the concept of wavelength and has evolved to pulmonary vein origin, mother rotor and spiral re-entry mechanisms. The discovery and subsequent development of the concept of atrial remodelling has significantly contributed to current AF management. Clinical trials has revealed the importance of anticoagulation and posted a warning on conventional antiarrhythmic drug usage. Most recently, genetic studies have provided new insights into AF and its molecular profile. Understanding these fundamental achievements will no doubt contribute to effective management of AF patients and guide future AF research.

References

Chen, Y.H., *et al.* (2003) KCNQ1 gain-of-function mutation in familial atrial fibrillation. *Science*, **299**, 251–254. http://www.ncbi.nlm.nih.gov/pubmed/12522251

Haïssaguerre, M., *et al.* (1998) Spontaneous initiation of atrial fibrillation by ectopic beats originating in the pulmonary veins. *New England Journal of Medicine*, **339**, 659–666. http://www.nejm.org/doi/full/10.1056/NEJM199809033391003

Li, D., *et al.* (1999) Promotion of atrial fibrillation by heart failure in dogs: atrial remodelling of a different sort. *Circulation*, **100**, 87–95. http://circ.ahajournals.org/cgi/content/full/100/1/87

Li, D., *et al.* (2001) Effects of angiotensin-converting enzyme inhibition on the development of the atrial fibrillation substrate in dogs with ventricular tachypacing-induced congestive heart failure. *Circulation*, **104**, 2608–2614. http://circ.ahajournals.org/cgi/content/full/104/21/2608

Mandapati, R., *et al.* (2000) Stable microreentrant sources as a mechanism of atrial fibrillation in the isolated sheep heart. *Circulation*, **101**, 194–199. http://circ.ahajournals.org/cgi/content/full/101/2/194

Moe, G.K., *et al.* (1964) A computer model of atrial fibrillation. *American Heart Journal*, **67**, 200–220. http://www.ncbi.nlm.nih.gov/pubmed/14118488

Petersen, P., *et al.* (1989) Placebo-controlled, randomised trial of warfarin and aspirin for prevention of thromboembolic complications in chronic atrial fibrillation. *The Copenhagen AFASAK study. Lancet*, **1**, 175–179. http://www.thelancet.com/journals/lancet/article/PIIS0140-6736(89)91200-2/Abstract

Rensma, P.L., *et al.* (1988) Length of excitation wave and susceptibility to reentrant atrial arrhythmias in normal conscious dogs. *Circulation Research*, **62**, 395–410. http://circres.ahajournals.org/cgi/reprint/62/2/395

Wijffels, M.C., *et al.* (1995) Atrial fibrillation begets atrial fibrillation: a study in awake chronically instrumented goats. *Circulation*, **92**, 1954–1968. http://circ.ahajournals.org/cgi/content/full/92/7/1954

Wyse, D.G., *et al.* (2002) Atrial Fibrillation Follow-up Investigation of Rhythm Management (AFFIRM) Investigators: a comparison of rate control and rhythm control in patients with atrial fibrillation. *New England Journal of Medicine*, **347**, 1825–1833. http://www.ncbi.nlm.nih.gov/pubmed/12466506

7 Asthma

Tak H. Lee and Leonard Siew

Division of Asthma, Allergy and Lung Biology, Kings College London, London, UK

Introduction

Asthma as a disease has been recognised since antiquity and accounts of it can be found in texts from ancient China up to modern times. Its symptoms of intermittent episodes of shortness of breath associated with wheeze have been well documented.

Asthma was thought to be a neurosis in the 1800s, until William Osler published his *Principles and Practice of Medicine* in 1892[1]. His theory on the aetiology of asthma (attributing asthma to spasm of the bronchial muscles, swelling of the bronchial mucous membrane and inflammation of the smaller bronchioles) was a groundbreaking revelation inspiring researchers to move away from the concept that asthma is a neurosis and to look for pathological causes. Shortly thereafter S.J. Meltzer published his research suggesting that asthma is an allergic phenomenon using a guinea-pig model[2], while F.M. Rackemann published his case series of the aetiology of asthma in 150 patients[3]. He recognised that there were extrinsic and intrinsic trigger factors for asthma and subdivided asthma into 'extrinsic asthma' and 'intrinsic asthma'. These terms are still used today, although they have become equated with atopic and non-atopic asthma.

The Pathophysiology of Asthma
Role of Immunoglobulins

The first major breakthrough in the understanding of the pathology of asthma came in the 1960s with the discovery of a new immunoglobulin, provisionally called IgND, by Hans Bennich and S. Gunnar Johansson, and the γE-globulin by Kimishige and Teruko Ishizaka.

Johansson, Lancet (1967)

The immunoglobulin IgND discovered by Bennich and Johansson[4] had characteristics similar to reagins (antibodies found in the blood of persons who have allergies). Johansson investigated the distribution of IgND in sera of 38 unselected patients with asthma. Johannson classified patients with asthma who had a positive skin and provocation test to be 'allergic type' and those who had negative skin and provocation tests to be 'non-allergic type'. The serum concentrations of immunoglobulins A, D, G, M and ND were also measured. Johansson found that the serum concentrations of IgND in patients with allergic-type asthma were 6 times higher when compared patients with non-allergic-type asthma. There was, however, no difference in the concentrations of immunoglobulin A, D, G and M.

Understanding Medical Research: The Studies that Shaped Medicine, First Edition. Edited by John A. Goodfellow. © 2012 John Wiley & Sons, Ltd. Published 2012 by John Wiley & Sons, Ltd.

The Ishizakas reported in 1966 their discovery of a unique immunoglobulin, which had reaginic activity against ragweed antigen E, which they provisionally designated γE-globulin[5]. Collaboration between Johansson and Ishizaka led to the discovery that the antigenic structure and characteristics of the immunoglobulin IgND and the γE-globulin were similar. This led them to propose a fifth new class of immunoglobulin designated immunoglobulin E (IgE). The World Heath Organisation in 1968 ratified this proposal leading to the discovery of the final class of immunoglobulin.

The discovery of IgE and its relation to atopic asthma validated the theories of Osler and the findings of Meltzer and Rackemann. It was the first step in the understanding of the immunological mechanisms of asthma. IgE is now recognized to play a key role in the pathophysiology of asthma and has been a target for rational drug development[6]. Nevertheless, aside from its well-established role in promoting acute asthma exacerbations in allergic subjects through triggering degranulation of mast cells and basophils, the full spectrum of the pathophysiological actions of IgE in asthma remains even now to be defined.

Role of Leukotrienes in Asthma
First described by Feldberg and Kellaway in 1938, Slow Reacting Substances of Anaphylaxis (SRS-A) were recognised to produce slow onset sustained smooth muscle contraction in anaphylactic responses[7]. This was in contradistinction to the effects of histamine which were rapid and evanescent. The structure and function of SRS-A were investigated by many eminent scientists, each one of them providing key steps in this arduous task. After a period of 40 years of research, the key constituents of SRS-A were finally uncovered.

Murphy et al., Proceedings of the National Academy of Sciences of the USA (1979)
Murphy and colleagues stimulated murine mastocytoma cells with the calcium iono-phore A23187 and found that they produced a 'slow reacting substance' (SRS), which caused smooth muscle contraction. Murphy purified the SRS using reverse-phase high-performance liquid chromatography (HPLC) and demonstrated that it had biological activity, using a guinea-pig ileum contraction assay. Using radiolabelled precursors, they demonstrated that both arachidonic acid and cysteine were precursors of the purified SRS and that it was a substrate for the enzyme lipoxygenase. They found that the chemical structure of the SRS was related to a compound recently designated as leukotriene B. Their newly identified substance was designated leukotriene C. Murphy and colleagues proposed that both leukotriene B and leukotriene C were derived from leukotriene A, of which arachidonic acid and cysteine are precursors.

Murphy's proposed mechanism of the derivation of leukotriene C in murine mastocytoma cells was also found to be applicable to the production of leukotriene C in humans. Elucidation of the structure–function characteristics of the cysteinyl leukotrienes was a critical step in developing leukotriene receptor antagonists that are now available for treatment of asthma.

Laitinen et al., Lancet (1993)
Collaborative studies between investigators in Helsinki, Finland and London, England investigated the capacity of leukotriene E_4 to recruit inflammatory cells in asthma. In this

study endobronchial biopsies were obtained from asthmatic patients at fibreoptic bronchoscopy. Later these same patients underwent bronchial provocation with either leukotriene E_4 or methacholine at random. A bronchoscopy was then repeated 4 hours later to generate further biopsies which were then analysed using transmission electron microscopy.

Despite causing a similar degree of bronchoconstriction the two substances caused substantially different inflammatory cellular infiltration into the bronchial mucosa. Inhalation of leukotriene E_4 caused an influx of eosinophils and neutrophils into the bronchial mucosa which was not seen with methacholine. The inflammation caused by leukotriene E_4 was predominantly eosinophilic with tenfold greater numbers of these cells compared with neutrophils. The numbers of mast cells, lymphocytes, plasma cells and macrophages were not affected by either leukotriene E_4 or methacholine.

The discovery that leukotrienes were able to promote eosinophilic inflammation, the pathological hallmark of asthma, further encouraged the development of anti-leuko-trienes for treatment of asthma for their bronchodilator, anti-inflammatory and corticosteroid-sparing effects.

T-Cell Eosinophilic Axis (Role of Cellular Inflammation in Asthma)

By the late 1980s it was well known that eosinophils were involved in asthmatic airways inflammation. The involvement of T lymphocytes was, however, poorly appreciated. Corrigan and colleagues sought to clarify the involvement of T lymphocytes in asthmatic inflammation.

Corrigan et al., Lancet (1988)

In this study the authors recruited patients with acute severe asthma with the aim of examining the involvement of T lymphocytes in the pathogenesis of asthma. Patients with evidence of chest infection were excluded. The participants were then treated on admission with a standard regimen of nebulised β2-agonist, intravenous aminophylline and oral or parenteral corticosteroids. Peripheral venous blood samples were obtained on the day of admission and on days 3 and 7 after admission. They also obtained peripheral venous blood from normal healthy volunteers and patients with mild asthma and chronic obstructive pulmonary disease (with an infective exacerbation) to act as control groups. Peripheral blood mononuclear cells were isolated and stained for markers of T cell subtypes and activation and analysed by flow cytometry.

To assess T lymphocyte activation the cell surface expression of the class II histo-compatibility antigen HLA-DR, the interleukin 2 receptor (IL-2R) and the very late activation antigen (VLA-1), were measured (T lymphocyte activation is associated with an increased expression of these markers). They found that the percentages of T lymphocytes expressing all three activation markers increased during an acute exacerbation of asthma. As the patients improved clinically the percentages of T lymphocytes expressing the activation marker HLA-DR and IL-2R reduced. The percentages of CD4+, CD8+ T lymphocytes as well as the CD4/CD8 ratio did not differ between patients with an acute exacerbation and the control groups. Subgroup analysis of the activated T lymphocytes in acute severe asthma revealed that the activated cells were predominantly of the CD4+ phenotype. Corrigan and colleagues had identified for the first time that T helper lymphocytes are involved in the pathogenesis of asthma.

In the late 1990s Hamid and colleagues elegantly demonstrated that there is an influx of T cells and eosinophils into the airways of patients with asthma, and that cellular inflammation was similar, be it more severe, in the peripheral airways compared to the central airways[8].

It has long been recognised that a subgroup of asthmatic patients shows resistance to corticosteroid therapy. These patients have persistent symptoms despite being maintained on high dosages of corticosteroids which are effective for the majority of patients. Apart from a difference in glucocorticoid responsiveness, the natural history and symptoms of this subgroup of patients are the same as that of glucocorticoid-sensitive patients. Following the identification of T helper lymphocytes as a key mediator in asthmatic inflammation, Corrigan and colleagues sought to determine if T helper lymphocytes were also involved in corticosteroid resistance. In 1991 they demonstrated that the inhibitory effect of dexamethasone on peripheral blood T lymphocyte proliferation was attenuated in corticosteroid resistant asthmatics with a shift in the dexamethasone dose response curve compared to corticosteroid sensitive asthmatics[9]. They also demonstrated that steroid resistance in asthma was not due to a difference in plasma clearance or glucocorticoid receptor expression by lymphocytes or monocytes. A correlation between the clinical response in lung function following prednisolone treatment and the degree of inhibition of T lymphocyte proliferation by dexamethasone was also demonstrated. The exact nature of the defect causing this resistance is still unknown and the answers are currently being sought at the genomic level by investigators throughout the world.

The confirmation that T cells played a key role in the pathogenesis of asthma and in the response to corticosteroid therapy was critical. This opened up an entire field of research into asthma; from investigating immune regulation in asthma to developing new molecular compounds to target T cells and their products in asthma.

Airway Remodelling and Airway Smooth Muscle

For years histological studies have demonstrated that there are changes in the structure of the airways in asthma. These changes correlate loosely with disease severity and are termed 'remodelling'. Remodelling is characterised by sub-epithelial fibrosis, reticular basement membrane thickening, angiogenesis, increased mucus production and smooth muscle hyperplasia and hypertrophy. Understanding the interplay of structural cells and cellular inflammation took a massive leap in the late 1990s.

John et al., Journal of Immunology (1997)

Up to this point in time, airway smooth muscle was known to have a contractile function and to respond, by hyperplasia and hypertrophy, to cytokines and growth factors. John and colleagues hypothesised that airway smooth muscle is not only a structural cell responding to pro-inflammatory stimuli in asthma but also an effector cell. They cultured human airway smooth muscle cells obtained from lobar or main bronchi of lung resections from patients undergoing surgery for carcinoma of the bronchus. They found that airway smooth muscle stimulated with tumour necrosis factor-alpha (TNF-α) secreted RANTES a chemokine for monocytes, memory T lymphocytes and eosinophils and that the addition of interferon-γ (IFN-γ) synergistically increased this. The release of RANTES by airway smooth muscle cells was found to be inhibited by dexamethasone and T helper 2 (Th2) cytokines, interleukin-4 (IL-4), interleukin-10 (IL-10) and interleukin-13 (IL-13).

In order to determine if RANTES released by cultured airway smooth muscle was functional, John and colleagues purified RANTES using reverse-phase HPLC from concentrated culture medium following stimulation of the airway smooth muscle cells. The purified RANTES was able to induce eosinophil chemotaxis in a concentration-dependent manner and neutralising antibodies inhibited this activity. In addition to RANTES John and colleagues also found that stimulated airway smooth muscle was able to produce other chemokines; in particular, the eosinophil chemoattractant eotaxin and the chemokine macrophage-inflammatory protein-1α.

The identification for the first time that airway smooth muscle is able to function as an effector cell changed our understanding of the pathogenesis of asthma. This highlighted that asthma is not purely an allergic inflammatory disease, but that the interplay between structural cells and inflammatory cells is also crucial in its pathogenesis.

The Mast Cell and Airway Smooth Muscle

Infiltration of eosinophils into the airway submucosa is characteristic of both asthma and eosinophilic bronchitis. A key clinical characteristic of asthma is variable airflow obstruction and bronchial hyper-responsiveness which is not present in eosinophilic bronchitis despite a similar inflammatory profile. Brightling and colleagues discovered a possible reason for this difference.

Brightling et al., New England Journal of Medicine (2002)

The investigators hypothesised that the mechanism may not be so much in differences in the numbers of inflammatory cells in the airways between eosinophilic bronchitis and asthma but in their localisation. To test this they recruited patients with asthma, eosinophilic bronchitis and healthy controls and performed fibreoptic bronchoscopy to obtain endobronchial biopsies.

Patients who had asthma were found to have bronchial hyper-responsiveness, while those who had eosinophilic bronchitis and healthy subjects did not. Immunohisto-chemical analysis of biopsies showed that there was no difference in eosinophil counts or the thickness of the basement membrane and lamina reticularis in the bronchial submucosa of patients with asthma and eosinophilic bronchitis, although these features were increased compared with healthy controls. Furthermore there was no difference in total T lymphocyte and mast cell count in the bronchial submucosa between the two groups of patients. However, the numbers of mast cells localised within the airway smooth muscle was strikingly greater in asthma compared to both eosinophilic bronchitis and healthy controls. The numbers of mast cells infiltrating the airway smooth muscle correlated with bronchial hyper-responsiveness.

Sutcliffe and colleagues in 2006 reported that cultured airway smooth muscle of asthmatic phenotype stimulated by Th2 cytokines releases chemotactic factors for mast cells[10]. They also showed that mast cell chemotaxis was inhibited by supernatants from cultured airway smooth muscle of non-asthmatic phenotype stimulated by Th2 cyto-kines. Thus a plausible mechanism has been identified by which the mast cell is recruited to airway smooth muscle.

Treatment of Asthma
Corticosteroids

The first report of the successful treatment of asthma using a corticosteroid was by Carryer in 1950[11]. This led to the routine use of prednisolone and hydrocortisone for the treatment of asthma. The use of oral corticosteroids, however, results in adverse systemic side effects. Delivery of a glucocorticoid directly to the airways could potentially solve this problem. Drugs delivered directly to the airways had to be given by nebulisation until 1956 when the first metered dose inhaler was introduced. Topical delivery of hydrocortisone and dexamethasone was unsuccessful in reducing the incidence of systemic side effects. The search for an inhaled corticosteroid which had limited systemic absorption reached a major breakthrough with the development of beclometasone.

Clark, Lancet (1972)

Clark recruited patients with asthma approximately half of whom were on systemic corticosteroids while the other half were not. He measured forced expired volume in one second (FEV_1) and vital capacity before and after commencement of beclomethasone delivered by a metered dose inhaler. Adrenal function was assessed by measuring morning plasma hydrocortisone levels and a tetracosactrin (synacthen) test.

He found that in patients not taking corticosteroids before commencement of treatment inhaled beclomethasone resulted in a sustained increase in lung function as measured by FEV_1. Furthermore, there was no evidence of adrenal suppression in these patients.

In patients who were taking oral corticosteroids before commencement of treatment, conversion of treatment to beclomethasone was not associated with a fall in FEV_1. Further, these patients showed reversal of adrenal suppression caused by the oral corticosteroid as evidenced by a rise in morning plasma hydrocortisone levels to within the normal range.

Adrenal function testing performed on patients while on inhaled beclomethasone was normal. Clark had shown that beclomethasone not only is effective in treating airways obstruction in asthma but also had a low systemic absorption as evident by the lack of adrenal suppression seen with systemic corticosteroids.

The use of inhaled corticosteroids changed the treatment of asthma forever, as there was now an effective treatment for asthma with minimal adverse systemic side effects. Inhaled corticosteroids have since been shown to be able to reduce airway inflammation in asthma and some aspects of remodelling.

Long-Acting B2 Agonist in Combination with Inhaled Corticosteroids

Salmeterol, a long acting β2 adrenoceptor agonist, was developed in the 1980s. Salmeterol has a duration of action of approximately 12 hours whereas that of short acting β2 adrenoceptor agonists is 4 to 6 hours. Guidelines for the management of asthma in the early 1990s recommended that patients who were uncontrolled on low-dosage inhaled corticosteroids should have this dosage increased or have a long acting β2 adrenoceptor agonist introduced. Greening and colleagues conducted a clinical trial to determine which of these two treatment strategies was more efficacious.

Greening et al., Lancet (1994)

The authors recruited 429 patients with asthma who remained symptomatic despite taking 200 μg of beclomethasone dipropionate twice daily. Patients were randomised to

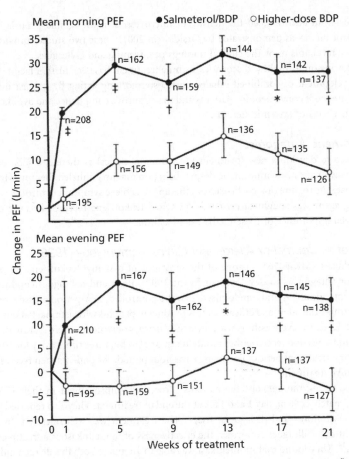

Figure 7.1 Changes from baseline (±SE) in mean morning and evening peak expiratory flow (PEF) during 6 months' study treatment. Reprinted from Greening *et al.*, *The Lancet*, Copyright (1994), with permission from Elsevier.

receive either 200 µg of beclomethasone dipropionate twice daily and salmeterol 50 µg twice daily or 500 µg of beclomethasone dipropionate twice daily and placebo for a period of 6 months. They found that patients receiving beclomethasone and salmeterol had a greater increase in mean morning and evening peak expiratory flow rates compared to patients receiving higher dosage beclomethasone (Figure 7.1). There was also a greater reduction in the median peak expiratory flow diurnal variation, night time awakening and asthma symptom scores in patients receiving beclomethasone and salmeterol. The findings of Greening and colleagues resulted in important changes in the guidelines for asthma management and to further investigation of the mechanisms for the synergistic effect of salmeterol combined with inhaled corticosteroids.

Li and colleagues in 1999 demonstrated that the addition of salmeterol to regular inhaled corticosteroid therapy reduced the eosinophil count in the lamina propria of endobronchial biopsies in asthmatics[12]. This reduction was not seen with an increased dosage of inhaled corticosteroids. The addition of salmeterol to regular inhaled corticosteroid also reduced the density of microvessels in the lamina propria of the asthmatic airway as demonstrated by Orsida[13] in 2001. These two studies provide one putative mechanism for the clinical findings of Greening and colleagues.

Following on from these discoveries, asthma treatment has been further facilitated by the development of combined inhaled corticosteroid/long-acting β2 agonist inhalers which are more convenient for patients and may improve compliance and avoidance of the side effects of systemic steroids.

Leukotriene Antagonist

The need to develop a new treatment for asthma is critical as there is a subgroup of patients who are still symptomatic despite being on maximal inhaled therapy. Many of these patients require oral corticosteroid therapy to achieve symptom control. A steroid sparing agent was sought targeting the cysteinyl leukotriene receptor because of the perceived importance of these mediators in asthma.

Reiss et al., Journal of Allergy and Clinical Immunology (1996)

Montelukast (MK-0476) was one of the most potent cysteinyl leukotriene$_1$ (CysLT$_1$) receptor antagonists in development in the 1990s. Reiss and colleagues conducted a multicentre double-blind, randomised, placebo controlled, two-period crossover study to determine the safety and efficacy of this product in patients with asthma. Patients who had moderate to severe asthma with reversible airways obstruction were recruited. They were randomised to receive either montelukast or placebo, three times a day for 10 days, in the first treatment period. Following a washout period, the patients then received the alternative treatment.

While taking montelukast the patients showed an improvement in their FEV$_1$ of approximately 10% on day 1 and 14% at the end of treatment. They also reported fewer asthma symptoms and β2-agonist usage. The treatment was well tolerated. In 1999 Diamant and colleagues confirmed the effectiveness of montelukast as a treatment for asthma[14]. They found that montelukast was able to attenuate both the allergen induced early and late asthmatic response in patients with mild asthma.

The successful development of montelukast not only increased the repertoire of treatments available to treat asthma, but also confirmed the importance of cysteinyl leukotrienes in the pathogenesis of asthma. Montelukast and zarfirlukast, both leukotriene CysLT$_1$ receptor antagonists, are currently used to treat patients who have moderate to severe asthma and are uncontrolled on inhaled corticosteroids and long acting β2-agonist. Nevertheless these drugs have not proven to be the panacea of asthma therapy that it was once thought they might be. This might be related to the fact that they block only one of the two identified receptors for the cysteinyl leukotrienes and the mounting evidence that further, perhaps more functionally relevant, receptors for these molecules exist.

Monoclonal Antibodies

Since the late 1960s, when IgE was discovered and identified as a key mediator in the pathogenesis of asthma, scientists and clinicians have been searching for a treatment which is able to interfere with the action and production of IgE. A breakthrough came in the late 1990s when a humanised, recombinant monoclonal antibody against the F$_c$ portion of IgE was engineered and developed for clinical use.

Milgrom et al., New England Journal of Medicine (1999)

This antibody, called rhuMAb-E25 (omalizumab), was engineered to bind to IgE at a site adjacent to that involved in binding of IgE to its high affinity receptor (FcɛRI). It forms complexes with free IgE in the circulation and over a period of weeks causes dissociation of IgE from its cellular receptors, thus attenuating IgE-mediated activation processes such as allergen-induced mast cell degranulation. In 1997 Fahy and colleagues[15] and Boulet[6] and colleagues demonstrated that rhuMAb-E25 was able to attenuate both the early and late allergen induced asthmatic response. Following this, the above large multicentre, randomised, placebo-controlled, double-blind trial was conducted by Milgrom and colleagues to determine the efficacy of this new antibody in the treatment of asthma. The therapy was expensive and envisioned as being cost-effective only in patients with severe disease leading to frequent exacerbations requiring unplanned use of health services despite taking maximal conventional therapy. This trial was therefore directed at moderate and severe asthmatics.

Milgrom and colleagues recruited 317 patients with moderate to severe perennial allergic asthma who had daily symptoms despite substantial treatment. They received injections of either rhuMAb-E25 or placebo over a period of 20 weeks, and their corticosteroid therapy was gradually withdrawn during the last 8 weeks of treatment.

Serum-free IgE concentrations fell rapidly following the first dose of rhuMAb-E25 and were eventually reduced by more than 95% of baseline. Asthma symptom scores were significantly reduced in patients in the active treatment group compared with those given placebo, even during the corticosteroid withdrawal phase of the study. An improved quality of life was maintained during the corticosteroid withdrawal phase in patients receiving active treatment. Furthermore, there was a reduction in asthma exacerbations in patients receiving active treatment.

A higher percentage of patients who were taking oral corticosteroids at baseline and who received active treatment were able to reduce their dose of corticosteroids by at least 50% compared to those given placebo. There was, however, no significant difference between active treatment and placebo in the numbers of patients who had their inhaled corticosteroids withdrawn.

Milgrom and colleagues had demonstrated that omalizumab was effective in treating patients with moderate to severe asthma who remained symptomatic despite being on treatment. Humbert and colleagues confirmed these findings in 2005 when they showed that, in patients with severe persistent asthma who were uncontrolled despite being on high-dose inhaled corticosteroids and long acting β2 agonist, omalizumab significantly reduced severe asthma exacerbation rate and emergency services visit rate[16]. It also improved asthma quality of life, symptom scores and morning peak expiratory flow.

This new modality of treatment has been a major advance in the treatment of patients with severe asthma, although its use is limited by its cost because it is potentially a lifelong treatment. Furthermore, not all patients respond well and work is in progress to identify poor responders *a priori*. A significant number of patients with severe atopic asthma with uncontrolled symptoms despite being on conventional therapy are now able to achieve better control with the introduction of omalizumab into their therapy regimen.

Summary and Conclusions

Our understanding of the pathogenesis of asthma has accelerated tremendously over the past 50 years. This has been due to key discoveries of IgE, inflammatory mediators, inflammatory cell subtypes and a change in our view of the role that structural cells play in asthma. Nevertheless these observations have not explained precisely what causes the symptoms of asthma on a day to day basis. The challenge for the future is to understand the interplay between inflammatory cells, structural cells and the day-to-day symptoms. While significant progress has been made, there is still an unmet need and a significant proportion of asthmatics remain symptomatic despite being on all currently available treatment modalities. Further research is still urgently required to inform development of new treatment modalities for these patients.

Key Outstanding Questions

1. What are the mechanisms of different phenotypes of asthma?
2. What are the relative contributions of genetic, epigenetic and environmental factors to the development of asthma?
3. How do you prevent the development of asthma and allergy?
4. How and why does asthma resolve spontaneously?
5. What controls asthma severity on a day-to-day basis?
6. Is asthma curable?

Key Research Centres

1. MRC & Asthma UK Centre in Allergic Mechanisms of Asthma. King's College London, Guy's Hospital and Imperial College London, United Kingdom
2. Institute for Lung Health, Department of Respiratory Medicine, Glenfield Hospital, Leicester, United Kingdom
3. Infection, Inflammation and Repair AIR Division, University of Southampton, Southampton General Hospital, Southampton, United Kingdom
4. Firestone Institute for Respiratory Health, Firestone Research, St. Joseph's Health-care, Ontario, Canada
5. The Woolcock Institute of Medical Research, Glebe, Australia
6. National Heart and Lung Institute, London, United Kingdom
7. Centre for Allergy Research, Karolinska Institutet, Stockholm, Sweden
8. Division of Pediatric Allergy and Immunology, National Jewish Health, Denver, United States
9. Department of Medicine, Harvard Medical School, and Division of Rheumatology, Immunology, and Allergy, Brigham and Women's Hospital, Boston, United States

References

Brightling, C.E., et al. (2002) Mast-cell infiltration of airway smooth muscle in asthma. *New England Journal of Medicine*, **346**(22), 1699–1705. http://www.ncbi.nlm.nih.gov/pubmed/ 12037149

Clark, T.J.H. (1972) Effect of beclomethasone dipropionate delivered by aerosol in patients with asthma. *Lancet*, **1**(7765), 1361–1364. http://www.thelancet.com/journals/lancet/article/ PIIS0140-6736(72)91094-X/abstract

Corrigan, C.J., *et al.* (1988) T lymphocyte activation in acute severe asthma. *Lancet*, **1**(8595), 1129–1132. http://www.thelancet.com/journals/lancet/article/PIIS0140-6736(88)91951-4/abstract

Greening, A.P., *et al.* (1994) Added salmeterol versus higher-dose corticosteroid in asthma patients with symptoms on existing inhaled corticosteroid. Allen & Hanburys Limited UK Study Group. *Lancet*, **344**(8917), 219–224. http://www.thelancet.com/journals/lancet/article/PIIS0140-6736(94)92996-3/abstract

Johansson, S.G. (1967) Raised levels of a new immunoglobulin class (IgND) in asthma. *Lancet*, **2**(7523), 951–953. http://www.thelancet.com/journals/lancet/article/PIIS0140-6736(67)90792-1/abstract

John, M., *et al.* (1997) Human airway smooth muscle cells express and release RANTES in response to T helper 1 cytokines: regulation by T helper 2 cytokines and corticosteroids. *Journal of Immunology*, **158**(4), 1841–1847. http://www.jimmunol.org/content/158/4/1841.long

Laitinen, L.A., *et al.* (1993) Leukotriene E4 and granulocytic infiltration into asthmatic airways. *Lancet*, **341**(8851), 989–990. http://www.thelancet.com/journals/lancet/article/PII0140-6736(93)91073-U/abstract

Milgrom, H., *et al.* (1999) Treatment of allergic asthma with monoclonal anti-IgE antibody. rhuMAb-E25 study group. *New England Journal of Medicine*, **341**(26), 1966–1973. http://www.ncbi.nlm.nih.gov/pubmed/10607813

Murphy, R.C., *et al.* (1979) A slow-reacting substance from murine mastocytoma cells. *Proceedings of the National Academy of Sciences of the USA*, **76**(9), 4275–4279. http://www.ncbi.nlm.nih.gov/pmc/articles/PMC411556/?tool=pubmed

Reiss, T.F., *et al.* (1996) Effects of Montelukast (MK-0476), a new potent cysteinyl leukotriene (LTD4) receptor antagonist, in patients with chronic asthma. *Journal of Allergy and Clinical Immunology*, **98**(3), 528534. http://www.jacionline.org/article/S0091-6749(96)70086-6/fulltext

Additional References

1. Osler, W. (1892) Bronchial asthma. *The Principles and Practice of Medicine*, **1**, 497–501.
2. Meltzer, S.J. (1910) Bronchial asthma as a phenomenon of anaphylaxis. *Journal of the American Medical Association*, **55**(12), 1021–1024.
3. Rackemann, F.M. (1918) A clinical study of one hundred and fifty cases of bronchial asthma. *Archives of Internal Medicine*, **22**(4), 517–552.
4. Bennich, H.H., *et al.* (1968) Immunoglobulin E, a new class of human immunoglobulin. *Bulletin of the World Health Organization*, **38**, 151–152.
5. Ishizaka, K., *et al.* (1966) Physicochemical properties of reaginic antibody V. Correlation of reaginic activity with gamma-E-globulin antibody. *Journal of Immunology*, **97**(6), 840–853.
6. Boulet, L.P., *et al.* (1997) Inhibitory effects of an anti-IgE antibody E25 on allergen-induced early asthmatic response. *American Journal of Respiratory and Critical Care Medicine*, **155**(6), 1835–1840.
7. Feldberg, W., and Kellaway, C.H. (1938) Liberation of histamine and formation of lysocithin-like substances by cobra venom. *Journal of Physiology*, **94**(2), 187–226.
8. Hamid, Q., *et al.* (1997) Inflammation of small airways in asthma. *Journal of Allergy and Clinical Immunology*, **100**, 44–51.
9. Corrigan, C.J., *et al.* (1991) Glucocorticoid resistance in chronic asthma: Glucocorticoid pharmacokinetics, glucocorticoid receptor characteristics, and inhibition of peripheral blood T-cell proliferation by glucocorticoids in vitro. *American Review of Respiratory Disease*, **144**, 1016–1025.

10. Sutcliffe, A., *et al.* (2006) Mast cell migration to Th2 stimulated airway smooth muscle from asthmatics. *Thorax*, **61**(8), 657–662.

11. Carryer, H.M., *et al.* (1950) The effect of cortisone of bronchial asthma and hay fever occurring in subjects sensitive to ragweed pollen. *Journal of Allergy*, **21**(4), 282–287.

12. Li, X., *et al.* (1999) An antiinflammatory effect of salmeterol, a long-acting beta(2) agonist, assessed in airway biopsies and bronchoalveolar lavage in asthma. *American Journal of Respiratory and Critical Care Medicine*, **160**(5 Pt 1), 1493–1499.

13. Orsida, B.E., *et al.* (2001) Effect of a long-acting beta2-agonist over three months on airway wall vascular remodeling in asthma. *American Journal of Respiratory and Critical Care Medicine*, **164**(1), 117–121.

14. Diamant, Z., *et al.* (1999) The effect of Montelukast (MK-0476), a cysteinyl leukotriene receptor antagonist, on allergen-induced airways responses and sputum cell counts in asthma. *Clinical & Experimental Allergy*, **29**(1), 42–51.

15. Fahy, J.V., *et al.* (1997) The effect of an anti-IgE monoclonal antibody on the early- and late-phase responses to allergen inhalation in asthmatic subjects. *American Journal of Respiratory and Critical Care Medicine*, **155**(6), 1828–1834.

16. Humbert, M., *et al.* (2005) Benefit of omalizumab as add-on therapy in patients with severe persistent asthma who are inadequately controlled despite best available therapy (GINA 2002 step 4 treatment): INNOVATE. *Allergy*, **60**, 309–316.

8 Cystic Fibrosis

Andrew Bush

Imperial College London and Royal Brompton Hospital, London, UK

Introduction

Cystic fibrosis (CF) is an autosomal recessive disease now known to be caused by absent or abnormal function of the cystic fibrosis transmembrane regulator (CFTR), which is a multifunctional protein encoded by a gene on the long arm of chromosome 7. CF was first differentiated from other conditions such as coeliac disease only as recently as 1938[1]. Initially the picture was dominated by either or both of diarrhoea and failure to thrive, and recurrent respiratory infections, and death in infancy was usual. The following years were of steady progress with treating these problems, so that now in many parts of the world babies are diagnosed by newborn screening, and median survival for babies born today has been predicted to be around 50 years[1]. In the main this has been achieved by meticulous application of relatively small therapeutic advances rather than dramatic 'headline news breakthroughs'. However, as a result of longevity CF has been found to be a true multisystem disease with older CF patients facing insulin deficiency and diabetes as a result of endocrine pancreatic dysfunction, portal cirrhosis and varices, pathological fracture due to osteopenia, nasal polyps, electrolyte depletion, male infertility due to bilateral absence of the vas deferens, and stress incontinence[1].

As yet, basic science has largely failed in its promise of delivering new therapies for CF. There are many novel therapies under development, but a cure of even lung manifestations of CF is far away. There is also a disconnect between our understanding of the multiple functions of CFTR and the pathophysiology of CF lung disease. This is important, because if therapeutic efforts correct only an irrelevant function of CFTR, then nothing will be achieved.

This chapter will review how knowledge of treatment and pathophysiology of CF developed in parallel; in the early stages, clinical practice progressed largely independently of the scientific stream which was exploring the pathophysiology of the disease. Treatment advances were on the basis of clinical observations, reactive to a problem but not tackling the underlying disease process; however, they made an enormous difference to the patient. Encouragingly, these streams have come together to produce a bright future of novel, disease modifying treatments.

An Electrifying Finding: Abnormal Mucosal Potential Differences
Knowles et al., New England Journal of Medicine (1981)

Perhaps no group has done more than Chapel Hill to elucidate the pathophysiology of CF. In this manuscript, the potential difference (PD) across the nasal mucosa was

Understanding Medical Research: The Studies that Shaped Medicine, First Edition. Edited by
John A. Goodfellow. © 2012 John Wiley & Sons, Ltd. Published 2012 by John Wiley & Sons, Ltd.

measured using an exploring bridge in the nose and a reference electrode placed subcutaneously. They showed clearly that in CF the baseline PD was more negative by at least three standard deviation scores. Furthermore, when the mucosa was perfused with amiloride, a blocker of the sodium channel ENaC, there was a much bigger positive deflection in CF, suggesting that the more negative baseline was due to sodium hyperabsorption. They confirmed these findings with a very small number of lower airway measurements. Subsequent investigators have confirmed in a much larger series that lower airway PD can be measured at bronchoscopy[2].

Measurement of nasal PDs using sophisticated protocols are used clinically as the most sensitive test of CFTR function in the rare patients in whom the diagnosis is in doubt, but the major contribution remains in the research field. As a result of the demonstration of sodium hyperabsorption, the group went on to trial nebulised amiloride as a therapeutic agent. The initial results were promising[3], but when amiloride was added to standard therapy no benefit was seen[4], and today nebulised amiloride is little used in CF, and then mainly as part of complex regimes for multiply resistant organisms. It may be that amiloride cannot reverse established lung disease but is valuable in preventing its development. The results of this study also led to the generation of the 'low-volume' hypothesis (below) which is currently the most likely link between the molecular functions of CFTR and the respiratory manifestations of the disease. Finally, measurements of nasal and lower airway PD are still used as clinical trial endpoints to determine improvement or correction in CFTR function. The equipment and measurements are complex and sophisticated, and the technique is only available in very few centres, but nearly 30 years after it was published, this work is still at the cutting edge of CF research.

On the Shoulders of Giants: Chloride Permeability and CF
Quinton, Nature (1983)

As long ago as 1951, CF patients were noted to be particularly vulnerable to heat prostration, and it was suggested that this was because of loss of salts in the sweat. In this paper Paul Quinton microdissected sweat glands from skin biopsies of normal and CF patients and used a microperfusion technique to study the abnormal physiology. He found that there was a markedly more negative PD in CF as described in the airway mucosa by the Chapel Hill group. This finding could not have been due to the relatively minor changes in sodium transport, but he showed that chloride permeability was an order of magnitude higher in normals than in CF patients. He suggested that a generalised defect of chloride permeability may underlie CF, rather than increased sodium permeability as had been suggested by the Chapel Hill group.

How has this observation stood the test of time? Looking back it clearly establishes the scientific basis for one of the most useful tests in medicine; the sweat test. In all but 1–2% of CF patients who have atypical presentations, the sweat test, properly performed, is diagnostic. The few very rare conditions which are said to be characterised by a high sweat chloride are rarely a diagnostic issue in real life. These observations subsequently established the role of CFTR as a chloride channel. The fact that different functions of CFTR may be important in different organs was not appreciated, and to this day there is a lack of appreciation that an insight that produced a wonderful diagnostic test may not be relevant to disease pathophysiology in the lung; it remains possible if not probable that correction of chloride channel function on its own will be insufficiently important to improve CF lung disease. Nonetheless, as a result of this brilliant paper, the sweat test remains the bedrock of diagnosis of CF and measurement of sweat electrolytes has been used in trials to demonstrate the effects or otherwise of novel compounds on CFTR function.

Big Is Beautiful, and More Is Better
Corey et al., Journal of Clinical Epidemiology (1988)

In the early days of CF, children had diarrhoea and steatorrhoea due to exocrine pancreatic failure, and the standard advice was to have a low fat diet to try to control these distressing symptoms as well as pancreatic enzyme supplements. This paper emerged from the finding from registry data that Canadian CF patients were surviving longer than CF patients in the United States. The authors compared the results in two well-established CF centres, Toronto and Boston. The Toronto patients were taller and heavier and survived a mean of nearly 10 years longer (21 vs. 30 years median age of death), despite having very similar spirometry. This amounted to around 5,000 patient years in the population studied. The most important difference found was the dietary advice; in the 1970s in Boston the great Harry Shwachman had advocated a low-fat diet, whereas Douglas Crozier advocated for a high-fat diet with 20–30 capsules per meal in Toronto. This finding was key in the dietetic revolution in CF. High-fat diets were widely introduced, and their acceptability was enhanced with enteric-coated microsphere preparations of pancreatic enzymes. It was clear that optimising fat intake and absorption was pivotal to getting good survival. The realisation of the pivotal importance of nutrition has lead to the use of gastrostomy feeding for those in nutritional failure. Poor weight gain is no longer shrugged off as inevitable, but triggers a detailed review. Nearly 20 years later, clinics are increasingly using databases to compare their results with those of others nationwide. They identify where they are doing less well, and try to determine what practices need to change. This 'process improvement' is being used to drive up standards, although no longer are there the huge differences between clinics as reported in this manuscript. However, the history of CF is that much improvement comes from small gains applied meticulously, and the approaches used in this manuscript are just as relevant today.

A False Dawn? Finding the CF Gene
Rommens et al.; Kerem et al.; Riordan et al., Science (1989)

These three consecutive papers in *Science*, reporting that the CF gene had been localised, galvanised the CF world. In the first paper, chromosome walking and jumping localised the CF gene to a region on the long arm of chromosome 7 encompassing about 250,000 base pairs of genomic DNA. In the second, a deletion of three base pairs in the putative gene led to a deletion of phenylalanine in the protein. This is now known to be the commonest CF mutation in many white races, ΔF_{508}. The third described other mutations and some were linked to the presence of residual pancreatic function. The identification of the gene and thus the abnormal protein gave a tremendous fillip to CF research. From the standpoint of 20 years hindsight, what has been the gain from these three seminal papers?

Clearly there has been a huge expansion in basic knowledge of CFTR biology. The gene for CFTR is complex, comprising 27 exons which encode a protein comprising 1480 amino acids. The complex post-transcriptional processing of CFTR and the interactions of the nascent protein with numerous intracellular proteins and molecular chaperones have been elucidated. The structure of the protein with 12 membrane spanning domains, two nucleotide binding folds, and an R domain and the functions of some of the domains have been worked out in detail. Multiple functions of CFTR have been discovered; as predicted by Quinton, CFTR is a chloride channel in the apical cell membrane. Additionally it modulates the functions of other epithelial ion channels, including ENaC, reconciling the observations from Quinton and Chapel Hill. Furthermore, CFTR is also a channel for bicarbonate and glutathione.

When the gene was discovered, the medical community envisioned that gene therapy was going to cure CF within ten years; a series of brilliant experiments in rodents established that using viral vectors, CFTR could be expressed in the airway and work progressed to proof of concept studies in humans[5]. Some transient gene expression has been produced in the nose and lower airway in humans and a large study will shortly be starting in the United Kingdom, led by the CF Trust Gene Therapy Consortium. However, the challenges of safety and preventing immune recognition of the vector leading to its destruction are still very real. It would be a brave man who today predicted when the first prescription for gene therapy will be signed in the clinic.

Diagnostically, genetic studies have established that some patients with phenotypic CF but normal sweat tests are indeed affected by CF. There are now over 1600 mutations discovered[6], and as complete CF gene sequencing becomes more widely available, genetic studies will be able to rule out CF with increasing accuracy. The wider role of CFTR in CF-like disease has become appreciated by the finding of an increased carrier frequency in patients with non-alcoholic acute pancreatitis, bronchiectasis, pulmonary infection with atypical *Mycobacterial* species, severe sinusitis and azoospermia. Initially it was hoped that knowing the individual CF patient's genotype would help predict prognosis, but this is not the case. The most important determinant of prognosis in CF is socioeconomic status[7]; as with so many diseases, it is better to be ill and rich than ill and poor.

In summary, these brilliant papers have delivered much in the field of basic science, and promise much in the clinical arena. Recent studies suggest that delivery in the clinical field is imminent; however, there have been bitter disappointments on the road.

Treatment of Respiratory Infection: The Early Bird Catches the Worm
Valerius et al., Lancet (1991)

Respiratory failure is the cause of most of the mortality and morbidity of CF. Initially *Staphylococcus aureus* was the main pathogen, but as anti-staphylococcal treatment became more effective, *Pseudomonas aeruginosa* began to dominate with around 80% of CF patients eventually becoming chronically infected. The replacement of one infective threat by another is a recurring theme in CF. The use of nebulised antibiotics in CF patients chronically infected with *Pseudomonas aeruginosa* had been described in a randomised controlled trial in 1981[8]. By modern standards the pre-trial safety and efficacy testing of the nebulised antibiotics used was very inadequate and the size of the study small. Nonetheless clear symptomatic benefit was shown in this pioneering study and the foundation was laid for the use of the aerosol route to deliver antibiotics. Subsequent studies have amply confirmed the findings. The next step was to assess a strategy of early treatment of *Pseudomonas aeruginosa* to try to prevent chronic infection developing. The Copenhagen clinic used a strategy of nebulised colistin and oral ciprofloxacin at first isolation of *Pseudomonas aeruginosa*. This trial was not formally randomised, and also was small; patients were offered treatment and those who declined were the control group. The authors showed a substantial increase in time to establishment of chronic infection in the treated group. Subsequent work has confirmed these findings, and protocols of increasing therapeutic intensity have been developed, including the use of intravenous antibiotics. These have largely often only been tested against historical controls, but it is quite clear that a placebo controlled trial would now be unethical, and that the first isolation of *Pseudomonas aeruginosa* mandates urgent treatment.

The nebulised antibiotics used initially were the intravenous preparations put into a nebuliser cup and contained excipients that could potentially cause bronchoconstriction. In 1999 the United States caught on to the potential benefits of the nebulised route and a preservative-free solution of tobramycin (TOBI™) was developed and trialled in CF[9]. This was shown to be superior to placebo in CF patients infected with *Pseudomonas aeruginosa* in a very large double-blind trial. TOBI was also used as a single agent successfully to eradicate first isolations of *Pseudomonas aeruginosa*.

In summary, this study showed that early and aggressive treatment of first isolation of *Pseudomonas aeruginosa* can delay established infection, and others have shown the benefits of nebulised antibiotics in established infection.

Many a Slip! The First Animal Model of CF
Snouwaert et al., Science (1992)

The development of an animal model of CF was a major breakthrough. The Chapel Hill group disrupted the CFTR gene in exon 10 (S489X) in mouse embryonic cells to produce a truncated CFTR protein and the first 'CF mouse'. These mice have been used extensively in CF research, but the models have proved less useful than was at first hoped. Many of the initial mice died quickly from intestinal obstruction. Newborn intestinal obstruction due to meconium ileus is a well known clinical presentation of CF. The CF mouse appeared to have only minimal pancreatic disease, and subsequent studies have shown that it does not have a really good pulmonary phenotype either. The absence of a pulmonary phenotype is a major blow, given the importance of respiratory disease in man. Although the mice can be infected with *Pseudomonas aeruginosa* if the organisms are given in agarose beads, the relevance of this is doubtful. The problem may be that there are non-CFTR chloride channels which are highly active in the mouse lower airway, thus ameliorating the effects of CFTR dysfunction or absence. CFTR is a less important ENaC inhibitor in mice compared with humans. Another problem with the mouse lower airway is that it has no submucosal glands, where in humans more than half of airway CFTR is found. The mouse nose is more like the human airway in terms of PD responses at least, and CF murine sinusitis may be a better model for studying human lower airway CF infection.

Since this initial description, many other CF mice have been produced, including gut-corrected animals with longer survival. However, a large animal model is urgently needed, and there is recent report of a pig model, with an early onset gastrointestinal disease and normal lungs as birth[10]. It remains to be seen whether this will be an important animal model of CF.

No Such Thing as a Free Lunch: New Infections, New Problems
Govan et al., Lancet (1993)

In the late 1980s bacterial infection in the CF airway was considered to be due to a very few micro-organisms: typically *Staphylococcus aureus, Pseudomonas aeruginosa* and *Haemophilus influenza*. It was widely taught that CF patients presented no risk of infection to normal people or other CF patients, and infection was exclusively localised to the airway, never systemic. A series of events shattered most of these perceptions. Firstly, '*Cepacia* syndrome' came on the scene. *Burkholderia cepacia* (then known as *Pseudomonas cepacia*) was known to be highly prevalent in some clinics in North America. CF patients visiting North America acquired this organism, and many within a few months went from stability and moderately good health to death from fulminating sepsis[11]. *Burkholderia cepacia* was found to be readily transmissible between patients, virulent and resistant to multiple antibiotics. For the first time, it was clear that people with CF posed a risk of infection to their fellow patients. The debate about segregation came right to the top of the agenda.

The first response was to have dedicated *Burkholderia cepacia* clinics. Unfortunately, it was not then appreciated that there were different strains (genomovars) of *Burkholderia cepacia* and, as a result, some patients carrying a benign strain who were herded into the special clinics there acquired a more serious strain and died as a result. This current paper highlighted that segregation in the hospital setting was insufficient to prevent cross-infection. Epidemiological evidence pointed to attendance at shared fitness sessions, for example, as leading to cross-infection between patients.

At this time, CF holiday camps had brought together groups of patients, with much benefit in terms of mutual support. Patients with *Burkholderia cepacia* were excluded, but it was becoming increasingly clear that this was not the only problem organism, and person-to-person transmission of *Pseudomonas aeruginosa* was also occurring. The camps shut down, and CF patients were strongly advised not to meet at all. Today, most CF clinics have a strict segregation policy; usually, the patient is placed straight in a private room, and the professionals (physician, specialist nurse, dietician, physiotherapist and any others) enter the room to see the patient in turn. Meticulous attention is paid to basic hygiene and hand washing. Within the ward, CF patients occupy separate cubicles, and should not mix in the hospital school or anywhere else. These methods have probably reduced cross-infection, but have certainly increased the sense of isolation felt by many CF patients.

As the aggressive use of nebulised and intravenous antibiotics has reduced the threat of *Pseudomonas aeruginosa*, other organisms such as other members of the *Burkholderia* family, *Achromobacter, Pandoraea, Ralstonia, Stenotrophomonas and Acinetobacter* have been selected. It is also becoming clear from anaerobic cultures and molecular fingerprinting methods that there are multiple species of anaerobes growing in the CF airway.

What lessons can be learned in hindsight from the *Burkholderia cepacia* story? We are I believe still suffering from the consequences of precipitate and ill-thought-out actions. The concept of segregation in hospital and in the community sounds fine, but can it work in practice? There may be segregation in the clinic, but in the elevator, while waiting in pharmacy or the X-ray department? Just because two patients have the 'identical' organism (which may in fact have less than 90% genetic overlap) does not prove one has passed it on to the other. Alternative explanations are acquisition from a point source in the environment, or that a particular strain has genetic advantages making it ubiquitous in the environment, and the two patients acquired the organism from different places. It is clear that organisms like *Burkholderia cepacia* and methicillin-resistant *Staphylococcus aureus* are contagious and adversely affect prognosis. However, many patients carrying epidemic strains of *Pseudomonas aeruginosa* are doing no worse than non-infected patients. Should two CF children be in the same class at school? Or even in the same school? How is this affected by patient confidentiality, and will we drive CF underground? There is no question but that many CF patients feel like lepers as a result of one of the most profound upheavals in CF care patterns in recent years.

Catch Them Early, Treat Them Quickly: A Randomised Controlled Trial of Screening for CF
Farrell et al., New England Journal of Medicine (1997)

In parts of the world such as Australasia, screening for CF using a heel prick blood spot test in the newborn period has been going on for more than 20 years; within the last 3 years, universal newborn screening is in place for the whole of England. This happened only after hot debate of the merits of screening, in which parents of CF children, CF children and all professionals employed in the care of CF were in uniformly and unanimously in favour, and the controllers of the purse strings, for whom CF meant only a pair of initials, were resolutely in opposition.

Various different protocols have been used, usually a combination of the measurement of immunoreactive trypsin (iRT), and a selection of the common severe CFTR mutations. Diagnosis is always confirmed by sweat testing even if two known CF producing mutations have been found. The evidence in favour of screening has come largely from observational studies using historical controls, and this major randomised controlled trial from Wisconsin. This group measured iRT in 650,341 newborns, and in the latter half of the study, the presence of the ΔF_{508} mutation. Half of the infants with abnormal results were recalled for sweat testing, the remainder of the abnormal tests were not actioned. CF was diagnosed in 74 patients in the early sweat test group, including five missed by screening. 56 of this group, and 40 patients diagnosed late on symptoms, were evaluated after 10 years. This manuscript showed clear cut nutritional benefits, but there was little evidence for benefit in respiratory outcomes. Another paper from the same group showed that malnutrition and vitamin deficiency in the first 2 years of life, the time of most rapid head growth, was associated with neurocognitive defects at age 10 years[12]. Screening leading to early diagnosis and treatment will undoubtedly be beneficial, provided the child is referred for state-of-the-art management.

Pathophysiology of CF: The Low-Volume Hypothesis
Matsui et al., Cell (1998)

The link between the many functions of CFTR and CF lung disease, the most important contributor to morbidity and mortality, has been difficult to elucidate.

An early model suggested that the airway surface liquid in CF had a much higher sodium concentration than normal, and this high-salt environment resulted in activation of airway surface antibacterial cationic peptides such as the defensins and lactoferrin. By contrast, in this paper the Chapel Hill group hypothesised that the fundamental abnormality was sodium hyper-absorption by ENaC as a result of the lack of modulation by CFTR. This hypothesis suggests that there is airway surface dehydration, but that airway surface liquid is isotonic. As a result of loss of airway surface liquid, the periciliary layer loses height, cilia cannot function, and mucociliary clearance fails, leading to mucus impaction and chronic infection. In this paper, they could find no evidence in cell culture models that airway surface liquid was other than isotonic. Positively, they showed that in CF but not normal cells, airway surface liquid height declined over time, and that as a result mucociliary clearance failed. A subsequent manuscript showed that CF and normal cells behaved similarly in terms of airway surface liquid height when grown under conditions of phasic contraction, mimicking the effects of normal breathing on the airway, but that infection of CF but not normal cells with respiratory syncytial virus triggers reduction in airway surface liquid height.

There are clear therapeutic implications of this model. If it is correct, then adding fluid to the airway surface is a potentially beneficial strategy, whereas if the high-salt hypothesis is correct, then salt removal would be a better approach. Hypertonic saline has been used with therapeutic benefit in CF[13], and may have a sustained effect on mucociliary clearance; if the high-salt hypothesis was correct, one would predict that hypertonic saline would be deleterious.

Although the low-volume hypothesis is still the leading means of connecting the molecular actions of CFTR with CF lung disease, it is also not without its problems. Some studies have shown that nasal and peripheral airway mucociliary clearance is normal in CF[14]. Nonetheless, the important implication is that strategies should focus on ENaC as the root cause of lung disease, and suggests that chloride transport, although leading to a great diagnostic test for CF, is not relevant to lung pathology in CF. Thus therapeutic strategies that only correct chloride transport may ultimately fail to impact the morbidity and mortality of CF lung disease.

A True Dawn? The Modern Era of Mutation Specific Therapies
Wilschanski et al., New England Journal of Medicine (2003)

This final paper is an exemplar of how the scientific and clinical streams described above are increasingly combining to produce novel, disease modifying therapies. CF mutations have been divided into six classes. This classification has clinical utility; classes 1–3, the so-called severe mutations, are associated with pancreatic insufficiency and a worse outlook than the milder, class 4–6 mutations, although there is wide overlap between the groups[15].

Aminoglycoside antibiotics have been known to be able to over-ride premature but not physiological stop codons. In this paper the Hadasseh group showed that topically applied gentamicin nose drops were effective in patients carrying premature stop codons but not homozygous ΔF_{508} controls. This was measured in terms of partial correction of baseline PD and CFTR staining peripherally and on the surface of nasal epithelial cells. Subsequently, an orally active compound which over-rides premature stop codons, PTC$_{124}$ has been tested in a number of contexts. There were dramatic responses in a mouse model of Duchenne's muscular dystrophy (a disease whose pathogenesis involves premature stop codons), and a phase 2 trial by the Hadasseh group in CF was also promising[16]. Since around 30% of all genetic diseases are produced by premature stop codons, compounds like PTC$_{124}$ may mean we can go from a disease-specific approach to a mutation class specific approach to therapy.

Summary and Conclusions

This chapter has charted some of the major advances in the understanding of CF as we have progressed from a disease which was fatal in childhood as a result of malnutrition and respiratory infection, to a true multisystem disease of adult life; there will soon be more adult than paediatric CF patients. Many important areas have had to be passed over in the selection of papers, including the use of chest physical therapy, rhDNase, macrolide antibiotics, early and aggressive use of insulin therapy for insulin deficiency and insights into the pathophysiology of bone disease and other multi-organ complications.

Key Outstanding Questions

1. The biggest benefit to patients has come from the meticulous application of incremental improvements in basic care, especially nutritional and respiratory. How do we continue to ensure that best care is offered, benchmarking using databases to drive up standards?
2. Can we find biomarkers that are responsive to change, relate to long-term outcome in CF and can be used as endpoints in clinical trials?
3. Too much treatment in CF is not evidence based, and there are too many small and inconclusive trials. We need to develop a hierarchy of really important questions, and collaborate to provide definitive answers.
4. Which functions of CFTR are important in the pathophysiology of CF lung disease? Should we be targeting chloride transport or ENaC, or both?
5. Can we produce a large animal CF model with an airway phenotype that closely approximates the human CF airway disease?
6. How can we monitor the effects of early treatment which is now possible due to screening?
7. Finally and most challengingly, do we need a major paradigm shift in the way we treat CF? When the disease was rapidly fatal, ever more intensive treatment was appropriate. More was better. Now we have to consider the very long-term safety consequences of what we do. If for example a patient is treated with 3-month courses of intravenous antibiotics for four decades, this is amounts to 120 courses. There is risk of nephrotoxicity, allergy and selection of resistant organisms. More is no longer necessarily better; the challenge is not to lose the benefits of strategies which have so greatly improved the prognosis of CF, and to ensure that treatment is safe in the long term, and unnecessarily aggressive treatments are avoided. This will indeed be a difficult road to follow.

Key Useful Websites

1. US CF Foundation: http://www.cff.org/
2. UK CF Trust: http://www.cftrust.org.uk/
3. European CF Society: http://www.ecfs.eu/

References

Corey, M., *et al.* (1988) A comparison of survival, growth, and pulmonary function in patients with cystic fibrosis in Boston and Toronto. *Journal of Clinical Epidemiology*, **41**, 583–591. http://www.sciencedirect.com/science/article/pii/0895435688900637

Farrell, P.M., *et al.* (1997) Nutritional benefits of neonatal screening for cystic fibrosis. Wisconsin Cystic Fibrosis Neonatal Screening Study Group. *New England Journal of Medicine*, **337**, 963–969. http://www.ncbi.nlm.nih.gov/pubmed/9395429

Govan, J.R., *et al.* (1993) Evidence for transmission of *Pseudomonas cepacia* by social contact in cystic fibrosis. *Lancet*, **342**, 15–19. http://www.sciencedirect.com/science/article/pii/014067369391881L

Kerem, B., *et al.* (1989) Identification of the cystic fibrosis gene: genetic analysis. *Science*, **245**, 1073–1080. http://www.ncbi.nlm.nih.gov/pubmed/2570460

Knowles, M., *et al.* (1981) Increased bioelectric potential difference across respiratory epithelia in cystic fibrosis. *New England Journal of Medicine*, **305**, 1489–1495. http://www.ncbi.nlm.nih.gov/pubmed/7300874

Matsui, H., *et al.* (1998) Evidence for periciliary liquid layer depletion, not abnormal ion composition, in the pathogenesis of cystic fibrosis airways disease. *Cell*, **95**, 1005–1015. http://www.sciencedirect.com/science/article/pii/S0092867400817249

Quinton, P.M. (1983) Chloride impermeability in cystic fibrosis. *Nature*, **301**, 421–422. http://www.nature.com/nature/journal/v301/n5899/abs/301421a0.html

Riordan, J.R., *et al.* (1989) Identification of the cystic fibrosis gene: cloning and characterization of complementary DNA. *Science*, **245**, 1066–1073. http://www.ncbi.nlm.nih.gov/pubmed/2475911

Rommens, J.M., *et al.* (1989) Identification of the cystic fibrosis gene: chromosome walking and jumping. *Science*, **245**, 1059–1065. http://www.ncbi.nlm.nih.gov/pubmed/2772657

Snouwaert, J.N., *et al.* (1992) An animal model for cystic fibrosis made by gene targeting. *Science*, **257**, 1083–1088. http://www.ncbi.nlm.nih.gov/pubmed/1380723

Valerius, N.H., *et al.* (1991) Prevention of chronic Pseudomonas aeruginosa colonisation in cystic fibrosis by early treatment. *Lancet*, **338**, 725–726. http://www.thelancet.com/journals/lancet/article/PII0140-6736(91)91446-2/abstract

Wilschanski, M., *et al.* (2003) Gentamicin-induced correction of CFTR function in patients with cystic fibrosis and CFTR stop mutations. *New England Journal of Medicine*, **349**, 1433–1441. http://www.ncbi.nlm.nih.gov/pubmed/14534336

Additional References

1. Hodson, M., *et al.* (2007) *Cystic fibrosis.* 3rd ed. Hodder Arnold, London.
2. Davies, J.C., *et al.* (2005) Potential difference measurements in the lower airway of children with and without cystic fibrosis. *American Journal of Respiratory Critical Care Medicine*, **171**, 1015–1019.
3. Knowles, M.R., *et al.* (1990) A pilot study of aerosolized amiloride for the treatment of lung disease in cystic fibrosis. *New England Journal of Medicine*, **322**, 1189–1194.
4. Graham, A., *et al.* (1993) No added benefit from nebulized amiloride in patients with cystic fibrosis. *European Respiratory Journal*, **6**, 1243–1248.

5. Alton, E.W., *et al.* (1999) Cationic lipid-mediated CFTR gene transfer to the lungs and nose of patients with cystic fibrosis: a double-blind placebo-controlled trial. *Lancet*, **353**, 947–954. http://www.genet.sickkids.on.ca/cftr/app

6. Schechter, M.S., *et al.* (2001) The association of socioeconomic status with outcomes in cystic fibrosis patients in the United States. *American Journal of Respiratory Critical Care Medicine*, **163**, 1331–1337.

7. Hodson, M.E., *et al.* (1981) Aerosol carbenicillin and gentamicin treatment of *Pseudomonas aeruginosa* infection in patients with cystic fibrosis. *Lancet*, **2**, 1137–1139.

8. Ramsey, B.W., *et al.* (1999) Intermittent administration of inhaled tobramycin in patients with cystic fibrosis. Cystic Fibrosis Inhaled Tobramycin Study Group. *New England Journal of Medicine*, **340**, 23–30.

9. Rogers, C.S., *et al.* (2008) Disruption of the CFTR gene produces a model of cystic fibrosis in newborn pigs. *Science*, **321**, 1837–1841.

10. Ledson, M.J., *et al.* (1998) Cross infection between cystic fibrosis patients colonised with *Burkholderia cepacia*. *Thorax*, **53**, 432–436.

11. Koscik, R.L., *et al.* (2004) Cognitive function of children with cystic fibrosis: deleterious effect of early malnutrition. *Pediatrics*, **113**, 1549–1558.

12. Elkins, M.R., *et al.* (2006) National Hypertonic Saline in Cystic Fibrosis (NHSCF) Study Group: a controlled trial of long-term inhaled hypertonic saline in patients with cystic fibrosis. *New England Journal of Medicine*, **354**, 229–240.

13. McShane, D., *et al.* (2004) Normal mucociliary clearance in CF children: evidence against a CFTR-related defect. *European Respiratory Journal*, **24**, 95–100.

14. McKone, E.F., *et al.* (2003) Effect of genotype on phenotype and mortality in cystic fibrosis: a retrospective cohort study. *Lancet*, **361**, 1671–1676.

15. Kerem, E., *et al.* (2008) Effectiveness of PTC124 treatment of cystic fibrosis caused by nonsense mutations: a prospective phase II trial. *Lancet*, **372**, 719–727.

9   Chronic Obstructive Pulmonary Disease

Paul A. Ford and Peter J. Barnes

Airway Disease Section, National Heart and Lung Institute, Imperial College London, London, UK

Introduction

In 1959 at a CIBA guest symposium of physicians, the terms 'chronic bronchitis' and 'emphysema' were formally defined. It is believed the term 'chronic obstructive pulmonary disease' (COPD) was first encapsulated by William Briscoe in discussion at the Ninth Aspen Emphysema Conference in 1965. Today this is the preferred name for the disease. In reality COPD is an 'umbrella term' and describes a heterogeneous group of diseases with similar manifestations – including overlapping disease processes such as chronic bronchitis, emphysema, asthma, bronchiectasis and bronchiolitis.

Modern consumption of cigarettes is by far the leading cause of COPD, but the disease has existed under various guises for centuries – long before smoking on an industrial scale became a worldwide pandemic. However, given the ever-increasing burden of COPD in terms of its rising prevalence (particularly in Indo-China) and socioeconomic cost, more accurate disease phenotyping together with a better understanding of the cellular and molecular mechanisms behind the nature of the airway inflammation should lead us to more effective treatment modalities.

The following original articles have been selected based on their importance with regard to aetiology, prognosis and treatment of COPD and are presented in chronological order.

The Dutch Hypothesis
Orie et al., Royal Van Gorcum (1961)

This was the first of three international symposia specifically organised to try and agree on an international consensus regarding the definition, primarily, of chronic bronchitis. Two 'camps' existed at the time; the 'British hypothesis' with mucous hypersecretion and pollution as the primary aetiological factors, and the 'Dutch hypothesis' – which considered asthma and bronchitis to be the expression of a common 'asthmatic constitution'. This Dutch hypothesis represents the origins of the concept of a genetically determined bronchial hyperreactivity in COPD.

Orie, supporting the Dutch stance, was so convinced of this at the time that he went on to say: 'Bronchitis and asthma may be found in one patient at the same age but as a rule there is a fluent development from bronchitis in youth to a more asthmatic picture in adults, which in turn develops in to bronchitis of elderly patients.' We now know this was, in part, a manifestation of airway remodelling leading to fixed airflow obstruction.

Understanding Medical Research: The Studies that Shaped Medicine, First Edition. Edited by John A. Goodfellow. © 2012 John Wiley & Sons, Ltd. Published 2012 by John Wiley & Sons, Ltd.

With the advent of inhaled steroids and their use in early asthmatic inflammation this is now rarely seen in the developed world. However, Orie's belief that chronic bronchitis can exist hand in hand with increased bronchial hypereactivity rings true to a certain extent.

We now know that those patients with COPD who have a demonstrable significant increase in bronchial hyperreactivity do worse clinically and will probably benefit from the bronchoprotective effect of inhaled steroids as opposed to the majority of COPD patients who do not. Future trials examining the effects of therapies upon the natural history of COPD will need to carefully quantify their patient population as we now recognise this as a heterogeneous population. Not only is it important to delineate the degree of emphysema, small airways disease and expiratory flow limitation and mucous hypersecretion, but also it is imperative to identify those patients who have *only* COPD with increased bronchial hyperreactivity.

Quantifying Lung Resistance in Small Airways Disease
Hogg et al., New England Journal of Medicine (1968)

Using a pioneering retrograde catheter technique for measuring airway resistance first developed in living dogs, the authors of this study examined airway resistance from the post-mortem lungs of 14 human subjects (5 normal, 7 emphysema, 1 bronchiectatic and 1 bronchiolitic). Bronchography was also performed after measurement of airway resistance using finely particulated lead.

The authors presented three main conclusions:

1. 'In normal lungs only about one quarter of the total [lung] resistance is in the small airways' (<2 mm in diameter).
2. 'In the [nine] diseased patients the peripheral airways are the major site of resistance in obstructive lung disease.'
3. 'In the early stages of bronchitis and emphysema, R_P [peripheral lung resistance] may be markedly increased, with a relatively insignificant effect on R_L [total lung resistance]. It is therefore entirely possible for a patient with chronic cough and sputum to have considerable small-airway obstruction and an increase in R_P and yet have virtually normal total airway resistance.'

The study eloquently showed that the resistance in the small airways of patients with emphysema could be up to 44-fold higher than the average for the five normal patients – or up to 93% of the total airway resistance (range 63–93%). This compared to an average R_P of 25% in the normal patients.

Thus, for the first time, the true intrinsic nature of small airways narrowing in emphysema was accurately quantified. The authors also discussed how this fits within the context of the morphological changes seen in the post-mortem bronchograms. These early descriptions of small airway tapering and tortuosity have allowed the reader to marry anatomy with functionality thereby greatly enhancing our understanding of small airway inflammation.

Assessing Decline in FEV_1
Fletcher and Peto, British Medical Journal (1977)

Perhaps the most widely quoted paper in respiratory medicine, this manuscript is actually a review and summarises the then complex statistical analyses performed by Richard Peto from a trial published by Charles Fletcher one year earlier.

In 1960 the MRC commissioned a prospective study to look at how smoking interacts with other factors in causing airflow obstruction, in particular mucous hypersecretion and respiratory infections, and how this would stack up with the British hypothesis.

From an initial sample of 1136 working men (30–59 years) taken in 1961 from West London, 792 were seen regularly enough over the next 8 years to be included in the data analysis (18 further men were excluded at the end of the trial).

Mucous hypersecretion (sputum volume), frequency of bronchial infections and FEV_1 (forced expiratory volume in one second) measurements were taken at 6-monthly intervals. The authors presented four main conclusions:

1. 'FEV_1 declines continuously and smoothly over an individual's life'.
2. 'Nonsmokers lose FEV_1 slowly and almost never develop significant airflow obstruction'.
3. 'Many smokers lose FEV_1 almost as slowly as nonsmokers'.
4. And, perhaps most importantly, 'a susceptible smoker who stops smoking will not recover lost FEV_1, but the subsequent rate of loss of FEV_1 will revert to normal'.

The FEV_1 decline slopes used in the figures were averages of clusters of men and are therefore estimates, but they do indicate clearly that there is a range of susceptibility to the effects of cigarette smoke. This 'holy grail' has still proved elusive, and the search for an accurate biomarker to predict this is seemingly no nearer than it was over 30 years ago. The paper also signalled the end of the 'British hypothesis', the authors concluding that 'neither mucous hypersecretion nor bronchial infection cause chronic [lung] obstruction to progress more rapidly.'

It has become clear that both the amount one smokes and continued smoking into later life are associated with higher prevalence rates of COPD than demonstrated by Fletcher and Peto, and that accelerated decline in FEV_1 may still occur after quitting smoking (with continued airway inflammation). However, this paper was way ahead of its time; carefully planned prospective longitudinal studies of this nature are the cornerstone of modern medical research.

Exercise Training in COPD
McGavin et al., Thorax (1977)

Pulmonary rehabilitation had been mainly overlooked within the United Kingdom until the publication of this paper. Whilst there was evidence of improvement in various parameters in a number of independent trials, firm conclusions were difficult to formulate. This was due to small sample sizes, heterogeneity of diagnostic criteria and both short periods of training and testing and a lack of placebo-controlled data.

McGavin and colleagues randomised 28 subjects with severe airflow obstruction to one of two groups. The exercise group underwent an intensive home stair-climbing programme, whilst the control group carried on as normal and were reviewed at monthly intervals. The only possible flaw in the methodology was that final exercise testing took place at 14 weeks in the control group and 19 weeks in the exercise group. The authors cite '[subjects] in an optimal state of health' as the reason for this – it seems those undergoing the exercise programme were ill more frequently than in the control group. It is not clear whether they received more supplementary prednisolone during this time though the authors do state that some of the events were unconnected with their airways disease.

Twenty-four subjects completed the study (12 in each group). Those undergoing the stair climbing programme could walk significantly further as judged by a 12-minute walking test (an increase of 64 m in the exercise group compared to a deterioration of 19 m in the control group). Subjects in the exercise group could also manage a significantly greater maximal workload based on a cycle ergometer test.

The authors presented three main conclusions:

1. 'There was a considerable subjective benefit'.
2. 'There was objective evidence of increased exercise tolerance'.
3. 'This [points 1 and 2] is not accompanied by any change in ventilator function tests'.

Whilst these conclusions had previously been accepted in various guises, McGavin and colleagues were the first to proffer them after performing tests which seemingly proved them in a robust, placebo-controlled manner.

Pulmonary rehabilitation is now a cornerstone of treatment for patients with COPD, and initial pioneering trials such as this one have paved the way for future progress using exercise-based treatment modalities.

Supplementary O_2 Therapy in COPD
[American] Nocturnal Oxygen Therapy Trial Group, Annals of Internal Medicine (1980)
[UK]Report of the Medical Research Council Working Party, Lancet (1981)

Two seminal trials published within a year of each other provide the rationale for supplementary O_2 therapy in patients with hypoxemic COPD. They are unlikely ever to be repeated due to ethical considerations.

The first and largest study was performed in six centres in the United States and Canada and randomised 203 subjects with severe COPD (FEV_1 30% predicted) into two groups – one receiving supplementary nocturnal O_2 (mean 12 hr/day), the other receiving continuous O_2 (mean 17.7 hr/day). Mean follow up was 19.3 months. Compared to the continuous O_2 group, the RR (relative risk) of death in the nocturnal group was 1.94. They also found that subgroups showing a high $PaCO_2$, haematocrit, pulmonary artery pressure or low FVC (forced vital capacity) and pH or severe disturbance of mood at entry to the trial appeared to derive the most benefit from continuous O_2.

The UK trial recruited 87 subjects with similar profiles to the US cohort from three centres with severe COPD (FEV_1 around 600 ml). In addition, they were all hypercapnic with evidence of congestive cardiac failure. Subjects were randomised to receive 15 hr/day of O_2 or no O_2 and followed for 5 years. The RR was lower than the American trial at 1.49 in favour of supplementary O_2 mainly due to the fact that in the 66 male subjects, the survival curves did not start to separate until the 500th day. In the small group of women (n=21), the RR at 3 years was an astonishing 6.1 in favour of supplementary O_2 – the effects becoming immediately apparent (Figure 9.1). The authors speculated that a rising $PaCO_2$ and red cell mass could predict mortality.

Whilst it is clear supplementary O_2 improves survival in hypoxaemic subjects with COPD and evidence of right heart failure, the trials inevitably raise more questions than they answer. For instance, what is the mechanism behind the improved survival? Is the profound effect in women real? What are the optimal time and dose of

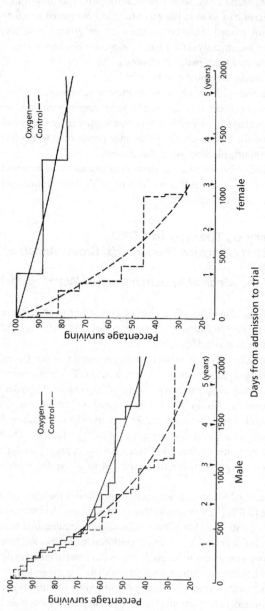

Figure 9.1 Mortality curves from males and females with and without LTOT. Note the disparity of mortality curve separation for males (500 days) and females (immediate). Adapted from Report of the Medical Research Council Working Party, *The Lancet* (1981), with permission from Elsevier.

supplementary O_2 therapy? At what level of hypoxemia should we start therapy? Unfortunately, it is unlikely we will ever know the answer to these questions – which is remarkable when you consider modern COPD treatment guidelines for supplementary O_2 are based on two trials performed more than 25 years ago.

Synchronised Smoking Cessation: Effect on Decline in FEV_1
Anthonisen et al., Journal of the American Medical Association (1994)

Conducted within ten centres in Canada and the United States, this trial (the Lung Health Study) was the first to assess the effect of large-scale synchronised smoking cessation on FEV_1 decline in subjects with mild airflow obstruction. Nearly 6000 subjects were randomised into three equal groups – usual care (UC), smoking intervention plus inhaled placebo (SIP), and smoking intervention plus inhaled ipratropium bromide (SIA). Subjects were followed up for 5 years with lung function measurements yearly. The trial is particularly noteworthy with regard to several parameters. Though the authors give no indication as to when recruitment was terminated, the rate at which this was achieved is astonishing. Smoking cessation rates were equally impressive (22% sustained quitters in the SI groups vs. 5% in the UC group) as was 5-year-follow up (71% of initial subjects provided a year 1 to year 5 FEV_1 comparison).

The authors presented three main conclusions:
1. 'Smoking cessation results in substantial benefit to lung function'
2. Though there was a small improvement in lung function with inhaled bronchodilator therapy at the end of the first year, this had no overall effect on lung function decline. Furthermore, when the bronchodilator was withdrawn at the end of the trial, this initial effect was reversed.
3. And, most importantly, when the authors compared sustained quitters versis continued smokers from each of the three groups (UC, SIP and SIA), the lung function decline curves actually *diverged*. The authors wrote: 'These results strongly support smoking cessation as the first and most important clinical intervention in smokers with mild airflow obstruction.'

For the first time in a well-conducted large-scale randomised trial, it was clear that smoking cessation is first-line treatment for COPD and that an inhaled anticholinergic given regularly has no effect whatsoever on lung function decline. A more recent trial examining the effects of tiotropium bromide (UPLIFT) upon lung function decline in COPD drew similar conclusions though effects upon lung function were much more impressive and other parameters (such as exacerbations and QOL) improved significantly. Anthonisen and his coauthors should be congratulated: by using intensive smoking cessation techniques, the Lung Health Study demonstrated that this is the only effective intervention that alters the natural history of lung function decline in COPD.

Breathlessness and Dynamic Hyperinflation
Tantucci et al., European Respiratory Journal (1998)

The concept of dynamic hyperinflation (DH) in patients with obstructive lung disease is a complex phenomenon. Simply, it is most easily understood if one takes in a deep breath, exhales partially and then breathes in again. Physiologically the term encompasses both the inability of the respiratory system to relax fully and an increasing end expiratory lung volume during exercise.

Using a pioneering negative expiratory pressure technique, which eradicated most of the technical problems with the then standard techniques, Tantucci and colleagues were able to more accurately quantify patients with COPD into those with expiratory flow limitation (EFL) and those without (NFL). They were then able to predict that those patients with EFL would respond to a bronchodilator by increasing inspiratory capacity, that is, reducing DH, making the work of breathing more efficient. Those without expiratory flow limitation did not respond in the same way and explains why only a *proportion* of patients with COPD will benefit from bronchodilatation and reduced dyspnoea, particularly during exercise.

Clearly the physiological concepts surrounding changes in lung volumes in patients with COPD, particularly during exercise, are very challenging. It remains to be seen if these measurements can be undertaken routinely and understandably in mainstream respiratory settings.

Effect of an Inhaled Steroid on FEV$_1$ Decline in Smokers with Mild COPD
Pauwels et al., New England Journal of Medicine (1999)

To this day the beneficial effect of inhaled steroids upon the natural history of lung function decline in COPD remains a contentious issue. Methodological issues surrounding trial designs, patient characteristics and follow-up arrangements make interpretation of results very difficult.

This was the first long-term study to assess treatment with an inhaled steroid in a large group of subjects with mild COPD who continued to smoke. It is noteworthy for its meticulous selection criteria and relatively long run-in period. Starting in 1992 and continuing for 18 months, over 2000 subjects were initially screened. Of these, 1695 were enrolled in a smoking cessation program for 3 months and 10% stopped smoking. The remaining subjects were then assessed for compliance with inhaled placebo medication for a further 3 months. 1277 subjects were then randomised to either 3 years treatment with inhaled budesonide or placebo (the subjects were therefore *relatively* steroid naive at trial entry having not taken any inhaled steroid for at least 6 months). Mean FEV$_1$ was 77% predicted for both groups with mean pack years smoking also identical at 39 years. The subjects were therefore very similar to those examined in the Lung Health Study. 71% of subjects randomised completed the study. Approximately 10% of subjects stopped smoking during the trial but cessation rates were equal in both treatment groups. Potential steroid side effects were also assessed including bone mineralisation using plain X-ray and densitometry measurements in a subset of subjects.

The authors came to one very important conclusion: 'In persons with mild COPD who continue smoking, the use of inhaled budesonide is associated with a small one-time improvement in lung function but does not appreciably affect the long-term progressive decline.'

Inhaled steroids seemed to provide a short-lived improvement in FEV$_1$ but this effect dissipated after 6 months and rates of decline then became identical. However, the rate of decline of lung function in the initial run-in period was much greater than expected. It is therefore entirely possible that this short term effect was a consequence of the inevitable steroid withdrawal which occurs during such trials. A sub-analysis of reduced smoking burden (<36 pack years) implied a more beneficial effect of active treatment, though this did not reach statistical significance. Subjects on inhaled budesonide had more skin bruising and oropharyngeal candidiasis than control subjects, but no other increase in side effects or adverse events was reported.

Subsequent trials examining the effects of inhaled steroids continue to generate more questions than they answer. The increased use of inhaled steroids has meant that many trials without adequate run-in periods are in fact assessing the effects of steroid withdrawal given that over 50% of subjects were previously on them. The advent of the combination products Symbicort and Seretide has further complicated matters as the contribution of the long-acting beta-blocker within the combination is often not adequately addressed in the correct 2×2 factorial analyses. Until these fundamental questions are answered, it remains to be seen if inhaled steroids have any long-term beneficial effect.

The Nature of Persistent Airway Inflammation in Ex-Smokers with COPD
Rutgers et al., Thorax (2000)

Surprisingly, until this paper was published, no trial had investigated the effect of smoking cessation on airway inflammation in subjects with COPD and how this compares to a 'normal airway' in subjects age and smoking matched without COPD. Conventional wisdom proposed by Fletcher and Peto had dictated that those subjects with COPD who stopped smoking would arrest their accelerated lung function decline and return to the slope of the corresponding age-matched nonsmoker implying that the airway had somehow 'recovered'.

Rutgers and colleagues compared the induced sputum, bronchial washings and bronchial biopsies from 18 subjects with moderate COPD who had stopped smoking with identical samples from 11 age-matched and smoking history-matched subjects.

They found that the subjects with COPD had higher numbers of eosinophils and CD68+ T lymphocytes within the bronchial mucosa. They also found higher numbers of neutrophils and eosinophils within the induced sputum, together with increased expression of IL-8 and eosinophilic cationic protein.

It was clear that 'subjects with COPD who do not smoke have airways inflammation as shown by a significant increase in [inflammatory cells] compared to healthy [matched] controls'. The authors went to great length to exclude subjects with an asthmatic phenotype, and at the time the increases in eosinophilic numbers in the COPD subjects were difficult to explain. It has subsequently become clear that this effector cell may play a more pivotal role in COPD than previously thought and that the authors had stumbled on something of potentially great importance. This trial established that there is a persistent inflammatory milieu in the absence of the initial cigarette smoke-induced stimulus.

Small Airways Inflammation in COPD
Hogg et al., New England Journal of Medicine (2004)

Some 36 years after his original publication on small airways resistance in COPD, Hogg and colleagues published an observational paper outlining an assessment of the small airways in the surgically resected lungs of 159 patients with all stages of COPD. In essence, they formulated two main conclusions:

1. The small airways are filled with inflammatory exudates which contribute to occlusion and this rises with increasing severity of disease. This is associated with thickening of the airway wall by way of a complex remodelling process.
2. In more severe disease there is evidence of adaptive processes within the airway walls, particularly germinal centres which stain strongly for B cells. These are surrounded by T cells.

This paper has changed the way we think about inflammatory processes within COPD. Early aberrant innate inflammatory responses to tobacco smoke challenge are superseded by a more advanced 'memory' driven adaptive immune response; which continues long after the patient has stopped smoking. This process leads to derangements in the small airways which lead to hallmark increases in small airway resistance: a major cause of morbidity in the disease. It is quite possible that the inflammatory exudates which occur within the lumen of the small airways occur independently of large airway secretions and are therefore a separate entity from chronic bronchitis.

Exacerbations in COPD
Soler-Cataluna et al., Thorax (2005)

Prior to the publication of this paper several trials had identified an exacerbation, with or without admission to hospital, as a poor prognostic factor in COPD outcomes such as mortality and health status.

In a 5-year prospective cohort of 304 subjects with severe COPD, Soler-Cataluna and colleagues specifically examined the *independent* risk of prior exacerbation frequency on the future mortality of the subjects at the end of the 5 years. They divided the subjects into those with no prior exacerbations, 1–2 exacerbations and $\geq$3 exacerbations prior to the start of recruitment in 1998. During the 5 years, they also recorded subjects' ongoing exacerbation profiles.

The authors came to two main conclusions:

1. 'Severe acute exacerbations of COPD have a negative [independent] prognostic impact [on all-cause mortality]'.
2. 'Mortality increases with the frequency of severe exacerbations, particularly if these require admission to hospital'.

By adjusting for various predictors, the authors found prior exacerbation frequency to be just as powerfully predictive for mortality as age and $PaCO_2$.

It would seem obvious then that strategies which reduce exacerbation frequency should have a major impact on COPD disease progression. In the subsequent TORCH trial, it was disappointing that although exacerbation rates were significantly reduced, the all-cause mortality was unaffected although, as previously discussed, methodological issues with the analysis have made the results difficult to interpret.

Given the need for a follow-up period of several years *and* that combinations of different therapies will have to be used to influence all-cause mortality in COPD, it is highly unlikely these large trials will ever be done. Nonetheless any therapy which can target the increasing hyperinflation and airway inflammation which accompanies an exacerbation of COPD should have a major therapeutic impact; in particular on mortality, as Soler-Cataluna and colleagues have eloquently shown. Though largely forgotten, the British hypothesis may have had some bearing on the natural history of COPD after all, as increased mucous hypersecretion – the cornerstone of the hypothesis – often accompanies acute exacerbations.

Summary and Conclusions

The therapeutic nihilism surrounding treatment and prognosis of COPD is thankfully long gone. In the United Kingdom, many patients who were previously undetected are now being assessed and offered smoking cessation, pulmonary rehabilitation and/or treatment with bronchodilators and, in those with severe disease, inhaled steroids. However, we are on the verge of a global epidemic of COPD now that the tobacco industry has turned its attention to the growing yet socially vulnerable economies of Indo-China. Until the governments of these emerging economies act to counter this global addiction, the incidence of COPD will continue to grow apace. Any 'cure' is certainly a long way off as seemingly is any clear indicator of susceptibility to the effects of noxious inhaled particulates.

Key Outstanding Questions

1. What is the true nature of the small airways inflammation in COPD?
2. How is it best to sample, visualise and measure small airway function in COPD?
3. Can we develop a biomarker that can detect long-term susceptibility to inhaled particulates (particularly cigarette smoke)?
4. Is there any possibility of reversing the irreversible, that is, the permanent loss of respiratory tissue which occurs with advancing COPD?
5. What are the real effects of inhaled steroids?
6. Can we classify COPD into 'many little COPDs' so that treatment can be individually tailored and therefore more specific to patients' needs?

Key Research Centres

1. National Heart and Lung Institute, London, United Kingdom
2. UBC James Hogg Research Centre, Vancouver, Canada
3. Faculty of Pulmonary and Critical Care Medicine, Johns Hopkins, Baltimore, USA

References

Anthonisen, N., et al. (1994) Effects of smoking intervention and the use of an inhaled anticholinergic bronchodilator on the rate of decline of FEV_1. The Lung Health Study. Journal of the American Medical Association, 272(19), 1497–1505. http://www.ncbi.nlm.nih .gov/pubmed/7966841

Fletcher, C., and Peto, R. (1977) The natural history of chronic airflow obstruction. British Medical Journal, 1(6077), 1645–1648. http://www.ncbi.nlm.nih.gov/pmc/articles/PMC1607732/ ?tool=pubmed

Hogg, J., et al. (1968) Site and nature of airway obstruction in chronic obstructive lung disease. New England Journal of Medicine, 278(25), 1355–1360. http://www.ncbi.nlm.nih.gov/ pubmed/5650164

Hogg, J.C., et al. (2004) The nature of small-airway obstruction in chronic obstructive pulmonary disease. New England Journal of Medicine, 350(26), 2645–2653. http://www. ncbi.nlm.nih.gov/pubmed/15215480

McGavin, C.R., *et al.* (1977) Physical rehabilitation for the chronic bronchitic: results of a controlled trial of excersises in the home. *Thorax*, **32**(3), 307–311. http://www.ncbi.nlm.nih.gov/pmc/articles/PMC470605/?tool=pubmed

Nocturnal Oxygen Therapy Trial Group (1980) Continuous or nocturnal oxygen therapy in hypoxemic chronic obstructive lung disease: a clinical trial. *Annals of Internal Medicine*, **93**(3), 391–398. http://www.annals.org/content/93/3/391.abstract

Orie, N.G.M., *et al.* (1961) Bronchitis: an international symposium, April 27–29, 1960 Royal Van Gorcum, Assen.

Pauwels, R.A., *et al.* (1999) Long-term treatment with inhaled budesonide in persons with mild chronic obstructive disease who continue smoking. *EUROSCOP – European Respiratory Society Study on Chronic Obstructive Pulmonary Disease. New England Journal of Medicine*, **340**(25), 1948–1953. http://www.ncbi.nlm.nih.gov/pubmed/10379018

Report of the Medical Research Council Working Party (1981) Long term domiciliary oxygen therapy in chronic hypoxic cor pulmonale complicating chronic bronchitis and emphysema. *Lancet*, **1**(8222), 681–686. http://www.thelancet.com/journals/lancet/article/PIIS0140-6736(81)91970-X/abstract

Rutgers, R., *et al.* (2000) Ongoing airway inflammation in patients with COPD who do not currently smoke. *Thorax*, **55**(1), 12–18. http://www.ncbi.nlm.nih.gov/pmc/articles/PMC1745599/?tool=pubmed

Soler-Cataluna, J.J., *et al.* (2005) Severe acute exacerbations and mortality in patients with chronic obstructive pulmonary disease. *Thorax*, **60**(11), 925–931. http://thorax.bmj.com/content/60/11/925.abstract

Tantucci, C., *et al.* (1998) Effect of salbutamol on dynamic hyperinflation in chronic obstructive pulmonary disease patients. *European Respiratory Journal*, **12**(4), 799–804. http://erj.ersjournals.com/content/12/4/799.long

Additional References

1. Calverley, P.M., *et al.* (2007) Salmeterol and fluticasone propionate and survival in chronic obstructive pulmonary disease. *New England Journal of Medicine*, **356**(8), 775–789.

2. Lokke, A., *et al.* (2006) Developing COPD: a 25 year follow up study of the general population. *Thorax*, **61**(11), 935–939.

3. Menezes, A.M., *et al.* (2005) Chronic obstructive pulmonary disease in five Latin American cities (the PLATINO study): a prevalence study. *Lancet*, **366**(9500), 1875–1881.

4. Sherman, C.B., *et al.* (1992) Longitudinal lung function decline in subjects with respiratory symptoms. *American Review of Respiratory Disease*, **146**(4), 855–859.

5. Suissa, S., *et al.* (2008) Methodological issues in therapeutic trials of COPD. *European Respiratory Journal*, **31**(5), 927–933.

6. Tashkin, D.P., *et al.* (2008) A 4-year trial of tiotropium in chronic obstructive pulmonary disease. *New England Journal of Medicine*, **359**(15), 1543–1554.

10 Pneumonia

John M. Wrightson[1], Eleanor K. Mishra[1] and Robert J.O. Davies[2]

[1]Oxford Centre for Respiratory Medicine, University of Oxford, Oxford, UK
[2]Respiratory Medicine Group, Experimental Medicine Division, University of Oxford, Oxford, UK

Introduction

'Pneumonia' describes an inflammatory process within the parenchyma of the lung commonly caused by an infective aetiology. The radiological and histological endpoint are consolidation, in which the pulmonary airspaces become obliterated by inflammatory cells. There are also many types of non-infective pneumonia; these are less common and are outside the scope of this chapter.

In 1918 Sir William Osler described pneumonia as 'Captain of the Men of Death' when it was one of the leading causes of death. Almost a century later, the situation is unchanged; pneumonia remains a major global health problem, accounting for more than 6% of the total burden of all disease and causing the highest disease burden of all infectious diseases in both the developed and developing world[1]. It causes more disease than cancer, myocardial infarction, stroke, HIV/AIDS or malaria.

In spite of modern advances in healthcare, between 6% and 13% of patients admitted to hospital with community-acquired pneumonia (CAP) still die[2]. It is the United Kingdom's third leading cause of death in women, is the fifth leading cause of death in men and has an annual incidence in over 75-year-olds of 75 in 1000, with mortality peaking in the elderly and in childhood. One in three newborn infant deaths worldwide is caused by pneumonia.

Different classifications of pneumonia have been devised, most commonly based on a composite of location and method of acquisition. This schema subdivides pneumonia into CAP, hospital- (or healthcare-) associated pneumonia, ventilator-associated pneumonia or aspiration pneumonia. Such subdivision is particularly useful given that each group shares common features of their microbiology, required treatment and prognosis.

This chapter presents a selection of the key papers that have been pivotal in increasing our understanding of pneumonia; its prevention, identification and treatment and the association with other diseases such as the acquired immunodeficiency syndrome (AIDS).

Prevention of Pneumonia – Vaccination against *Streptococcus pneumoniae*
Huss et al., *Canadian Medical Association Journal (2009)*

Streptococcus pneumoniae (pneumococcus) is the commonest cause of bacterial pneumonia in the United Kingdom. Many developed countries currently recommend

---

Understanding Medical Research: The Studies that Shaped Medicine, First Edition. Edited by John A. Goodfellow. © 2012 John Wiley & Sons, Ltd. Published 2012 by John Wiley & Sons, Ltd.

vaccination against pneumococcus for those aged over 65 years or younger people who have an increased risk of pneumococcal disease with the pneumococcal polysaccharide vaccine (PPV). The current 23-valent PPV includes 23 serotypes accounting for 72–95% of invasive pneumococcal disease.

Despite such diverse use of PPV, the evidence of benefit from vaccination is lacking. A recent World Health Organisation (WHO)-funded meta-analysis of 22 PPV trials by Huss and colleagues found absolutely no evidence of protection of pneumococcal vaccination even among the populations for whom the vaccine is currently recommended. Within the double-blinded trials they examined, PPV was associated with a relative risk (RR) of 1.20 (95% confidence intervals (CI) 0.75–1.92) for presumptive pneumococcal pneumonia, 1.19 (95% CI 0.95–1.49) for all-cause pneumonia and 0.99 (95% CI 0.84–1.17) for all-cause mortality. Within all randomised trials, the relative risk of invasive pneumococcal disease (IPD) was 0.90 (95% CI 0.46–1.77).

This was a startling result, given that a 2008 Cochrane review by Moberley and colleagues[3], and other previous meta-analyses[4], had shown 'strong evidence of PPV efficacy against invasive pneumococcal disease' with an odds ratio of 0.26 (95% CI 0.15–0.46) although inconclusive evidence against all-cause pneumonia.

Such an alarming discrepancy between meta-analyses presents a salutary tale in selection strategies used to combine trial data: both studies examined similar, but critically not identical, trial sets. Huss and co-workers used the most stringent techniques to assess the methodological quality of studies. They restricted inclusion to randomised trials and examined for sources of trial heterogeneity, critically considering whether double blinding and allocation concealment were employed. By stratifying studies using these methods of assessing trial quality all positive effects of vaccination vanished.

Predictably Huss' findings are contentious[5]. Such contention demonstrates that the role for pneumococcal vaccination remains to be defined and may not necessarily be the same in the developing and developed world.

Recognising the Patient with Pneumonia
Heckerling et al., Annals of Internal Medicine (1990)
The symptoms and examination signs of pneumonia have been recognised for many years. Maimonides (1138–1204 AD) described the basic symptoms as 'acute fever, sticking pain in the side, short rapid breaths, serrated pulse and cough, mostly with sputum.' Other symptoms include myalgia, haemoptysis and malaise. However cough and breathlessness are common symptoms in patients presenting to general practitioners or emergency care physicians and are also symptoms of many other common conditions such as bronchitis, upper respiratory tract infections, asthma and exacerbations of COPD. In order to reduce unnecessary investigations and guide correct treatment, it is important to perform a careful clinical assessment of the patient presenting with suspected pneumonia.

Heckerling and colleagues presented a clinical rule for determining which patients presenting to an emergency department with suspected pneumonia were subsequently found to have radiographically confirmed pneumonia. The authors found that a temperature $>37.8°C$, heart rate >100 beats per minute, rales (crackles heard on chest auscultation), decreased breath sounds and the absence of asthma were significant predictors of confirmed pneumonia.

In validation studies, patients presenting with all five of these findings had a ~90% chance of chest X-ray confirmed pneumonia. Conversely, pneumonia could be virtually excluded when none of these features were present. This prediction rule has clinical applicability for community general practitioners and emergency department physicians in determining which patients should undergo further diagnostic testing beyond clinical examination.

Despite the usefulness of this predictive rule, it is important to recognise that no single feature on history or examination is sufficient to diagnose or exclude pneumonia and eliminate the need for chest X-ray. Furthermore, physician examination concordance is relatively poor for the presence or absence of physical signs. Given the myriad of symptoms and signs attributable to pneumonia, physicians should always take a holistic assessment of a patient in determining the appropriateness of further investigations.

Determining Where to Treat the Patient Diagnosed with Pneumonia
Fine et al., New England Journal of Medicine (1997)

The treating physician needs to balance considerations of physical, psychological and economic cost of treatment and hospital admission with the potential mortality of inadequately treated pneumonia. Admission to hospital is important in patients with a high mortality to allow the opportunity for intravenous antibiotics, close observation and expeditious admission to the intensive care unit (ICU) if necessary.

Fine and colleagues developed a prediction rule for risk of death within 30 days of presentation with CAP. They initially analysed data on 14,199 adults admitted to hospital with CAP to develop a prediction rule, the Pneumonia Severity Index (PSI), which divided patients into five groups with distinct mortalities. This rule was subsequently validated using data from over 40,000 further patients, including patients in the Pneumonia Patient Outcomes Research Team (PORT) cohort study.

The PSI assigns a variable number of points for each of the following clinical parameters assessed at presentation:

Age in years

Nursing home resident

Coexisting disease (e.g. neoplastic disease or liver disease)

Abnormal physical findings – altered mental status, respiratory rate ≥ 30 breaths per minute, temperature <35 or $\geq 40°C$, pulse ≥ 125 and systolic blood pressure <90 mmHg

Abnormal laboratory and radiographic findings (e.g. pH <7.35, urea concentration ≥ 11 mmol/L, sodium concentration <130 mmol/L and presence of a pleural effusion)

Based on the results of the PSI, patients are assigned a class of I (none of the clinical parameters described above) to class V. Patients in class I had a mortality of only 0.1–0.4%, whereas class V patients had a mortality of ~30%. Given the low mortality of patients in classes I–III, physicians suggest that such patients may be able to be treated as an outpatient with oral antibiotics whereas patients in classes IV and V require hospital admission.

Although the PSI has been proved to be a useful predictor of mortality in patients presenting to hospital with CAP, its use has been limited because of the complexity of PSI score calculation and its requirement for laboratory blood tests to fully assess the patient. This has led to the development of another severity score, CRB65[6], which can be used without the need for blood tests by general practitioners in the community. CRB65 assigns one point each for the risk factors of confusion, respiratory rate $\geq$30 breaths per minute, blood pressure systolic <90 mmHg and/or diastolic $\leq$60 mmHg and age $\geq$65. Patients with a score of 0 can usually be managed in the community with oral antibiotics. Those with a score of 1–2 should be considered for assessment in hospital. Those with a score of 3 have severe pneumonia and should be urgently admitted to hospital and treated with intravenous antibiotics without delay.

The development of severity scores for the assessment of patients with pneumonia at presentation helps to avoid hospital admissions whilst also recognising the sickest patients who require aggressive therapy. Such scores will never, however, replace the clinical judgement of an experienced physician.

Surviving Sepsis: Reducing the Mortality of Patients with Severe Pneumonia
Rivers et al., New England Journal of Medicine (2001)

A common complication of pneumonia is sepsis, defined as a systemic inflammatory response syndrome (SIRS) to infection. SIRS is characterised by the presence of 2 or more of tachycardia, hypothermia or fever, tachypnoea, and leukopaenia or leukocytosis. A subset of those with sepsis also suffers with hypotension despite adequate fluid resuscitation and are said to have septic shock. These patients have a high mortality, and should be considered for admission to an ICU. Despite an increase in the incidence of septic shock, modern medicine had not, prior to the publication of Rivers' study, consistently adopted a robust approach to aggressively treating sepsis.

The authors conducted a randomised trial comparing standard therapy with early goal-directed therapy (during the first 6 hours after recognition) in the emergency department for patients presenting with sepsis. The commonest cause ($\sim$40%) of sepsis was CAP. Early goal-directed therapy involved central venous oxygen saturation monitoring and specific targets for mean arterial pressure, urine output and central venous pressure. Patients were treated aggressively with fluid resuscitation, blood transfusion, vasoactive agents and ionotrope infusions, as required in a stepwise systematic fashion. They found that in-hospital mortality was reduced from 46.5% in the group who received standard care to 30.5% in the patients who received early goal-directed therapy. Other results were improved organ function and physiological parameters in the patients who received early goal-directed therapy. This study has been criticised, particularly for the use of blood transfusion and that the patients enrolled had particularly severe hypovolaemic sepsis[7,8]. However it remains the only good-quality, adequately powered, randomised trial that showed a clear improvement in mortality from sepsis.

The high mortality from sepsis and results from this study formed the basis for the Surviving Sepsis campaign, which aims to decrease mortality by improving sepsis recognition, thereby allowing initiation of timely treatment. The campaign has been coordinated by several international critical care and infectious disease organisations, which together have developed sepsis management guidelines[9]. As well as early goal-directed therapy, specific recommendations include appropriate diagnostic studies to identify infective organisms prior to antibiotic treatment, early administration of broad-spectrum antibiotic therapy and guidelines for the management of the patient in the ICU.

Optimal Duration of Antibiotic Therapy
Li et al., American Journal of Medicine (2007)

Another major challenge to antibiotic therapy for pneumonia is the determination of an optimal duration of treatment for pneumonia. The physician needs to strike a balance in determining duration; longer courses of antibiotics pose a huge economic burden and increase the risks of antibiotic-associated side effects. Shorter courses of treatment risk inadequately treating the infection.

Li and colleagues conducted a meta-analysis of 15 randomised controlled trials totalling 2796 adult patients who received antibiotic monotherapy for mild to moderate CAP. Their primary outcome measure was failure to achieve clinical improvement or cure; secondary outcomes were mortality, bacteriological failure and adverse events. Trials were analysed on an intention to treat basis.

Overall there was no difference in the primary outcome (the risk of clinical failure) between short courses of antibiotics (≤ 7 days) and longer courses of antibiotics (>7 days) (relative risk 0.89, 95% CI 0.78–1.02), with about 9% in each arm suffering clinical failure. There was also no increase in the secondary outcome measures of mortality, bacteriological failure or adverse events.

Limitations of the trials included in the meta-analysis were that most 'short-course' antibiotics were different from 'long-course' antibiotics, making direct comparison for a particular antibiotic difficult. Furthermore, a monotherapy-based approach was used which is at odds with the current British Thoracic Society guidelines for moderate CAP. Patients with severe CAP were not included in any of the studies making extrapolation impossible.

In spite of the limitations, the results provide supporting evidence that a 7-day (or less) course of antibiotics is likely to be satisfactory for the majority of mild to moderate CAP. Specific exceptions exist, for example treatment of *Staphylococcus aureus* or Gram-negative enteric bacilli pneumonia, which normally requires a prolonged course of therapy.

Sequelae of Pneumonia: Pleural Space Infection
Maskell et al., New England Journal of Medicine (2005)

Even patients who do not die of pneumonia often experience major complications such as lung abscess or pleural infection/empyema (infection in the pleural space around the lung).

Pleural infection has a 20% mortality[10] and affects about 60,000 to 80,000 people annually in the United Kingdom and United States. Healthcare costs of pleural infection are high; median duration of inpatient care for pleural infection is 15 days, with 20% of cases requiring inpatient stays of one month or greater.

Standard management of pleural infection is with broad-spectrum antibiotics and pleural fluid drainage via a chest tube. Unfortunately there is often poor drainage associated with loculated pleural collections and thick pus such that up to 40% of patients require surgical management.

There has been much interest in adjunctive intrapleural agents to improve fluid drainage to improve overall outcome. Medicines with potential include intrapleural fibrinolytics, such as urokinase, streptokinase and tissue-plasminogen activator (tPA), which may aid in disrupting loculations, and intrapleural DNase, which may reduce fluid viscosity.

The first Multi-centre Intrapleural Sepsis Trial (MIST-1) by Maskell and colleagues was the largest randomised controlled trial investigating intrapleural streptokinase for the treatment of pleural infection. This trial enrolled 454 patients with pleural infection, who were randomised to either intrapleural streptokinase or placebo for 3 days. The primary outcome measures were death or requirement for surgery at 3 months. Interestingly, despite previous common physician practice, there was no clinically significant benefit to streptokinase use, with rates of death or surgical requirement of about 30% for each arm.

MIST-2 was a further double-blind, placebo-controlled trial using adjunctive intrapleural therapy[11]. A 2×2 factorial design using intrapleural tPA, intrapleural DNase and placebo in four arms was used in 210 patients. The initial results from this study have demonstrated that a combination of intrapleural tPA and DNase causes a significant improvement in the primary outcome: that of change of radiographic pleural effusion volume (29.7% improvement for combination therapy vs. 15.1-17.1% for the other three arms). Neither tPA nor DNase alone conferred any advantage although, curiously, more patients in the DNase-alone arm died or required surgery for pleural infection (45.1% vs. 12.7–17.3%).

Microbiology of Pneumonia
Marston et al., Archives of Internal Medicine (1997)

Despite the incidence and severity of pneumonia, the precise aetiology of pneumonia is often poorly characterised. Blood cultures are positive in only 5–14% of patients; sputum samples are unobtainable in about 40% of patients and are often contaminated by upper respiratory tract flora; and urinary antigen testing is specific to only two pathogens (*Streptococcus pneumoniae* and *Legionella pneumophila* serogroup 1). Furthermore, upper airway carriage of *Streptococcus pneumoniae* can give a false positive urinary antigen test.

One of the earlier studies to attempt to systematically characterise the aetiology of community acquired pneumonia was Marston and co-workers' paper. They performed an ambitious prospective cohort study in two counties in Ohio, United States, to attempt to capture the data from all adults admitted with CAP in 1 year. They recorded 2776 cases of community-acquired pneumonia during 1991, giving an overall incidence of about 270 per 100,000 population. The investigators identified causative organisms using a combination of blood and pleural fluid culture, increases in serum antibody titres, identification of bacteria from respiratory secretions and by urinary antigen testing.

Despite the framework of a clinical study, a 'definite' aetiology diagnosis was achieved in only 16.5%, a 'probable' diagnosis in 19.5% and a 'possible' diagnosis in 44.3%. These figures highlight the difficulty in ascertaining an aetiological diagnosis in routine clinical practice.

Mycoplasma pneumoniae (32.5%), *Streptococcus pneumoniae* (12.6%) and *Chlamydophila pneumoniae* (8.9%) were the commonest bacteria causing pneumonia. Other common bacteria were *Haemophilus influenzae* (6.6%), *Staphylococcus aureus* (3.4%) and other Gram-negative bacilli (4.5%), including *Escherichia coli* (1.2%) and

Pseudomonas species (1.7%). Respiratory viruses, including influenza A and B (9.6%) and respiratory syncytial virus (4.5%), were responsible for a smaller proportion of cases of pneumonia. Other studies have suggested *Streptococcus pneumoniae* to be the commonest cause of CAP[12].

Overall, Marston and co-workers were only able to diagnose a 'definite' or 'probable' aetiology in 36% of patients despite extensive testing. This has enormous practice implications. Difficulties in correctly identifying an organism with rapid testing usually requires physicians to treat patients with broad spectrum empirical antibiotics: a 'best guess' based on local pathogen prevalence and sensitivity patterns. The current British Thoracic Society guidelines[12] propose use of amoxicillin (a β-lactam) with clarithromycin (a macrolide) for moderate severity pneumonia or co-amoxiclav (a β-lactam/β-lactamase inhibitor) with clarithromycin for severe pneumonia.

Such a strategy necessarily means that most patients receive broad spectrum empirical antibiotics with an antibacterial coverage greatly in excess of what would be required if an aetiological diagnosis was possible. This has the effect of increasing antimicrobial drug resistance pressures, increasing drug costs and increasing rates of antibiotic-associated side effects such as *Clostridium difficile*-associated diarrhoea. Such problems are likely to pose huge problems in years to come.

Novel Approaches to Diagnosing an Aetiological Cause of Pneumonia
Briese et al., Emerging Infectious Diseases Journal (2005)

A strategy that may increase the rate of aetiological diagnoses and reduce reliance on empirical antibiotic therapy is the use of nucleic acid amplification techniques (NAAT), which employ the polymerase chain reaction to directly detect the nucleic acids of pathogens in clinical specimens. These have shown much promise in providing diagnoses within hours, rather than 24–72 hours typically required for conventional culture, providing results in a clinically meaningful timescale.

NAAT have already demonstrated clinical utility for the rapid detection of difficult to culture pathogens such as *Mycoplasma pneumoniae*, *Chlamydophila pneumoniae* and *Pneumocystis jirovecii*. However, such strategies have been limited to the detection of only a few pathogens in a single reaction and do not examine for a broad range of pathogens.

However, recent work by Briese and colleagues has given a glimpse of the potential applicability of NAAT for rapid diverse pathogen identification. This group used 22 primer sets in a 'multiplex' PCR reaction. Each primer was chemically joined to a different molecular 'tag', each with a different mass unit which gives a specific 'signature' rapidly detectable by a mass spectrometer. When a pathogen was present in the reaction mixture, the specific primers from a complementary primer set were incorporated into the replicated nucleic acid strands. The noncomplementary unincorporated primers are subsequently washed from the reaction mixture allowing detection of the pathogen-specific primers.

Other groups have used a variety of primers and different detection techniques, including primer-specific fluorescent beads, each specific to a pathogen and each with a specific fluorescent signature[13].

NAAT show great promise in the clinical arena but are still in evolution. Certain requirements are required prior to NAAT implementation in routine clinical diagnostic work, including validation of results with standard culture techniques, optimisation of PCR reactions and development of automation to allow high-throughput routine microbiology laboratory usage. Nevertheless this technology could identify a causative organism with such rapidity as to allow rational choice of narrow-spectrum antibiotics.

Clustering of *Pneumocystis jirovecii* The First Presentation of the Acquired Immunodeficiency Syndrome (AIDS)
Gottlieb et al., Morbidity and Mortality Weekly Report (1981)
Gottlieb et al., New England Journal of Medicine (1981)

In addition to the common pathogens that cause pneumonia in immunocompetent individuals, a variety of other pathogens can cause pneumonia in immunocompromised hosts. These particularly include viruses such as cytomegalovirus (CMV), fungi such as *Candida albicans*, *Aspergillus fumigatus* and *Pneumocystis jirovecii* (formally known as *Pneumocystis carinii*).

Until the 1980s *Pneumocystis jirovecii* had been sporadically isolated as a cause of pneumonia only in those with profound immunosuppression. However, in 1981 there was a spate of reports of *P. jirovecii* pneumonia in individuals not previously known to be immunosuppressed. Gottlieb and colleagues published the first such report in the weekly *Mortality and Morbidity Report* for Los Angeles. This report marked a crucial point in the description of what became known as AIDS.

Gottlieb's report was initially published in the *Morbidity and Mortality Weekly Report* of the CDC, and subsequently in the *New England Journal of Medicine*. They described four young, previously healthy homosexual men who developed *P. jirovecii* pneumonia, extensive mucosal candidiasis and severe viral infection. Each patient had been unwell for some months, often with fever and cachexia. One patient developed oesophageal and chest wall Kaposi's sarcoma.

Laboratory investigations found characteristic marked lymphopaenia, particularly of T-lymphocytes. Further analyses suggested that the CD4+ T-lymphocytes were particularly affected. The authors postulated that CMV may have been a major factor towards the patients' illnesses.

It soon became clear that there were an increasing number of similar, mostly homosexual, patients with a clinical syndrome suggestive of immunosuppression without an obvious aetiological factor: there were two further papers[14,15] and an editorial[16] on this subject in the same edition of the *New England Journal of Medicine*.

The subsequent identification of the causative virus: the human immunodeficiency virus (HIV) in 1983 by two separate groups (led by Gallo[17] and Montagnier[18]) earned Montagnier and Barré-Sinoussi the Nobel Prize for Medicine in 2008.

Legionnaires' Disease: an Epidemiological and Laboratory Mystery
Fraser et al., New England Journal of Medicine (1977)
McDade et al., New England Journal of Medicine (1977)

The term 'atypical' pathogens refers to pneumonia caused by *Mycoplasma pneumoniae*, *Chlamydophila pneumoniae*, *Chlamydophila psittaci*, *Coxiella burnetii* and *Legionella* species, which are not sensitive to β-lactam antibiotics. One of the most important and common atypical bacteria is *Legionella pneumophila*, the cause of Legionnaires' disease, responsible for between 3.6% to 17.8% of cases of CAP presenting to hospital in the United Kingdom[12]. This is commonly acquired from infected water sources, particularly air conditioning units or standing untreated water.

Despite its importance, Legionnaires' disease was only discovered as recently as 1976. Its first description was made in two landmark papers in the same edition of the *New England Journal of Medicine* by workers from the Center for Disease Control in Atlanta.

The articles by Fraser and McDade respectively discussed the epidemiological investigations and microbiological studies which led to the discovery of the causative novel Gram negative bacillus, subsequently named *Legionella pneumophila*.

The story unfolded during July and August 1976, when ~4400 attendees at the 58th American Legion state convention in Philadelphia, United States, experienced an sudden outbreak of pneumonia affecting 182 patients, of which 147 were hospitalised (and 29 died); the term 'Legionnaires' disease' was coined for the outbreak. The disease was characterised by pneumonia, dry cough, myalgia and gastrointestinal symptoms with organ failure in a few. Typically, illness began 7 days after arrival at the convention.

Histological findings from the lungs of those who died were highly suggestive of bacterial pneumonia along with diffuse alveolar damage, although a bacterial cause remained elusive on conventional Gram staining. Epidemiological data from patients showed that the disease primarily occurred in the Legionnaires who had attended the convention, particularly at the convention's headquarters, 'Hotel A'.

A breakthrough in proving a bacterial aetiology came when it was observed that guinea pigs and embryonated eggs succumbed to transmissible infection when inoculated with isolates from infected individuals. Furthermore, electron microscopy and the use of special staining (including Giménez staining), consistently demonstrated Gram negative rods in the guinea pigs and embryonated eggs along with morphologically identical bacteria within human lungs inspected post mortem[19]; these rods would become subsequently named *Legionella pneumophila*.

A subsequently developed fluorescent serological assay demonstrated that 101 of 111 patients had diagnostic increases in antibody titres. Serological investigations also suggested *Legionella* to be the aetiological cause of a prior outbreak of unexplained fever called 'Pontiac fever'.

Even in this first description of *Legionella*, the authors concluded that erythromycin and probably also tetracycline were associated with the most favourable outcome; indeed, these antibiotic classes are still currently used for *Legionella* treatment.

Investigations suggested that airborne transmission was likely to have occurred from an environmental source either in or near to the hotel lobby of Hotel A. Person-to-person transmission did not seem to have occurred, particularly as there was no clustering of cases in hotel rooms.

Curiously, only 1 of 400 hotel employees, an air conditioning mechanic, became unwell with the disease. However, serological studies of the employees suggested immunity, raising the possibility that the aetiological agent was likely to have been present for some time, perhaps in low concentration.

The environmental reservoir for *Legionella* is now known to often be water-containing systems in buildings such as untreated standing water and air conditioning systems.

Curiously, despite extensive investigations, the exact source of the Philadelphia outbreak was never identified.

Summary and Conclusions

There have been dramatic advances in our understanding of pneumonia in the past 40 years, including the identification of common novel causative agents and the discovery of AIDS. Critical progress has also been made in identifying causative pathogens and determining optimal treatment paradigms for pneumonia. However, despite all these advances, there has still been a one-third increase in the number of hospital admissions due to CAP in the last decade, and it remains a major killer throughout the world. We have not yet stripped pneumonia of its rank of Captain of the Men of Death despite a century of scientific advances.

Key Outstanding Questions

1. What is the optimal duration of antibiotic therapy?
2. Which organisms account for the cases of culture-negative pneumonia?
3. Will NAAT and other technologies allow for more rapid and specific antibiotic therapy?
4. Will new antibiotic development keep pace with emerging resistance?

References

Briese, T., *et al.* (2005) Diagnostic system for rapid and sensitive differential detection of pathogens. *Emerging Infectious Diseases Journal*, **11**(2), 310–313. http://www.cdc.gov/ncidod/EID/vol11no02/04-0492.htm

Fine, M.J., *et al.* (1997) A prediction rule to identify low-risk patients with community-acquired pneumonia. *New England Journal of Medicine*, **336**(4), 243–250. http://www.ncbi.nlm.nih.gov/pubmed/8995086

Fraser, D.W., *et al.* (1977) Legionnaires' disease: description of an epidemic of pneumonia. *New England Journal of Medicine*, **297**(22), 1189–1197. http://www.ncbi.nlm.nih.gov/pubmed/335244

Gottlieb, M.S., *et al.* (1981) Pneumocystis carinii pneumonia and mucosal candidiasis in previously healthy homosexual men: evidence of a new acquired cellular immunodeficiency. *New England Journal of Medicine*, **305**(24), 1425–1431. http://www.ncbi.nlm.nih.gov/pubmed/6272109

Gottlieb, M.S., *et al.* (1981) Pneumocystis pneumonia. *Los Angeles. Morbidity and Mortality Weekly Report*, **30**(21), 1–3. http://www.cdc.gov/mmwr/preview/mmwrhtml/june_5.htm

Heckerling, P.S., *et al.* (1990) Clinical prediction rule for pulmonary infiltrates. *Annals of Internal Medicine*, **113**(9), 664–670. http://www.ncbi.nlm.nih.gov/pubmed/2221647

Huss, A., *et al.* (2009) Efficacy of pneumococcal vaccination in adults: a meta-analysis. *Canadian Medical Association Journal*, **180**(1), 48–58. http://www.ncbi.nlm.nih.gov/pubmed/19124790

Li, J.Z., *et al.* (2007) Efficacy of short-course antibiotic regimens for community-acquired pneumonia: a meta-analysis. *American Journal of Medicine*, **120**(9), 783–790. http://www.ncbi.nlm.nih.gov/pubmed/17765048

Marston, B.J., *et al.* (1997) Incidence of community-acquired pneumonia requiring hospitalization. Results of a population-based active surveillance Study in Ohio. The Community-

Based Pneumonia Incidence Study Group. *Archives of Internal Medicine*, **157**(15), 1709–1718. http://www.ncbi.nlm.nih.gov/pubmed/9250232

Maskell, N.A., *et al.* (2005) U.K. controlled trial of intrapleural streptokinase for pleural infection. *New England Journal of Medicine*, **352**(9), 865–874. http://www.ncbi.nlm.nih .gov/pubmed/15745977

McDade, J.E., *et al.* (1977) Legionnaires' disease: isolation of a bacterium and demonstration of its role in other respiratory disease. *New England Journal of Medicine*, **297**(22), 1197–1203. http://www.ncbi.nlm.nih.gov/pubmed/335245

Rivers, E., *et al.* (2001) Early goal-directed therapy in the treatment of severe sepsis and septic shock. *New England Journal of Medicine*, **345**(19), 1368–1377. http://www.ncbi.nlm.nih.gov/ pubmed/11794169

Additional References

1. Mizgerd, J.P. (2006) Lung infection – a public health priority. *PLoS Medicine*, **3**(2), e76.
2. Kothe, H., et al. Outcome of community-acquired pneumonia: influence of age, residence status and antimicrobial treatment. *European Respiratory Journal*, **32**(1), 139–146.
3. Moberley, S.A., *et al.* (2008) Vaccines for preventing pneumococcal infection in adults. *Cochrane Database System Reviews* (1): CD000422.
4. Jefferson, T. (2009) Pneumococcal vaccines: confronting the confounders. *Lancet*, **373**(9680), 2008–2009.
5. Andrews, R. and Moberley, S.A. (2009) The controversy over the efficacy of pneumococcal vaccine. *Canadian Medical Association Journal*, **180**(1), 18–19.
6. Lim, W.S., *et al.* (2003) Defining community acquired pneumonia severity on presentation to hospital: an international derivation and validation study. *Thorax*, **58**(5), 377–382.
7. Marik, P.E. and Varon, J. (2002) Goal-directed therapy for severe sepsis. *New England Journal of Medicine*, **346**(13), 1025–1026.
8. Perel, A. and Segal, E. (2007) Management of sepsis. *New England Journal of Medicine*, **356**(11), 1178.
9. Dellinger, R.P., *et al.* (2008) Surviving Sepsis Campaign: international guidelines for management of severe sepsis and septic shock: 2008. *Critical Care Medicine*, **36**(1), 296–327.
10. Ferguson, A.D., *et al.* (1996) The clinical course and management of thoracic empyema. *QJM*, **89**(4), 285–289.
11. Rahman, N.M., *et al.* (2009) Primary Result of the Second Multicentre Intrapleural Sepsis (Mist2) Trial; Randomised Trial of Intrapleural tPA and DNase in Pleural Infection. *Thorax*, **64**, A1.
12. Lim, W.S., *et al.* (2009) BTS guidelines for the management of community acquired pneumonia in adults: update 2009. *Thorax*, **64** (Suppl. 3), iii1–55.
13. Mahony, J., *et al.* (2007) Development of a respiratory virus panel test for detection of twenty human respiratory viruses by use of multiplex PCR and a fluid microbead-based assay. *Journal of Clinical Microbiology*, **45**(9), 2965–2970.
14. Masur, H., *et al.* (1981) An outbreak of community-acquired Pneumocystis carinii pneumonia: initial manifestation of cellular immune dysfunction. *New England Journal of Medicine*, **305**(24), 1431–1438.
15. Siegal, F.P., *et al.* (1981) Severe acquired immunodeficiency in male homosexuals, manifested by chronic perianal ulcerative herpes simplex lesions. *New England Journal of Medicine*, **305**(24), 1439–1444.

16. Durack, D.T. (1981) Opportunistic infections and Kaposi's sarcoma in homosexual men. *New England Journal of Medicine*, **305**(24), 1465–1467.

17. Gallo, R.C., *et al.* (1983) Isolation of human T-cell leukemia virus in acquired immune deficiency syndrome (AIDS). *Science*, **220**(4599), 865–867.

18. Barre-Sinoussi, F., *et al.* (1983) Isolation of a T-lymphotropic retrovirus from a patient at risk for acquired immune deficiency syndrome (AIDS). *Science*, **220**(4599), 868–871.

19. Chandler, F.W., *et al.* (1977) Demonstration of the agent of Legionnaires' disease in tissue. *New England Journal of Medicine*, **297**(22), 1218–1220.

11 Stroke

Philip M.W. Bath and Nikola Sprigg

Division of Stroke, School of Clinical Sciences, University of Nottingham,
Nottingham, UK

Introduction

Stroke is the commonest cause of adult disability and dependency and the third commonest cause of death in the West. The clinical presentation is varied but typically involves one or more of hemiplegia, hemianaesthesia, dysphasia and hemianopia. It is vital to consider stroke as a syndrome and not a disease; pathologically it follows intracerebral infarction (ischaemic stroke, which explains about 85% of strokes in the West) or intracranial bleeding, the latter due to either intracerebral haemorrhage (10%) or subarachnoid haemorrhage (5%). The principal causes of ischaemic stroke are large artery disease; cardioembolism, often due to atrial fibrillation (AF) or recent myocardial infarction; or small vessel disease causing lacunar infarcts. Intracerebral haemorrhage is most commonly associated with hypertension or cerebral amyloid angiopathy. Key risk factors for stroke include increasing age, male sex, hypertension, smoking, diabetes mellitus and AF.

Stroke is devastating to patients resulting in permanent disability and dependency in 30% and death in another 25%; many of the remaining patients are left with permanent impairments. Recovery from stroke can be fraught with early complications such as pneumonia and venous thromboembolism; later complications include depression, anxiety and dementia. Approximately 40% of patients with a stroke suffer a recurrence within 5 years.

Although stroke, or apoplexy, was first described by Dunlison in 1846, and later by Thomas in 1875, it is only recently that a detailed understanding of the pathological, pathophysiological and biochemical mechanisms has been elucidated. As a result, interventions have been developed to treat acute ischaemic stroke and prevent recurrence. Although we could have chosen our 10 papers from those describing the causes and pathology underlying stroke, or even papers illustrating early historical advances, we prefer to focus our choice on matters of direct clinical importance to patients and doctors, specifically on classification, investigation and treatment; it is these which directly improve outcome and reduce recurrence. The papers are ordered as a patient might pass though the care pathway.

Classifying Stroke by Aetiological Subtype
Adams et al., Stroke (1993)

Stroke is a collection of symptoms and signs, resulting from several different diseases requiring different investigation and treatment. Within ischaemic stroke it has long

---

Understanding Medical Research: The Studies that Shaped Medicine, First Edition. Edited by
John A. Goodfellow. © 2012 John Wiley & Sons, Ltd. Published 2012 by John Wiley & Sons, Ltd.

been accepted that aetiology affects prognosis, outcome and management. Historically many different classifications existed making diagnosis and description difficult.

The Trial of Org 10172 in Acute Stroke Treatment (TOAST) classification was originally designed so that patients recruited into the TOAST trial of danaparoid,[1] a low molecular weight heparinoid, could be classified by their aetiology. The TOAST classification denotes five groups, based on clinical presentation and results of ancillary investigation,[1] these comprising (1) large artery atherosclerosis (LAA), (2) cardioembolism (CE), (3) small vessel occlusion (SVO), (4) stroke of other determined aetiology (SO) and (5) stroke of undetermined aetiology (SU). Twenty stroke patients were classified by two independent neurologists, following the results of ancillary investigations including computerised tomography (CT), magnetic resonance imaging (MRI), angiography, electrocardiogram (ECG), echocardiography and laboratory tests for prothrombotic states.

For patients to be classified as LAA, there had to be evidence of significant (>50%) stenosis of a large extracranial vessel. Cardioembolism was diagnosed if a potential source of embolism from the heart was found, such as AF or intraventricular clot following a myocardial infarction. SVO was diagnosed if there was both an absence of cortical dysfunction clinically and normal brain imaging or a stroke lesion of less than 1.5 cm in diameter; markers of LAA or CE also had to be absent. Stroke of other determined aetiology included patients with less common thrombotic, immunological or genetic causes. Patients with no determined cause, or with two or more potential causes of stroke (e.g. evidence of both LAA and CE), were classified as stroke of undetermined aetiology. During development the classification was easy to use and had good interrater reliability; the neurologists disagreed in only one patient but were unable to determine the aetiology of stroke in nine patients. This inability to classify some patients is a widely recognised limitation of the TOAST approach.

Despite limitations the TOAST classification has been adopted by the stroke community and is usually reported in the results of clinical trials so that the interaction between treatment and stroke subtype can be described. Clinically, TOAST is used to determine subsequent treatment decisions: patients with CE stroke usually need oral anticoagulation, and those with LAA may benefit from carotid endarterectomy.

The TOAST classification is often reported in parallel with the Oxford Community Stroke Project (OCSP) classification which comprises a set of clinical syndromes.[2] The OCSP is predictive in identifying clinical outcomes in first-ever acute strokes, and the four syndrome groups differ in prognosis, rates of stroke recurrence and disability.[3] Total anterior circulation syndrome (TACS) features the triplet of higher cortical dysfunction (such as dysphasia and/or neglect), visual defect (homonymous hemianopia) and motor and/or sensory defects. Partial anterior circulation syndrome (PACS) has features of higher cortical dysfunction, with or without motor and/or sensory defects. Lacunar syndrome (LACS) affects the small penetrating arteries supplying the deep regions of the brain, resulting in motor and/or sensory defect (and without cortical dysfunction or visual defects). Posterior circulation syndrome (POCS) has symptoms of brain stem involvement, such as isolated homonymous hemianopia, cerebellar ataxia and/or cranial nerve palsies.

The Brain Must Be Imaged Immediately after Arrival at Hospital
Wardlaw et al., Health Technology Assessment (2004)

Management of stroke is dependent on the accurate diagnosis of the underlying pathology since this will influence further investigation, treatment and outcome. CT and magnetic resonance (MR) are the techniques of choice for imaging the brain. but their timing has been controversial.

In this landmark paper, a decision analysis model was developed using data from two large international stroke trials [the International Stroke Trial (IST) and Chinese Acute Stroke Trial (CAST)], including 40,000 patients admitted to hospital with first stroke, to determine the cost-effectiveness of CT after stroke. In addition to patient data from the stroke trials, data from a hospital stroke registry and health economic modelling were used to assess a strategy of 'Scan all patients within 48 hours' against 12 other scan strategies, including 'Scan all immediately'. Outcomes included functional status, accuracy of diagnosis and effect of diagnosis on quality-adjusted life years (QALYs).

The study confirmed that clinicians are unable to reliably exclude stroke mimics or differentiate between haemorrhage and ischaemia. CT is very sensitive and specific for haemorrhage in the first 8 days but is unreliable if used later. Overall the use of immediate scanning was most cost-effective as it allowed the early use of aspirin in ischaemic stroke, avoided aspirin in haemorrhage, and led to appropriate early management of those who had not had a stroke.

Diagnostic questions persist about indications for MR in acute stroke and on-going studies are assessing the ability of imaging to detect perfusion–diffusion mismatch in potentially salvageable tissues in the ischaemic penumbra surrounding the infarct core.

The timing of investigation for an underlying cause in haemorrhage is also controversial; some centres advocate immediate imaging of the vasculature with angiography, whilst others perform interval scanning a few weeks later once the haematoma has resolved.

Stroke Units Save Lives
Langhorne et al., Lancet (1993)

It had long been noted that specialist stroke care improved recovery but the critical effect of this on outcome was only quantified by a systematic review of the available trial data.

This systematic review and meta-analysis of 10 small randomised controlled trials of stroke unit care included 1586 patients with stroke, 766 allocated to a stroke unit and 820 to general wards. Patients treated on a stroke unit had a 28% reduction in mortality as compared to those treated on a general ward [odds ratio (OR) 0.72; 95%, confidence intervals (CI) 0.56–0.92], an effect that was sustained at 12 months. Although two of the trials did not use a strict randomisation protocol, the reduction in mortality was still present in the remaining eight trials. In addition, the odds of being in an institution at 12 months were also reduced in those managed on a stroke unit. Unfortunately the use of different functional outcome measures in the trials prevented a direct assessment of disability. A common theme for stroke wards was the presence of organised, specialist care coordinated by a multidisciplinary team comprising medical, nursing, physiotherapy, occupational therapy, speech therapy, psychology, dietetic care and access to other services such as podiatry, orthoptics and orthotics.

Importantly, care in a stroke unit appeared to reduce length of stay and did not necessarily require an increase in resources. As a result, the total cost is probably less if patients are managed on a stroke unit.

The benefit of stroke unit care has been regularly updated as new trials have become available, as published in the *Cochrane Database of Systematic Reviews*. The most recent update[4] includes 26 trials (5592 patients) and confirms the above findings as well showing that functional outcome (assessed as death or dependency) is also improved by stroke unit care. It is important to recognise that stroke unit care is relevant to, and can benefit, all patients with stroke, which contrasts with medical and surgical interventions discussed later in this chapter.

The First Definitive Drug Treatment for Acute Ischaemic Stroke
The NINDS rt-PA Stroke Study Group, New England Journal of Medicine (1995)

The publication in 1995 of the results of the National Institute of Neurological Disorders and Stroke (NINDS) trial provided the first clear evidence that functional outcome could be improved after acute ischaemic stroke. This landmark trial involved 624 patients from North America with hyper-acute stroke whose symptoms had started within 3 hours of treatment. Following a plain CT scan to exclude intracranial bleeding, intravenous alteplase (rt-PA) was given. In comparison with placebo, alteplase reduced combined death or dependency by absolute 12% (giving a number needed to treat [NNT] of 9). This efficacy takes account of the 6% absolute increase in symptomatic intracerebral haemorrhage. All the more remarkable was the inclusion of half the patients within 90 minutes, no mean feat since this time includes presentation, transfer to hospital, clinical assessment, CT scanning and administration of the bolus injection of alteplase. The NINDS trial led to the licensing of alteplase, first in the United States and then elsewhere in the world. In Europe a conditional license was awarded dependent on completion of a second confirmatory trial and a post-marketing surveillance study. Uptake around the world has been disappointing, reflecting the need for significant infrastructure to deliver hyper-acute treatments in stroke.

The beneficial effects of alteplase were confirmed in 2008 with the positive ECASS III trial[5] which studied 821 patients with stroke 3 to 4.5 hours prior to treatment. This trial should fulfil licensing requirements so that the treatment time window can be expanded to 4.5 hours post stroke onset. Importantly, treatment should always be started as early as possible since efficacy declines with time, as shown in Figure 11.1. The favourable balance between efficacy and safety across all thrombolysis trials is summed up in a *Cochrane* systematic review.[6] On-going trials are assessing whether the time window can be further extended, whether thrombolysis is safe and effective in people over 80 years of age and whether other thrombolytics such as desmoteplase show similar efficacy.

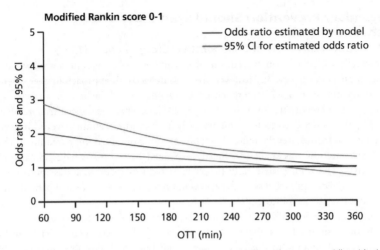

Figure 11.1 'Time is lost brain'; the treatment effect of alteplase decreases rapidly with time, reflecting that approximately 1.9 million neurones die per minute in untreated ischaemic stroke. Adapted from Lees *et al.*, *The Lancet* (2010), with permission from Elsevier.

Hemicraniectomy Saves Lives in Malignant Cerebral Infarction without Increasing the Numbers of Severely Disabled Survivors
Vahedi et al., Lancet Neurology (2007)

Cerebral oedema is a common complication of large middle cerebral infarction and has a mortality rate as high as 80%. Hemicraniectomy, where a large segment of skull overlying the stroke is removed, facilitates the relief of raised intracranial pressure. Whilst this is a relatively simple neurosurgical technique that has been documented to prolong life in case series, definitive randomised evidence was not available until 2007.

Three small European randomised controlled trials, Decompressive Craniectomy in Malignant Middle Cerebral Artery Infarcts (DECIMAL),[11] Decompressive Surgery for the Treatment of Malignant Infarction of the Middle Cerebral Artery (DESTINY)[12] and Hemicraniectomy after Middle Cerebral Artery Infarction with Life-Threatening Edema Trial (HAMLET),[13] have been completed and their data presented in a prospective pooled analysis (Vahedi *et al.*, 2007). The trials had similar inclusion criteria and trial design; specifically, patients were eligible if they had an ischaemic stroke, were age 18–60 years, had decreased consciousness and had imaging confirming infarction of >50% of the middle cerebral artery territory and mass effect within 45 hours of symptom onset. Together the trials enrolled 93 patients with 51 randomised to decompressive surgery and 42 to conservative treatment. Surgery significantly reduced the chances of a bad outcome [modified Rankin Scale (mRS) 5–6], NNT 2, and of a poor outcome (mRS 4–6), NNT 4. Importantly surgery did not increase the number of survivors who were severely disabled (mRS 5). Time to treatment is important and the overall results of HAMLET, where some patients were treated up to 96 hours after stroke, were less favourable. The use of hemicraniectomy in patients older than 60 years remains uncertain.

Secondary Prevention Should Start Early after Ischaemic Stroke
International Stroke Trial Collaborative Group, Lancet (1997)

Historically, the prevention of recurrent events after a stroke has commenced weeks or even months after the event. However, the IST changed this approach forever when it found that oral aspirin, when commenced within 48 hours of the onset of an ischaemic stroke, reduced recurrence over the following 14 days. This was a mega-trial involving 19,435 patients designed to test whether early aspirin administration would improve functional outcome after the index event; however, the observed improved function of 1.1% at 6 months was small and mostly explained by the 0.7% reduction in early recurrence. The finding that early prophylaxis reduces recurrence has motivated a change in trial design so that secondary prevention trials now try to recruit patients early after stroke, as seen in PRoFESS.[7]

Running in parallel with IST was another mega-trial, the Chinese Aspirin Stroke Trial, which found similar favourable results for aspirin.[8,9] Although the beneficial effect of aspirin is small in an individual, its universal availability and ultra-low cost mean that aspirin has a massive public health effect at the world level, and it is now used globally in patients with a recent ischaemic stroke.

Utilising a factorial design IST also tested a second question, namely, whether subcutaneous unfractionated heparin would improve functional outcome. Heparin failed to change outcome and it increased secondary haemorrhagic stroke and extra-cranial bleeding. These negative aspects more than offset a reduction in pulmonary embolism. Taken together, these effects of heparin have been mirrored in other trials of early anticoagulation, including low molecular weight heparins such as tinzaparin.[10] Whether newer anticoagulants such as factor Xa inhibitors or direct thrombin inhibitors will have more success in acute ischaemic stroke remains to be seen.

Preventing Recurrent Stroke in Those with Atrial Fibrillation
EAFT Study Group, Lancet (1993)

Atrial fibrillation is the leading cause of cardio-embolic ischaemic stroke and typically leads to large cortical infarcts and a poor outcome. Although previous trials had shown that anticoagulation reduced the risk of first stroke, it was the European Atrial Fibrillation Trial (EAFT) that led to a step change in secondary prevention. 669 patients (108 sites, 13 countries) with nonrheumatic AF and a recent minor ischaemic stroke or transient ischaemic attack (TIA) were randomised to receive open oral anticoagulation (warfarin or equivalent), double-blind treatment with aspirin (300 mg per day) or placebo. During a mean follow-up of 2.3 years, the annual rate of vascular death, stroke, myocardial infarction or systemic embolism was reduced by 53% from 17% in patients taking placebo to 8% in those assigned to anticoagulation. Similarly, the risk of stroke was reduced from 12% to 4% with anticoagulation. The annual incidence of major bleeding was low at 2.8% for anticoagulation.

However, vitamin K antagonists such as warfarin need regular monitoring and changes in dose, and they suffer from numerous drug and food interactions and alternatives have been sought. Recently, the RE-LY mega-trial compared dabigatran, a new oral direct thrombin inhibitor, with warfarin in patients with AF and a risk of stroke (including previous stroke).[14] High-dose dabigatran (150 mg twice day) was superior to warfarin in preventing stroke or systemic embolism and had a similar rate of major bleeding; in comparison with warfarin, lower dose dabigatran (110 mg twice daily) was associated with a similar rate of stroke or embolism and a lower rate of major bleeding. With other new anticoagulants also being developed for stroke prophylaxis in AF (e.g. rivaroxaban), it is likely that warfarin will be replaced eventually in routine clinical practice for stroke prophylaxis in patients with AF.

Preventing Recurrent Stroke in Those with Severe Carotid Artery Stenosis
European Carotid Surgery Trialists Collaborative Group, Lancet (1998)

Patients with atherosclerosis and stenosis of the carotid artery are at high risk of recurrent stroke. The role of carotid endarterectomy (CEA), which removes the atherosclerotic core of the internal carotid artery, has been studied in two landmark trials in Europe and North America.

The European Carotid Surgery Trial (ECST) recruited 3024 patients with TIA or mild ischaemic stroke between 1981 and 1994, and from 97 centres in 12 countries. Stenosis of the internal carotid artery, categorised in bands of 0–29%, 30–69% and 70–99%, was confirmed by conventional contrast angiography prior to enrolment. Patients were randomised to undergo CEA as soon as possible or to avoid surgery if at all possible. 50% of patients allocated to early surgery underwent this within 14 days, and the mean follow-up was 6 years. The primary outcome (major stroke or death) did not differ between the groups; 37% with surgery and 36.5% in the control group. The risk of ipsilateral major stroke in unoperated patients was related to the severity of stenosis, and was greatest if stenosis exceeded 70%, a risk that persisted for only 2–3 years. When assessed by severity of stenosis, surgery was hazardous in patients with mild stenosis (0–29%), neutral in those with stenosis of 30–69% and beneficial in severe (70–99%) stenosis.[15]

The North American Symptomatic Carotid Endarterectomy Trial (NASCET),[16] which recruited 2885 patients between 1987 and 1996 in 106 centres across the United States and Canada, reported similar results, although it did not include patients with mild stenosis (0–29%). A pooled analysis of data from ECST and NASCET revealed that 15 (95% CI 10 to 31) patients with severe stenosis needed to be operated on to prevent one disabling stroke or death over 2–6 years follow-up.[17] Further, the benefit of surgery was greatest in the first 2 weeks after stroke.

Improvements in best medical treatment and variability in surgical quality have led to questions about the modern application of the ESCT and NASCET results. A number of studies have compared stenting with carotid endarterectomy, and meta-analysis shows that stenting is associated with a worse outcome.[18]

Lowering Blood Pressure to Reduce the Risk of Recurrence after Stroke
PROGRESS Collaborative Group, Lancet (2001)

The value of lowering an elevated blood pressure for preventing first stroke and myocardial infarction is fundamental in community practice. The results of multiple trials show that it is the magnitude by which blood pressure is lowered that is critical rather than the type of antihypertensive agent. Because atherosclerosis and stenosis in large extracranial or intracranial arteries are common in people who have had an ischaemic stroke, concerns were widespread in the 20th century that lowering blood pressure chronically after stroke would increase recurrence through reducing cerebral blood flow (i.e. causing a 'haemodynamic stroke'). As a result randomised evidence was needed to assess whether lowering blood pressure reduced recurrence, as predicted from primary epidemiology, or increased stroke.

The Perindopril Protection against Recurrent Stroke Study (PROGRESS) enrolled 6105 patients with previous ischaemic or haemorrhagic stroke from 172 centres in Asia, Australasia and Europe. Individuals were randomised to a flexible regimen based on perindopril (4 mg daily) or placebo; the investigator could choose between monotherapy (perindopril versus placebo) or dual therapy (perindopril and indapamide versus double placebo). Patients were enrolled an average of 8 months after stroke. Over 4 years of follow-up, active treatment reduced blood pressure (BP) by 9/4 mmHg, stroke recurrence (the primary outcome) by 28% (relative risk reduction, 95% CI 17–38%) and major vascular events by 26% (95% CI 16–34%). Dual antihypertensive therapy was more effective at reducing both BP (12/5 mmHg) and stroke recurrence (RRR 43%, 95% CI 30–54%) than monotherapy which lowered BP (5/3 mmHg) but not stroke. Significant reductions in stroke were seen irrespective of baseline BP in patients enrolled with ischaemic and haemorrhagic stroke.

Other trials have shown that lowering BP also reduces stroke recurrence, notably the Chinese Post-Stroke Antihypertensive Treatment Study (PATS) trial.[19] A meta-analysis of PROGRESS, PATS and other relevant studies confirms that active lowering of BP, rather than just treatment of hypertension, reduces the risk of further stroke and other vascular events;[20] as in primary prevention, the magnitude of BP reduction appears to be the primary driver in prophylaxis. PROGRESS also provides the first indication that lowering BP may also reduce post-stroke dementia, an effect that appears to be mediated, in part, through reducing further macroinfarction.[21]

Lowering Blood Lipids to Reduce the Risk of Recurrence after Stroke
SPARCL Investigators, New England Journal of Medicine (2006)
The relationship between blood cholesterol levels and stroke has always been more complex than that between BP and stroke not least because high cholesterol appears to be associated with increased ischaemic stroke but reduced haemorrhagic stroke. Nevertheless, trials of pravastatin and simvastatin suggested that they reduced the risk of stroke in patients with other vascular disease and moderate to high cholesterol levels.

The answer to whether lowering cholesterol levels would reduce recurrent stroke came from the Stroke Prevention by Aggressive Reduction in Cholesterol Levels (SPARCL) trial. The study randomised 4731 patients within 1–6 months of an ischaemic stroke, intracerebral haemorrhage or transient ischaemic attack to atorvastatin (80 mg daily) or placebo. Baseline cholesterol levels ranged from 2.6 to 4.9 mmol/l (100–190 mg/dl). Over a median of 4.9 years follow-up, the statin lowered LDL cholesterol (1.9 mmol/l

[73 mg/dl] versus 3.3 mmol/l [129 mg/dl]), combined fatal or nonfatal stroke by 16% (95% CI 1 to 29%, the primary outcome) and major vascular events by 20% (95% CI 8–31%). The effect on stroke varied by its pathology; ischaemic stroke was reduced by 22% (95% CI 6–34%), whereas haemorrhagic stroke rose by 66% (95% CI 8–155%). Elevated liver enzyme levels were more common in those on atorvastatin.

The prophylactic effects of statins in patients with prior vascular disease (including 3280 patients with cerebrovascular disease) were also seen in the Heart Protection Study (HPS) mega-trial.[22] Treatment with simvastatin was associated with a 25% (95% CI 15–34%) reduction in stroke, an effect also explained by a reduction in ischaemic but not haemorrhagic stroke. Both SPARCL and HPS recruited patients whose stroke was months or years before enrolment into the trial, and the question of when to start treatment remains. Only one small trial, Fast Assessment of Stroke and Transient Ischaemic Attack to Prevent Early Recurrence (FASTER),[23] assessed the effect of early statin and found a nonsignificant increase in stroke recurrence by 90 days. Nevertheless, it is standard practice to start statins early after an ischaemic cerebrovascular event for long-term secondary prophylaxis.

Key Outstanding Questions

1. Can ischaemic brain cells be protected?

   Numerous trials, some involving thousands of patients, have tested whether 'neuroprotectants' can protect neurones and other cells in the brain from ischaemia. To date, all strategies have failed, and the relevance of preclinical findings to clinical development is now being questioned. Nevertheless, several putative neuroprotectants remain in clinical development.

2. How can intracerebral haemorrhage be treated?

   Despite significant advances in the treatment of ischaemic stroke, there remains a dearth of effective treatments for haemorrhagic stroke. The use of procoagulants is being examined following suggestive, but nondefinitive, data in studies of factor VIIa.

3. Can the brain be assisted in repairing itself after stroke?

   Neuroreparative approaches are being developed using stem cell technology, either with transplanted exogenous stem cells or through mobilising endogenous stem cells. Neuropharmacological approaches are testing stimulant drugs (e.g. amphetamine) to see if they can improve functional recovery.

Key Research Centres

1. Geoff Donnan and Steve Davis, Melbourne, Australia
2. Markku Kaste, Helsinki, Finland
3. Pierre Amarenco, Paris, France
4. Werner Hacke, Heidelberg, Germany
5. Michael Hennerichi, Mannheim, Germany
6. Nils-Gunnar Wahlgren, Stockholm, Sweden
7. Martin Dennis, Peter Sandercock and Joanna Wardlaw, Edinburgh, United Kingdom
8. Peter Langhorne and Ken Lees, Glasgow, United Kingdom
9. Alistair Buchan and Peter Rothwell, Oxford, United Kingdom

10. Philip Gorelick, Chicago, United States
11. Ralph Sacco, Miami, United States
12. Greg Albers, Stanford, United States

References

Adams, H.P., *et al.* (1993) The TOAST Investigators: classification of subtype of acute ischemic stroke. Definitions for use in a multicenter clinical trial. *Stroke,* **24**, 35–41. http://stroke.ahajournals.org/cgi/reprint/24/1/35

European Atrial Fibrillation Trial (EAFT) Study Group (1993) Secondary prevention in non–rheumatic atrial fibrillation after TIA or minor stroke. *Lancet,* **342**, 1255–1262. http://www.thelancet.com/journals/lancet/article/PII0140-6736(93)92358-Z/abstract

European Carotid Surgery Trialists Collaborative Group (1998) Randomised trial of endarterectomy for recently symptomatic carotid stenosis: final results of the MRC European Carotid Surgery Trial (ECST). *Lancet,* **351**, 1379–1387. http://www.ncbi.nlm.nih.gov/pubmed/9593407

International Stroke Trial Collaborative Group (1997) The International Stroke Trial (IST): a randomised trial of aspirin, subcutaneous heparin, both, or neither among 19435 patients with acute ischaemic stroke. *Lancet,* **349**, 1569–1581. http://www.ncbi.nlm.nih.gov/pubmed/9174558

Langhorne, P., *et al.* (1993) Do stroke units save lives? *Lancet,* **342**, 395–398. http://www.ncbi.nlm.nih.gov/pubmed/8101901

NINDS rt-PA Stroke Study Group (1995) Tissue plasminogen activator for acute stroke. *New England Journal of Medicine,* **333**, 1581–1587. http://www.ncbi.nlm.nih.gov/pubmed/7477192

PROGRESS Collaborative Group (2001) Randomised trial of a perindopril-based blood-pressure-lowering regimen among 6105 individuals with previous stroke or transient ischaemic attack. *Lancet,* **358**, 1033–1041. http://www.ncbi.nlm.nih.gov/pubmed/11589932

Stroke Prevention by Aggressive Reduction in Cholesterol Levels (SPARCL) Investigators (2006) High-dose atorvastatin after stroke or transient ischemic attack. *New England Journal of Medicine,* **355**, 549–559. http://www.ncbi.nlm.nih.gov/pubmed/16899775

Vahedi, K., Decimal D., Hamlet investigators, *et al.* (2007) Early decompressive surgery in malignant infarction of the middle cerebral artery: a pooled analysis of three randomised controlled trials. *Lancet Neurology,* **6**, 215–222. http://www.ncbi.nlm.nih.gov/pubmed/17303527

Wardlaw, J.M., *et al.* (2004) What is the best imaging strategy for acute stroke? *Health Technology Assessment,* **8**(1), III, ix–x, 1–180. http://www.hta.ac.uk/execsumm/summ801.htm

Additional References

1. The Publications Committee for the Trial of ORG 10172 in Acute Stroke Treatment (TOAST) Investigators (1998) Low molecular weight heparinoid, ORG 10172 (danaparoid), and outcome after acute ischemic stroke. *Journal of the American Medical Association,* **279**, 1265–1272.
2. Bamford, J.S.P., *et al.* (1991) Classification and natural history of clinically identifiable subtypes of cerebral infarction. *Lancet,* 1521–1526.

3. Aerden, L., *et al.* (2004) Validation of the Oxfordshire Community Stroke Project syndrome diagnosis derived from a standard symptom list in acute stroke. *Journal of the Neurological Sciences*, **220**, 55–58.

4. Stroke Unit Trialists' Collaboration (2004) Organised inpatient (stroke unit) care for stroke (Cochrane Review). *The Cochrane Library* (3)

5. Hacke, W., *et al.* (2008) Thrombolysis with alteplase 3 to 4.5 hours after acute ischemic stroke. *New England Journal of Medicine*, **359**, 1317–1329.

6. Wardlaw, J.M., *et al.* (2009) Thrombolysis for acute ischaemic stroke. *Cochrane Database of Systematic Reviews*.

7. The PROFESS Study Group (2008) Aspirin and extended-release dipyridamole versus clopidogrel for recurrent stroke. *New England Journal of Medicine*, **359**, 1238–1251.

8. Chinese Acute Stroke Trial (CAST) Collaborative Group (1997) CAST: randomised placebo-controlled trial of early aspirin use in 20,000 patients with acute ischaemic stroke. *Lancet*, **349**, 1641–1649.

9. Chen, Z.M., *et al.* (2000) On behalf of the CAST and IST Collaborative Groups. Indications for early aspirin use in acute ischemic stroke – a combined analysis of 40 000 randomized patients from the Chinese Acute Stroke Trial and the International Stroke Trial. *Stroke*, **31**, 1240–1249.

10. Bath, P., *et al.* (2001) Tinzaparin in acute ischaemic stroke (TAIST): a randomised aspirin-controlled trial. *Lancet*, **358**, 702–710.

11. Vahedi, K., *et al.* (2007) D Sequential-design, multicenter, randomized, controlled trial of early decompressive craniectomy in malignant middle cerebral artery infarction (DECIMAL Trial). *Stroke*, **38**, 2506–2517.

12. Jüttler, E., *et al.* (2007) Decompressive Surgery for the Treatment of Malignant Infarction of the Middle Cerebral Artery (DESTINY): a randomized, controlled trial. *Stroke*, **38**, 2518–2525.

13. Hofmeijer, J., *et al.* (2009) Surgical decompression for space-occupying cerebral infarction (the Hemicraniectomy After Middle Cerebral Artery infarction with Life-threatening Edema Trial [HAMLET]): a multicentre, open, randomised trial. *Lancet Neurology*, **8**, 326–333.

14. Connolly, S.J., *et al.* (2009) Dabigatran versus warfarin in patients with atrial fibrillation. *New England Journal of Medicine*, **361**(12), 1139–1151.

15. European Carotid Surgery Trialists' Collaborative, Group., (1991) MRC European Carotid Surgery Trial: interim results for symptomatic patients with severe (70–99%) or with mild (0–29%) carotid stenosis. *Lancet*, **337**, 1235–1243.

16. North American Symptomatic Carotid Endarterectomy Trial Collaborators (1991) Beneficial effect of carotid endarterectomy in symptomatic patients with high-grade carotid stenosis. *New England Journal of Medicine*, **325**, 445–453.

17. Cina, C, *et al.* (1999) Carotid endarterectomy for symptomatic carotid stenosis. *Cochrane Database of Systematic Reviews*.

18. Asymptomatic Carotid Surgery Trial (ACST-2) (N.d.) [Study website]. http://www.acst.org.uk/protocol/ACST2protocol.php.

19. PATS Collaborating Group (1995) Post-stroke antihypertensive treatment study. A preliminary result. *Chinese Medical Journal*, **108**, 710–717.

20. Rashid, P., *et al.* (2003) Blood pressure reduction and the secondary prevention of stroke and other vascular events: a systematic review. *Stroke*, **34**, 2741–2479.

21. Tzourio, C., *et al.* (2003) Progress Collaborative Group. Effects of blood pressure lowering with perindopril and indapamide therapy on dementia and cognitive decline in patients with cerebrovascular disease. *Archives of Internal Medicine*, **163**, 1069–1075.

22. Heart Protection Study Collaborative Group (2004) Effects of cholesterol-lowering with simvastatin on stroke and other major vascular events in 20536 people with cerebrovascular disease or other high-risk conditions. *Lancet*, **363**, 757–767.
23. Kennedy, J., *et al.* for the FASTER Investigators (2007) Fast assessment of stroke and transient ischaemic attack to prevent early recurrence (FASTER): a randomised controlled pilot trial. *Lancet Neurology*, **6**, 961–969.

12   Parkinson's Disease

Edward J. Newman and Donald G. Grosset

Greater Glasgow Movement Disorder Clinic, Institute of Neurological Sciences,
Southern General Hospital, Glasgow, UK

Introduction

Parkinson's disease (PD) is a common neurodegenerative disorder with a prevalence of around 1% in the population over 65 years. Most commonly it presents with brady-kinesia, tremor and/or rigidity and is pathologically characterised by degeneration of dopaminergic neurones within the substantia nigra pars compacta of the midbrain.

Describing the Condition
Parkinson, London, 1817

James Parkinson is an unlikely candidate to posthumously bear the name of the most famous neurological eponym. He was born in Shoreditch, London in 1755, son of an apothecary and surgeon. He practised surgery and was a fellow of the Medical Society of London. He was an accomplished and well-published geologist, amassing one of the largest collections of fossils in Britain at that time. He was a founding member of Geological Society of London. He was also a radical political pamphleteer, writing under the pseudonym 'Old Hubert' and actively supporting parliamentary and electoral reform. He died shortly following a stroke in 1824, aged 69 years.

He wrote about many conditions including gout and appendicitis, but his major work is the 66-page monograph entitled *An Essay on the Shaking Palsy*. In this, Parkinson delivers a remarkably clear clinical description of 'paralysis agitans' or the 'shaking palsy'. He describes six male cases aged over 50 years, of whom three had been assessed clinically, two had been 'casually met on the street', and one had been seen from afar. He described tremor (or agitation), stooping of posture, propulsion ('a propensity to bend the trunk forward and to pass from walking to a running pace'), constipation, speech and swallowing difficulties and drooling. He noted asymmetry of signs in one case and recognised the gradual progression of symptoms over time with marked differences between early and late stages of the disease. He also argues that the tremor should be distinguished from that caused by alcohol, tea and coffee abuse and old age.

There were some things that Parkinson got wrong. He thought there was motor weakness in the limbs, asserted 'that the senses and cognitive functions remain unim-paired' and speculated that the pathological changes were located in the cervical cord extending up towards the medulla. He acknowledged the lack of clinicopathological correlates and hoped that pathologists would turn their attention towards this condition.

Understanding Medical Research: The Studies that Shaped Medicine, First Edition. Edited by
John A. Goodfellow. © 2012 John Wiley & Sons, Ltd. Published 2012 by John Wiley & Sons, Ltd.

Parkinson's achievement was in writing an original description and recognition of a constellation of motor symptoms where others had thought these separate entities.

It was another 40 years before paralysis agitans was referred to in clinical lectures on paralysis by Robert Bentley Todd. Armand Trousseau then recognised cognitive disturbance and developed the concept of bradykinesia, describing this as progressive slowing of repeated hand opening. It was Jean-Martin Charcot who not only published a definitive clinical account, but also the first to refer to the condition as *la maladie de Parkinson* or Parkinson's disease. He recognised nontremulous forms, axial and limb rigidity and distinguished slowness of movement from weakness, and described the characteristic pill-rolling tremor as 'when a pencil or paper ball is rolled between [the thumb and index finger] ... or as if crumbling bread'.

Drug Treatments in Parkinson's Disease
Cotzias et al., New England Journal of Medicine (1967)

In 1910 the Wellcome laboratories in London first synthesized an aromatic amine called dopamine (or 3,4-dihydrophenylalanine) that could cross the blood–brain barrier. The functions of dopamine as a sympathomimetic agent were known for many years before its recognition as a neurotransmitter. L-dopa, a dopamine isomer, was isolated from fava bean seeds (*Vicia faba*) in 1913. In 1938, the DOPA decarboxylase enzyme, which converts L-dopa to biologically active dopamine, was discovered.

By 1959 it was recognised that nearly all brain dopamine in dogs and humans was located within the basal ganglia, and it soon became evident that dopamine was involved in the control of motor functions. Severe striatal dopamine loss was then found at autopsy in PD patients. Accordingly, it was postulated that PD motor features resulted from dopaminergic deficiency, and that L-dopa could replenish it therapeutically.

The initial administration of L-dopa was intravenous, and allowed a dramatic but short-lived improvement in motor function. In 1967 George Cotzias reported treating ten PD patients with oral D,L-dopa in New York. Very low initial doses were titrated gradually, thereby avoiding the previous experience of dose-limiting side effects (nausea and vomiting). Marked improvement was seen in eight of his patients. Granulocytopenia was reported in four patients, but did not occur 2 years later when Cotzias used oral L-dopa, with similar efficacy.

L-dopa still remains the mainstay of PD drug management more than 40 years later. Although not all parkinsonian symptoms are fully dopa-responsive (e.g. postural instability, swallowing disturbance), the dramatic improvement in bradykinesia and rigidity, at a time when no effective treatment was available, was revolutionary. This sparked much research interest in PD and gave neurology an exciting efficacious treatment at a time when much of the specialty was purely diagnostic. L-dopa therapy remains an isolated example of therapeutic replacement of a deficient neurotransmitter.

Assessing Disease Severity
Hoehn and Yahr, Neurology (1967)

By the late 1960s interest in PD was blossoming with an emerging new therapy. Given its varied presentation, scales for measuring severity or progression of PD are essential for clinical trials and helpful in assessing an individual's response to medication.

Table 12.1 Hoehn and Yahr staging system for Parkinson's disease

Stage	Clinical findings
1	Unilateral symptoms only
1.5	Unilateral and axial symptoms
2	Bilateral symptoms; no impairment of balance
2.5	Bilateral symptoms; recovery on pull test
3	Impaired balance; mild to moderate disease; physically independent
4	Severe disability; able to mobilise without assistance
5	Unable to stand or mobilise without assistance

Source: Hoehn and Yahr (1967).

In 1967 Margaret Hoehn and Melvin Yahr published a study of PD patients followed in New York during the pre-L-dopa era of 1948 – 1964. They reported age at onset, initial symptoms and cause of death. Their somewhat arbitrary but practical 5-point (1 through 5) scale of motor disability was used to document degree of disability and therefore disease progression (see Table 12.1). The evolution of the disease is captured in their scale and soon became widely used. It was later modified to include intermediate steps.

Scales for measuring disease severity have since become more complicated. For example, the increased recognition of disabling nonmotor symptoms is captured in the Non-Motor Scale Questionnaire (NMSQuest). The most widely used clinical scale is the Unified Parkinson's Disease Rating Scale (UPDRS), introduced in 1987 and updated in 2008 by the Movement Disorder Society. This is divided into four sections (nonmotor symptoms, motor symptoms, motor examination and motor complications) and includes functional measures of daily living. Quality of life scores, such as the Parkinson's Disease Quality of Life (PDQ39) scale, also combine motor and functional components. Such scales remain an essential element in contemporary clinical trails.

Developing Animal Models
Langston, Science (1983)
Research interest into the pathophysiology and pharmacological basis of PD grew as neurologists sought to optimise treatment and seek out the underlying causes. Animal models of PD are now invaluable in understanding cellular mechanisms of dopaminergic cell degeneration and in development of new drugs. The most faithful and widely used animal model, MPTP (or 1-methyl-4-phenyl-1, 2, 3, 6-tetrahydropyridine), was discovered by accident. In 1983 J. William Langston and Philip Ballard reported the local outbreak of acute severe parkinsonism among young intravenous drug abusers in northern California. Those affected responded clinically to L-dopa and dopamine agonists and rapidly developed motor complications. The responsible neurotoxin was MPTP, which had been inadvertently produced in the illicit manufacture of MPPP (or 1-methyl-4-phenyl-4-propionoxy-piperidine). Later, pathological studies in three affected patients found dopaminergic cell loss in the substantia nigra, as seen in idiopathic disease, although characteristic Lewy bodies were absent.

Nonhuman primates are also sensitive to MPTP and develop parkinsonism and pathological dopaminergic cell loss following systemic injection. It was found that the MPTP metabolite MPP+ (or 1-methyl-4-phenylpyridium) was actually the neurotoxic agent. It is taken up specifically by monoaminergic neurones, inhibits mitochondrial complex 1, and then depletes ATP resulting in cell death. Dopaminergic neurones are the most vulnerable to these damaging effects of MPP+. Although it was not the first animal model of PD, it had the distinction over previous models of conferring permanent rather than temporary motor symptoms. The primate model responds to L-dopa and motor complications develop later. Most rodent species are insensitive to MPTP, so the primate MPTP model became the most important and widely used in research.

The MPTP model has been used to evaluate dopaminergic and nondopaminergic drugs, neuroprotective agents and neurosurgical techniques. The vast majority of symptomatic drugs trialled in primate models have correctly predicted human drug efficacy. However, perhaps because of the rapidity of nigral cell degeneration in the MPTP model compared with human PD, neuroprotection in the model has not been replicated in patient studies.

Parkinson's Disease Surgery
Benabid et al., Applied Neurophysiology (1987)

Although surgery has been used as a treatment for PD in thousands of patients since the 1950s, the introduction of a reproducible animal model moved the technique into the laboratory and then back into the clinic as a more detailed understanding of its neuroanatomical basis became established. Thalamotomy was known to improve tremor and pallidotomy to improve motor symptoms and dyskinesia. Benabid and colleagues first described deep brain stimulation (DBS) in 1987. During stereotactic thalamotomy they observed that high-frequency (100Hz) stimulation of the thalamic ventralis intermedius (VIM) nucleus improved tremor. Patients with bilateral tremor, resistant to drug therapy, underwent radiofrequency VIM thalamotomy ('lesioning') on the more affected side, and continuous VIM stimulation on the other side using stereotactically implanted electrodes connected to subcutaneous stimulators. VIM thalamotomy relieved the tremor whilst stimulation only reduced the tremor. During the 1990s, this technique was refined. Advances in stereotactic techniques allowed identification of the subthalamic nucleus (STN) as the best target. STN DBS has now largely replaced ablative surgery.

DBS involves the insertion of electrodes bilaterally into the STN. These electrodes emerge through small burr holes and are connected to pulse generators implanted superficially in the upper anterior chest wall. The procedure improves motor function, reduces dyskinesia and time spent in an 'off' state, and allows reduction of the L-dopa dose. Unfortunately speech, swallowing, postural instability and gait disturbance are not improved and continue to deteriorate. Patients require follow-up particularly in the first few months for adjustment of stimulator settings.

It is essential that patients are carefully selected for surgery. Patients must be L-dopa responsive with poor control of motor complications despite optimised medical therapy (earlier surgery is advocated in some centres, especially for tremor). Gait impairment, dementia and other psychiatric disturbance are contraindications for surgery, and presurgical psychological evaluation is recommended. Older age (>70 years) is a relative contraindication.

Establishing the Diagnosis

Hughes et al., Journal of Neurology, Neurosurgery and Psychiatry (1992)

The clinical diagnosis of PD was historically based on clinical signs and symptoms known to characterise the disease: tremor, rigidity and bradykinesia. While this proved to be a relatively easy basis for making clinical diagnoses and starting treatment, it was recognised to lack specificity. As clinical trials increasing sought to become more sophisticated, controlled and precise, diagnostic accuracy became a major concern for the PD community. Brain bank studies on autopsies of patients carrying a clinical diagnosis of PD found an error rate in around a quarter of cases. This resulted in the development of more robust clinical diagnostic criteria. The most influential and widely applied are the UK Brain Bank criteria, which require three steps:

Step 1: Confirmation of parkinsonism, which is defined as bradykinesia (slowness in the initiation of voluntary movement with progressive reduction in speed and amplitude of repetitive movements) plus one of the following: postural instability, muscular rigidity or a 4–6 Hz resting tremor.

Step 2: Exclusion of other causes of parkinsonism (e.g. vascular, drug-induced and Parkinson-plus disorders).

Step 3: Presence of supportive features (e.g. unilateral onset, prominent rest tremor, good L-dopa response and dyskinesia).

Hughes and colleagues described post-mortem findings in 100 consecutive cases diagnosed as PD in life, collected between 1987 and 1990. Seventy-six cases were pathologically confirmed as PD. Underlying diagnoses in the remaining 24 cases included progressive supranuclear palsy, multiple system atrophy, Alzheimer's disease, post-encephalitic parkinsonism and one case that was pathologically normal. This meant that patients were being given inaccurate prognostic information, started on medication that was unlikely to improve their symptoms and entered into clinical trials inappropriately. Diagnostic accuracy improves to above 90% when patients are assessed by movement disorder specialists, Brain Bank diagnostic criteria are strictly applied, and there is sustained clinical follow-up.

Such studies should be interpreted with some caution. Most are retrospective and patients with atypical features, more rapid progression, and those who have died in hospital are over-represented. Studies assessing diagnosis in the community yield even higher rates of misdiagnosis, with a greater likelihood of more benign tremor disorders (e.g. essential tremor), Alzheimer's disease and vascular parkinsonism.

Benamer et al., Movement Disorders (2000)

Clinicopathological and community studies consistently demonstrate inaccuracies in diagnosing PD, especially early in the disease course. 'Parkinson plus' disorders, vascular parkinsonism, Alzheimer's disease and benign tremor disorders are frequently mis-diagnosed as PD. Appropriate imaging ligands allow assessment of presynaptic dopa-minergic function which is disrupted in degenerative parkinsonism. Scanning techni-ques *in vivo* use either single photon emission computerized tomography (SPECT) or positron emission tomography (PET). 18F-dopa PET scanning was first used to image the dopaminergic system in 1983, but SPECT is more widely available.

The dopamine transporter (DAT) is a sodium chloride-dependent protein on presynaptic nerve terminals in the striatum and controls dopamine levels in the synaptic cleft by active reuptake of dopamine after it acts at the post-synaptic receptor. Imaging DAT gives an indirect measure of dopaminergic neuronal degeneration, which allows *in vivo* testing of clinical diagnostic accuracy. DAT-SPECT demonstrates asymmetrical reduced striatal uptake even in early PD, and this correlates with disease duration and motor severity. Striatal DAT uptake is also abnormal in dementia with Lewy bodies and 'Parkinson plus' disorders, and is unable to differentiate between causes of degenerative parkinsonism. However, DAT-SPECT imaging is normal in benign tremor disorders, drug-induced parkinsonism and psychogenic parkinsonism. A proportion of patients is clinically diagnosed incorrectly as PD and has normal DAT-SPECT imaging; anti-parkinson medication can be safely withdrawn without clinical deterioration in these patients. In addition, vascular parkinsonism (which shows either normal DAT-SPECT or 'punched-out' lesions matching areas of infarction) can be differentiated from PD. FP-CIT is a commercially available radioligand used for DAT-SPECT imaging.

In this European multicentre study, Benamer and colleagues performed FPCIT SPECT in patients with a clinical diagnosis of parkinsonism or essential tremor and healthy controls. Striatal FP-CIT uptake was normal in all 27 essential tremor cases, 34/35 healthy volunteers and abnormal (reduced) in 154/158 parkinsonism cases. In the four cases showing parkinsonism but with normal SPECT scans, the diagnosis was subsequently revised to nondegenerative disorders.

Dopaminergic imaging has become a valuable tool in the differentiation of patients presenting with parkinsonian features or tremor disorders. In a research setting it can measure the rate of disease progression and can identify preclinical or very early (premotor) disease, for example first-degree relatives of young-onset PD patients.

The concept and importance of a more robust basis for the diagnosis of PD have thus become firmly established in the research community, and most major studies now require clear and validated diagnostic criteria. In addition, dopaminergic imaging now allows for trials targeting 'pre-symptomatic' or early PD which potentially opens up the disease to early, aggressive or novel therapies.

Motor Complications
Fahn et al., New England Journal of Medicine (2004)

Soon after L-dopa was found to be efficacious in PD, it was realised that continued treatment resulted in progressively more troublesome motor complications – 'on-off' fluctuations and dyskinesia. Furthermore it was noted that young-onset (<40 or 45 years) patients developed these problems sooner. Debate followed as to whether L-dopa actually advanced neurodegeneration by increasing oxidative stress in dopaminergic neurones and, if so, whether the problem related to treatment duration or the L-dopa dose used. The lower rate of motor complications in those treated with dopamine agonists lent support to the benefits of more continuous dopaminergic stimulation (due to their longer half-life than L-dopa).

In the ELL-DOPA trial 361 drug-naive PD patients were randomised to placebo or low-dose (150 mg/day), medium-dose (300 mg/day), or high-dose (600 mg/day)

L-dopa for 40 weeks. Drugs were then tapered, and there was a 2-week washout period. Patients were assessed using the motor component of the Unified PD Rating Scale (UPDRS). Motor function was worse in the placebo group throughout, compared to all groups receiving L-dopa. The persistence of benefit after the washout period (in L-dopa treated cases, and not placebo cases) raised the possibility of neuroprotection, or (more likely) that washout was incomplete (referred to as the 'long-duration L-dopa effect'). Motor complications were greatest in the group receiving the highest L-dopa dose, indicating that such doses should be avoided during the first year of anti-Parkinson therapy

In contrast with these clinical findings, SPECT scans in a subgroup of 116 patients showed less decline in dopamine transporter (β-CIT) uptake in L-dopa treated patients compared with the placebo group at 40 weeks, which indicates either a protective effect of L-dopa, or an interaction between L-dopa and the SPECT technique. Nineteen patients had normal β-CIT uptake and were excluded from this analysis. Such cases, clinically diagnosed as PD but with normal dopaminergic imaging, are labelled 'subjects with scans without evidence of dopaminergic deficit' (SWEDDs). In these cases, alternative nondegenerative diagnoses (e.g. essential tremor and dystonic tremor) are likely.

Rascol et al., New England Journal of Medicine (2000)

Dopamine agonists have been used in the treatment of PD since the 1970s. They exert their action by stimulating the striatal postsynaptic dopamine receptors and have longer half-lives than L-dopa. Older ergot-derived agonists (e.g. Pergolide, Bromocriptine, Cabergoline and Lisuride) are associated with lung, cardiac valve and retroperitoneal fibrosis with longer term usage, whilst newer non-ergot agonists (e.g. Ropinirole, Pramipexole, Rotigotine and Apomorphine) are not. In addition to dopaminergic side effects, daytime somnolence, ankle swelling, pathological gambling and other impulse control disorders have been reported with non-ergot agonists. They are currently available in oral, transdermal and subcutaneous forms. While dopamine agonists are not as efficacious as L-dopa in the treatment of motor symptoms, they are useful as monotherapy in early disease, although most patients will require the addition of L-dopa treatment within 3 years.

This double-blind study randomised patients with early PD to either Ropinirole or L-dopa. The primary endpoint was the proportion developing dyskinesia over 5 years. Previous studies had suggested that the agonists were less likely to cause dyskinesias and thus presented neurologists with a troublesome treatment dilemma. Doses were increased according to clinical response, and patients were allowed supplemental open-label L-dopa as necessary. Largely as a result of adverse events, completion rates for both groups were low (around 50%). The incidence of dyskinesia in patients on Ropinirole monotherapy (i.e. without supplemental L-dopa) for 5 years was 5%, compared to 45% in the L-dopa group. It was concluded that early use of Ropinirole-delayed motor complications, and that L-dopa should be avoided initially. However, including patients in the Ropinirole group who required L-dopa supplementation increased the dyskinesia rate to 20%. Some observers have concluded that any dyskinesia sparing benefit from initial dopamine agonist monotherapy is rapidly lost when L-dopa is inevitably added. A further analysis of the above study with longer follow-up did not support this, but only a small proportion of the originally entered patients were available for analysis. The study is representative of other clinical trials comparing dopamine agonists with L-dopa in early PD, which also showed a delayed onset of motor complications when dopamine agonists are used. However, the treatment choice depends on additional factors, as the control of motor symptoms is better for L-dopa, and there are tolerability issues for dopamine agonists, and the risk of developing dyskinesia is lower in older-onset PD patients.

Redefining the Pathology
Braak et al., Neurobiology of Aging (2003)

The pathological hallmark of PD is degeneration of dopaminergic neurones within the substantia nigra pars compacta of the midbrain. Patients do not develop motor symptoms until more than 50% of these dopaminergic neurones have been lost. There is also widespread deposition of alpha-synuclein-containing Lewy bodies throughout the central and autonomic nervous system. The exact role of alpha-synuclein is unclear, but PD results when this protein forms toxic intracellular aggregates.

Based on semiquantitative post-mortem analysis of lesions from 413 patients (PD patients and age-matched controls), Braak and colleagues proposed a novel pathological staging system in 2003, based on the topographical extent of Lewy body lesions. These six stages predict a gradual caudo-rostral progression of PD pathology, correlating with evolving clinical features; this has become known as the Braak hypothesis.

Stages 1 and 2 are considered preclinical and suggestive of incidental Lewy body disease. These lesions initially occur within the lower medulla: the efferent motor nucleus of the glossopharyngeal and vagal nerves and the anterior olfactory nucleus (which explains why patients often lose their sense of smell years before diagnosis). In stages 3 and 4, lesions are found within the locus ceruleus, amygdala, limbic system and substantia nigra; these are associated with motor symptoms. In stages 5 and 6, lesions become widely distributed within the cortex, initially within the anteromedial temporal mesocortex and then spreading to temporal and frontal cortices; this is associated with cognitive impairment.

This study was the first pathological staging system to describe lesion progression in PD. Subsequent clinicopathological studies largely confirm the Braak hypothesis, but a proportion of cases do not show the ascending propagation of lesions. In addition, overlapping pathological features of dementia with Lewy bodies and Alzheimer's disease are often found, in addition to the Parkinson changes.

Understanding the Genetics
Healy et al., Lancet Neurology (2008)

Most cases of PD are sporadic; however, having an affected first-degree relative increases an individual's risk of developing the disease around threefold. An underlying genetic cause is more common in patients with young-onset disease. Since 1997 mutations within eight genes have been strongly associated with development of PD, accounting for around 5% of cases. Identified first was the A53T mutation within the alpha-synuclein gene (chromosome 4), recognised within a large Greek-Italian family known as the Contursi kindred. Other mutations and duplications within this gene were then described. Identification of gene mutations in sporadic and familial disease has greatly improved our understanding of disease pathogenesis. The fact that dysfunction within multiple genes can result in such a similar phenotype is suggestive of a common final pathway.

The most significant genetic cause identified to date is mutation within the leucine-rich repeat kinase 2 (LRRK2, pronounced 'LARK 2') gene, located on chromosome 12, which is autosomal dominant. LRRK2 encodes dardarin that has a role in cellular vesicle dynamics and secondary messenger signalling. The clinical phenotype of LRRK2-associated PD resembles idiopathic disease and most neuropathological studies show classical Lewy body pathology. The international LRRK2 consortium reported 1045 patients with LRRK2 mutations from 133 families in 24 populations worldwide. They examined the LRRK2 clinical phenotype, identified six separate mutations (G2019Ser being the most common) and estimated that the lifetime penetrance was up to 74%. The G2019Ser mutation accounts for 1% of sporadic and 4% of familial disease. The frequency of LRRK2 mutation is considerably higher in southern Europe and the Middle East. Studies of North African Arab populations have reported prevalence of G2019Ser mutations in up to 41% of families with apparently sporadic disease.

Genetic testing for common mutations is not routinely performed in sporadic disease. Patients with a strong family history or those of North African Arabic or Ashkenazi Jewish origin may undergo gene testing (with counselling), but presently the treatment approach does not differ according to gene test results.

Summary

There has been great advance in our understanding of PD over the past 200 years. Drugs for the management of PD have been available for less than 50 years. Each year, millions of pounds are spent in anti-Parkinson drug development and clinical trials. Contemporary movement disorder specialists now approach PD from medical and surgical perspectives, have genetic considerations and insights and have sophisticated imaging modalities available for diagnostically challenging cases. PD is likely to remain a key area of neurological research.

Key Outstanding Questions

1. Mutations within different genes result in a similar clinical appearance of PD. What are the underlying pathophysiological processes in genetic PD, and are these relevant to sporadic PD? What factors influence penetrance, and can these be manipulated to delay disease expression?
2. Can therapeutic targets be identified for prevention and/or treatment of motor complications?
3. Which stem cell approach will achieve the greatest and most sustained therapeutic benefit?
4. Can new therapeutic targets be identified for prevention and/or treatment of dementia and other nonmotor symptoms?
5. Can a biomarker (preferably a blood test) be developed for diagnosis and disease monitoring in PD?

Key Research Centres

Increasingly PD research is multicentre. Therefore, we suggest the following five research groups:

1. European Parkinson's Disease Association, Kent, United Kingdom
2. The Michael J. Fox Foundation for Parkinson's Research, New York, United States
3. The Movement Disorder Society, Wisconsin, United States
4. National Parkinson Foundation, Florida, United States
5. Parkinson's Disease Society of the United Kingdom, London, United Kingdom

References

Benabid, A.L., *et al.* (1987) Combined (thalamotomy and stimulation) stereotactic surgery of the VIM thalamic nucleus for bilateral Parkinson disease. *Applied Neurophysiology*, **50**(1–6), 344–346. http://www.ncbi.nlm.nih.gov/pubmed/3329873

Benamer, H.T., *et al.* (2000) Accurate differentiation of parkinsonism and essential tremor using visual assessment of [123I]-FP-CIT SPECT imaging: the [123I]-FP-CIT study group. *Movement Disorders*, **15**(3), 503–510. http://onlinelibrary.wiley.com/doi/10.1002/1531-8257 (200005)15:3%3c503::AID-MDS1013%3e3.0.CO;2-V/abstract

Braak, H., *et al.* (2003) Staging of brain pathology related to sporadic Parkinson's disease. *Neurobiology of Aging*, **24**(2), 197–211. http://www.ncbi.nlm.nih.gov/pubmed/12498954

Healy, D.G., *et al.* (2008) Phenotype, genotype, and worldwide genetic penetrance of LRRK2-associated Parkinson's disease: a case-control study. *Lancet Neurology*, **7**(7), 583–590. http://www.ncbi.nlm.nih.gov/pubmed/18539534

Cotzias, G.C., *et al.* (1967) Aromatic amino acids and modification of Parkinsonism. *New England Journal of Medicine*, **276**(7), 374–379. http://www.ncbi.nlm.nih.gov/pubmed/5334614

Fahn, S., *et al.* (2004) Levodopa and the progression of Parkinson's disease. *New England Journal of Medicine*, **351**(24), 2498–2508. http://www.ncbi.nlm.nih.gov/pubmed/15590952

Hoehn, M.M. and Yahr, M.D. (1967) Parkinsonism: onset, progression and mortality. *Neurology*, **17**(5), 427–442. http://www.neurology.org/content/17/5/427.full.pdf+html?sid=2f0e537a-f1a4-49f4-b18d-7e5b7db3eebc

Hughes, A.J., *et al.* (1992) Accuracy of clinical diagnosis of idiopathic Parkinson's disease: a clinico-pathological study of 100 cases. *Journal of Neurology, Neurosurgery and Psychiatry*, **55**(3), 181–184. http://www.ncbi.nlm.nih.gov/pubmed/1564476

Langston, J.W., *et al.* (1983) Chronic Parkinsonism in humans due to a product of meperidine-analog synthesis. *Science*, **219**(4587), 979–980. http://www.ncbi.nlm.nih.gov/pubmed/6823561

Parkinson, J. (1817) *An essay on the shaking palsy*. London. http://neuro.psychiatryonline.org/cgi/content/full/14/2/223

Rascol, O., *et al.* (2000) A five-year study of the incidence of dyskinesia in patients with early Parkinson's disease who were treated with ropinirole or levodopa. 056 Study Group. *New England Journal of Medicine*, **342**(20), 1484–1491. http://www.ncbi.nlm.nih.gov/pubmed/10816186

Additional References

1. Charcot, J.M., and Sigerson, G.,trans. (1877) On paralysis agitans. In: *Lectures on diseases of the nervous system*. 129–156. New Sydenham Society, London.
2. Chaudhuri, K.R., et al. (2006) International multicenter pilot study of the first comprehensive self-completed nonmotor symptoms questionnaire for Parkinson's disease: the NMSQuest study. *Movement Disorders*, **21**(7), 916–923.

3. Cotzias, G.C., et al. (1969) Modification of Parkinsonism-chronic treatment with L-dopa. *New England Journal of Medicine*, **280**(7), 337–345.

4. Gandhi, S. and Wood, N.W. (2005) Molecular pathogenesis of Parkinson's disease. *Human Molecular Genetics*, **14**(18), 2749–2755.

5. Garnett, E.S., et al. (1983) Dopamine visualized in the basal ganglia of living man. *Nature*, **305**(5930), 137–138.

6. Gibb, W.R., and Lees, A.J. (1988) The relevance of the Lewy body to the pathogenesis of idiopathic Parkinson's disease. *Journal of Neurology, Neurosurgery and Psychiatry*, **51**(6), 745–752.

7. Goetz, C.G., et al. (2008) Movement Disorder Society-sponsored revision of the Unified Parkinson's Disease Rating Scale (MDS-UPDRS): scale presentation and clinimetric testing results. *Movement Disorders*, **23**(15), 2129–2170.

8. Horykiewicz, O. (1966) Dopamine (3-hydroxytyramine) and brain function. *Pharmacological Reviews*, **18**(2), 925–964.

9. Hughes, A.J., et al. (2002) The accuracy of diagnosis of parkinsonian syndromes in a specialist movement disorder service. *Brain*, **125**(4), 861–870.

10. Hulihan, M.M., et al. (2008) LRRK2 Gly2019Ser penetrance in Arab-Berber patients from Tunisia: a case-control genetic study. *Lancet Neurology*, **7**(7), 591–594.

11. Jenner, P. (2003) The contribution of the MPTP-treated primate model to the development of new treatment strategies for Parkinson's disease. *Parkinsonism and Related Disorders*, **9**(3), 131–137.

12. The Parkinson Study Group 2000 (2000) Pramipexole vs levodopa as initial treatment for Parkinson disease: a randomized controlled trial. *Journal of the American Medical Association*, **284**(15), 1931–1938.

13. Pearce, J.M. (1989) Aspects of the history of Parkinson's disease. 1989 *Journal of Neurology, Neurosurgery and Psychiatry*, **June**(Suppl.), 6–10.

14. Rajput, A.H., et al. (1991) Accuracy of clinical diagnosis in parkinsonism – a prospective study. *Canadian Journal of Neurological Science*, **18**(3), 275–278.

15. Rascol, O., et al. (2006) Development of dyskinesias in a 5-year trial of ropinirole and L-dopa. *Movement Disorders*, **21**(11), 1844–1850.

13 Epilepsy

Fergus J. Rugg-Gunn

Department of Clinical and Experimental Epilepsy, National Hospital for Neurology and Neurosurgery, Queen Square, London, UK

Introduction and Historical Perspective

Epilepsy is the commonest serious neurological disorder affecting children and young adults with approximately 450,000 affected in the United Kingdom and 30,000 new cases every year. The lifetime incidence of experiencing a single seizure is surprisingly high at 1 in 20. Epilepsy represents an enormous burden on healthcare resources and has significant additional indirect costs such as unemployment and increased mortality.

The oldest detailed description of epilepsy, a Babylonian text, dates from the second millennium BC. Despite having no understanding of the pathophysiological basis of epilepsy or brain function as a whole, the accounts of each seizure type, such as a generalised tonic-clonic, complex partial or Jacksonian motor seizure, are well documented and are mostly accurate descriptions. At this time demonic possession was considered the most likely cause. The first line of the text states:

> If epilepsy falls once upon a person or falls many times, it is the result of possession by a demon or a departed spirit.

In the fifth century, the Greeks considered epilepsy to be the 'sacred disease'; they rejected the erroneous belief of a supernatural aetiological basis and considered the condition to be due to a disorder of the brain.

> The brain is the seat of this disease, as it is of other very violent diseases.

In 1849 Robert Bentley Todd was the first to develop an electrical theory of brain function and believed seizures were the result of aberrant electrical discharges in the brain. Eighty years later Berger developed the human electroencephalograph; which remains one of the principal investigations used today in the evaluation of patients with a suspected seizure disorder[1].

Early 'medications' tended to be substances that were rarely of significant benefit, with minimal medicinal value and frequent toxic and unpleasant adverse effects. The introduction of bromides in the mid-19th century by Sir Charles Locock was a major advance as there was a clear response in terms of reducing seizure frequency in up to 50% of patients. The use of bromides was adopted widely, although the general standard of therapeutics was limited and inappropriately high dosing was commonplace. Enthusiasm waned by the early 20th century as it became clear that bromides were ineffective in a significant proportion of patients. The introduction of phenytoin in the late 1930s

Understanding Medical Research: The Studies that Shaped Medicine, First Edition. Edited by John A. Goodfellow. © 2012 John Wiley & Sons, Ltd. Published 2012 by John Wiley & Sons, Ltd.

curtailed its use dramatically, but it was not until the 1970s, with the development of carbamazepine and sodium valproate, that its use in Western countries virtually ceased. Arguably the most important milestone in the treatment of epilepsy was the development and widespread use of phenobarbitone. It was introduced 100 years ago, and in terms of volume and numbers of patients it remains the most prescribed drug for epilepsy in the world.

The Birth of Anti-Epileptic Medication
Hauptmann, Münch med Wochenschr (1912)

Phenobarbitone was the first worthwhile compound in epilepsy to result from the rapid development of synthetic chemistry, and in particular the discovery of the benzene ring by Friedrich Kekulé. In 1904, shortly after the earliest barbiturate derivatives were developed, 5-ethyl-5-phenylbarbituric acid (phenobarbitone, *Luminal*) was launched onto the market as a hypnotic and sedative. In early 1912 Alfred Hauptmann gave phenobarbitone to his epilepsy patients as a tranquiliser and noted that their seizures became less frequent. Following this chance observation Hauptmann systematically evaluated the efficacy of phenobarbitone in patients with chronic epilepsy who had not responded to bromides and for whom there were accurate records of seizure frequency. He noted that some patients with severe epilepsy became seizure free, at relatively modest doses. Harmful side effects were absent and he noted that phenobarbitone was also effective in status epilepticus, for which it is still used today. The first recorded use in the United Kingdom was by Dr F.I. Golla who subsequently published his experience with the drug at the National Hospital for Neurology and Neurosurgery in the *British Medical Journal*. Other case studies followed, and by the mid-1930s most patients with epilepsy were prescribed Luminal as first-line treatment with bromides used as either a substitute or adjunct in nonresponders. It was not until 1979 that the mechanism of action of phenobarbitone at the γ-aminobutyric acid (GABA)-A receptor was recognised, some 60 years after its introduction into clinical practice. Its efficacy has been demonstrated in both randomised controlled trials and observational studies, and it has been shown to be equivalent to phenytoin and carbamazepine in terms of reducing seizure frequency[2]. Despite its effectiveness in treating epilepsy, widespread availability and low cost, phenobarbitone has fallen out of favour in affluent societies, most likely as a result of a lack of specific pharmaceutical company support and the perceived side effects of sedation, drowsiness and behavioural disturbance. It is therefore prescribed most in developing countries, where the cost of modern anti-epileptic drugs (AEDs) is prohibitive.

When to Begin Anti-Epileptic Medication?
Marson et al., Lancet (2005)

The decision to commence medication in patients with few or infrequent seizures is not as straightforward as one might imagine. The potential benefits of treatment in terms of reducing the number of subsequent seizures and the impact of longstanding epilepsy need to be weighed against the adverse effects and costs of medication. Furthermore, approximately 50% of patients do not experience seizure recurrence after a single episode[3] suggesting that early treatment may be unnecessary in half of the treated patients. After a second seizure the recurrence rate increases to about 70% without medication. The recurrence rate is higher still in patients with a structural brain lesion or abnormal electroencephalogram (EEG) recording. However, a compelling case for starting treatment early in all patients, possibly after the first seizure, could be made if the long-term outcome was more favourable or seizure remission achieved earlier than if treatment was delayed. Additionally, studies of seizure recurrence in animal models have suggested that frequent electrical stimulation leads to a 'kindling' response where progressive structural changes result in the development of spontaneous seizures.

The largest and most important study examining when to start AEDs is the MESS trial (Multi-Centre Study of Early Epilepsy and Single Seizures) which studied 1443 patients, randomised to either early or deferred treatment and utilised an unmasked and pragmatic protocol. The participants included patients with single seizures, patients with infrequent tonic-clonic seizures and patients with seizures with minor symptomatology. Outcome measures were time to subsequent seizures, seizure freedom and time to 2-year remission. A measure of quality of life was also assessed. Despite immediate treatment increasing the time to a second seizure and reducing the time to achieve a 2-year remission of seizures, this did not translate into long-term seizure freedom, with 76% of patients in the immediate group and 77% of those in the deferred treatment being seizure free at 5 years. There were no differences in quality of life measures or frequency of serious complications of either treatment or disease between the two groups despite the deferred group experiencing more seizures. This is most likely as a result of the immediate treatment group having additional medication adverse effects. The number of patients with a single seizure needed-to-treat in order to prevent a single seizure recurrence within the first two years was 14. Overall it can be concluded that delaying medication does not increase the risk of developing chronic epilepsy and that unless there are additional risk factors for seizure recurrence treatment after a single seizure is unnecessary. However, there are often other lifestyle issues to consider with patients on an individual basis.

Which Anti-Epileptic Drugs to Start? The SANAD study
Marson et al., Lancet (2007a, b)

Starting treatment with an AED is a major event for a patient and should not be undertaken without consideration of the potential benefits and pitfalls, and only after careful discussion with the patient. Generally therapy is long term, at least 3 years, but it can be lifelong. The initial choice of treatment is therefore critically important and all the relevant patient factors including age, gender, epilepsy syndrome, seizure types, presence of comorbidities and coprescribed medication must be carefully considered[4]. The rationale for the SANAD (Standard and New Anti-epileptic Drugs) trial was that both well-established and novel medications need to be compared in a head-to-head protocol with both clinical and financial outcome measures so as to establish which should be first choice for appropriate groups of patients. This study has proved to be both useful and controversial in informing clinical practice, almost in equal measure!

SANAD Arm A compared the effectiveness of carbamazepine, taken as the standard treatment for partial onset seizures, with gabapentin, lamotrigine, oxcarbazepine and topiramate. One thousand seven hundred and twenty-one patients were recruited and randomly assigned to one of the drugs. Primary outcome measures were time to treatment failure (a composite of withdrawals due to adverse effects or inadequate seizure control) and time to achieve a 12-month remission. In summary, lamotrigine had the lowest treatment failure rates compared to all the other drugs except oxcarbazepine. Although lamotrigine had similar efficacy to carbamazepine, the treatment of choice at that time, it was better tolerated and hence possessed a lower treatment failure rate. The authors recommended that lamotrigine is a more cost-effective alternative to carbamazepine and should replace it as standard treatment for patients with focal epilepsy.

The second arm of the study compared sodium valproate, currently standard treatment for patients with generalised epilepsy, with lamotrigine and topiramate. Seven hundred and sixteen patients were recruited and randomly assigned to one of the treatments. Overall it was clear that sodium valproate was the most effective medication and was better tolerated than topiramate but not lamotrigine. The authors recommended that sodium valproate remain the standard treatment for generalised and unclassified seizures.

Generally the SANAD trial has been well received by the epilepsy community. The study was adequately powered to detect clinical important differences in efficacy and the duration of follow-up was sufficient to confirm the findings over a clinically meaningful period of time. Furthermore, the conception and analysis of the study was independent of the pharmaceutical industry and the pragmatic entry criteria and flexibility of management mirrored contemporary clinical practice. However, the study was not blinded and by the time of publication it was already partially outdated. Gabapentin, used in arm A, did not receive a monotherapy licence in the United Kingdom and during the studies three novel drugs were launched; Pregabalin, Zonisamide and Levetiracetam. It appears that approximately 10% of the patients in arm A were misclassified and actually had generalised seizures. This would tend to favour treatment with lamotrigine rather than carbamazepine which can exacerbate generalised epilepsy. In arm B, subgroup analysis of the idiopathic generalised epilepsy group was not reported. Topiramate has not been shown to be effective in absence seizures and lamotrigine can aggravate myoclonic jerks, thus artificially improving the apparent efficacy of sodium valproate in comparison. Other criticisms include, in arm A, the use of immediate-release carbamazepine rather than the now more widely used and better tolerated slow-release preparation and the aggressive escalation and dosing schedule of carbamazepine. These factors may have influenced the tolerability of carbamazepine, thus favouring lamotrigine in this arm of the trial.

The SANAD study is an outstanding and remarkable achievement; the culmination of a colossal amount of work and commitment. It is the landmark paper in this vitally important area of AED treatment and, despite the controversies, there is no doubt that the trial has informed the debate about which medications to recommend as first-line in patients with newly diagnosed epilepsy.

Early Identification of Refractory Epilepsy
Kwan and Brodie, New England Journal of Medicine (2000)

Most patients achieve seizure remission with their first or second AED. However, approximately 25–30% of patients continue to experience seizures. It is important to identify patients who respond poorly to medication early in order to plan rational combination therapy or preferably epilepsy surgery, which can be successful in achieving seizure freedom in up to 70% of selected patients. This paper by Kwan and Brodie was the first major attempt to consider whether it was possible to predict which patients would ultimately prove pharmacoresistant and then to ascertain which factors were most helpful prognostically. Five hundred and twenty-five patients were followed prospectively over a 13-year period. Normal epilepsy care was instituted and doses of medication were adjusted as clinical circumstances dictated. Sixty-three percent of patients became seizure free during treatment or after medication had been withdrawn, in line with other studies. There were no differences between the responders and drug-resistant patients in terms of sex, age at referral or onset of seizures or family history of epilepsy. Patients with a presumed genetic basis were more likely to become seizure free than those with either a structural lesion or those with an unknown underlying cause (74% versus 60%). A history of more than 20 seizures before starting medication or an inadequate response to initial treatment with AEDs was associated with refractory epilepsy. Forty-seven percent became seizure free during treatment with their first medication and 14% with the second or third drug, and it appears that with every new medication that a patient tries there is a smaller chance of a good response. This paper is important therefore in prompting clinicians to contemplate alternative therapeutic strategies earlier in a patient's epilepsy journey, including the option of epilepsy surgery. Furthermore, it has led to the formulation of a consensus definition of drug-resistant epilepsy by the International League against Epilepsy (ILAE) as 'failure of adequate trials of two tolerated, appropriately chosen and used antiepileptic drug schedules to achieve sustained seizure freedom'. In 2007, Luciano and Shorvon published a study evaluating the effect of adding a previously unused anti-epileptic drug to the treatment regimen of patients with pharmacoresistant epilepsy[5]. In total, 265 drug additions were made in 155 adult patients. Interestingly, about 16% of all drug introductions resulted in seizure freedom and overall, almost 30% of patients became seizure free after one or more medication changes. This was higher than expected given the earlier study by Kwan and Brodie. Nevertheless, it was clear that the patients most likely to become seizure free were those who had tried fewer medications previously, in line with the study by Kwan. Due to ethical considerations, the study was not placebo controlled or randomised, and it is possible therefore that selection bias by the physician may have influenced enrolment. Follow-up was only for a median of 19 months, and it is not clear whether the results can be translated to long-term seizure freedom. Nevertheless, the results are encouraging and the regrettable tendency to offer no new therapy to patients with difficult epilepsy should be resisted and physicians should take an active and explorative approach in trying to attain the important goal of seizure freedom.

Anti-Epileptic Drug Withdrawal
MRC Anti-Epileptic Drug Withdrawal Study Group, Lancet (1991)

The ultimate goal is to become seizure free without the need to take anti-epileptic medication. In addition to the serious adverse effects of AEDs, subtle deficits in fine motor control or cognition may be evident on detailed testing[6]. Additionally patients may wish to stop taking medication for personal reasons including the consideration of pregnancy. Despite these issues, many seizure-free patients continue to take medication due to concerns regarding seizure relapse and the sequelae of driving restrictions and lifestyle changes. It is important to be able to advise patients on the relative benefits and disadvantages of stopping or continuing medication, and to be able to support this dialogue with sound trial data. The earliest studies in this area consisted of small numbers of patients and nonrandomised observations and did little to inform clinical practice. A much larger and more comprehensive study was undertaken by the MRC Anti-Epileptic Drug Withdrawal Study Group. This prospective, multicentre randomised study compared seizure free rates between patients maintained on AEDs with patients who had medication gradually withdrawn over 6 months. Of the 1013 patients recruited, 78% of the medication maintained group and 59% of the treatment withdrawal group remained seizure free at 2 years. Thereafter, the difference between the groups diminished but did not reach equivalence, even after 5 years of follow-up (Figure 13.1). The most important factors determining a seizure-free outcome were longer seizure-free periods before treatment withdrawal, monotherapy prior to withdrawal and absence of generalised tonic clonic seizures. This landmark study has helped quantify the risk of seizure recurrence, and patients and their physicians are now better equipped to make the difficult decision as to whether to withdraw medication. Recently Class I evidence of the benefits and risks of drug withdrawal has emerged in a small, controlled, prospective, randomised, double-blind trial[6]. One hundred and sixty patients were randomised to medication withdrawal or nonwithdrawal. After 12 months there was no significant difference between the groups with a 15% seizure relapse rate in the drug withdrawal group versus 7% in those patients continuing. After 41 months of

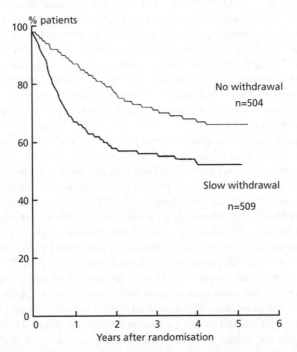

Figure 13.1 Actuarial percentage seizure-free among randomised groups. Reprinted from MRC Study Group, *The Lancet* (1991), with permission from Elsevier.

follow-up, the seizure relapse rate was 27% in the drug withdrawal group. Data from the nonwithdrawal group is not available as following completion of the 12-month study period, almost all the patients still on medication decided to withdraw their drugs as well! Overall the study is small, probably underpowered and of inadequate duration to be truly informative clinically. It does, however, provide further reassurance that the risk of seizure relapse following treatment withdrawal is small in well-selected patients.

Genetics and Epilepsy
Berkovic et al., Lancet Neurology (2006)

Large-scale vaccination programmes have probably saved more lives and prevented more disability than any other medical intervention. However, public opinion has often been vocal in its opposition. Despite evidence that the risk of developing permanent neurological complications is much greater with pertussis infection (1 in 1,200 to 12,000) than following vaccination (1–3 cases per million vaccinations), specific concerns persist. In 1942, with the introduction and widespread use of the combined diphtheria, pertussis and tetanus (DPT) whole-cell vaccines, serious public controversies arose. A small number of vaccinated children experienced febrile or afebrile seizures and a very small proportion developed much more severe neurological complications, including *vaccine-related encephalopathy*. As a result the National Childhood Encephalopathy Study (NCES) was established in 1976. The study provided over 5 million child-years of observation during which time 2 million doses of DPT vaccine were administered. Of the 1182 children who developed neurological disease during this period, 39 (3.3%) presented within one week of a DTP vaccination. It was concluded that the rate of permanent neurological deficit after immunisation was 1 in 330,000. The rate of neurological disability was less in children who received only diphtheria and tetanus vaccinations thus implicating the pertussis component. The study was criticised on methodological ground, but vaccination rates in the United Kingdom and other European countries fell dramatically and pertussis epidemics emerged. Attempts to replicate this finding in the United States failed to demonstrate an association, and other studies have also proved negative.

In 2006 Berkovic and colleagues published a pivotal study which suggested a genetic rather than environmental basis for the development of 'pertussis vaccine-related encephalopathy'. Ninety-six cases of children with unexplained encephalopathy and epilepsy were identified. Of these, 14 had the onset of symptoms within 72 hours of receiving the pertussis vaccine. The clinical presentation of 11 of these children bore a striking resemblance to the phenotype for severe myoclonic epilepsy of infancy (SMEI, or Dravet syndrome) which is often caused by spontaneous mutations in the SCN1A gene[7]. Eleven of the 14 children with presumed vaccine-related encephalopathy, and 10 of the 11 with the SMEI phenotype, had mutations in this gene. The mutations were not present in the normal population or the other three cases. These findings strongly suggested that many cases of apparent vaccine-related encephalopathy could be SMEI and due to an inherent genetic defect rather than the pertussis vaccination directly. The findings of this study are important, not only with regard to the pertussis vaccination but also from a wider perspective, as they may do much to improve the public's understanding of the true risks and safety of vaccination programmes as a whole.

Leppert et al., Nature (1989)
Steinlein et al., Nature Genetics (1995)

The common idiopathic generalised epilepsy (IGE) syndromes tend to display a complex inheritance pattern and are probably influenced by variation in several susceptibility genes. The genetic analyses of these conditions are complicated, and there is poor concordance between the over 50 association studies that have been performed[8].

The first of the Mendelian-inherited seizure disorders to be localised by linkage analysis was the rare, autosomal dominant idiopathic epileptic syndrome, benign familial neonatal convulsions (BFNC), which was first described in 1963. In this condition seizures occur in otherwise well neonates from the second or third postpartum day and remit by week 2–3. The seizures manifest as tonic posturing with ocular and autonomic features, followed by a clonic phase with motor automatisms. Prognosis is favourable although approximately 10% of patients subsequently develop seizures in later life. The first locus to be identified was EBN1 on chromosome 20q. The gene for EBN1, subsequently named KCNQ2, was identified by characterisation of a submicroscopic deletion on chromosome 20q13.3 in affected individuals and showed significant homology with a voltage-dependent delayed rectifying potassium channel gene, KCNQ1[9].

Patients with autosomal dominant nocturnal frontal lobe epilepsy (ADNFLE) present with seizures arising exclusively from sleep. Patients retain awareness and often report a somatosensory or psychic aura and are neurologically and cognitively intact. Segregation analysis performed in five families supported an autosomal dominant inheritance pattern with 69% penetrance and variable expression. Linkage studies assigned the gene to chromosome 20q13.2-q13.3, the same region as EBN1[10]. The neuronal nicotinic acetylcholine receptor α4 subunit (CHRNA4) maps to the same region, and the gene is expressed in all layers of the frontal cortex. Steinlein and colleagues screened affected family members for mutations within CHRNA4 and found a missense mutation that replaces serine with phenylalanine at codon 280. The mutation was present in all 21 available affected family members and in four obligate carriers but not in 333 healthy control subjects. Additional mutations within CHRNA4 have been described in other affected families. These findings led to a search for candidate genes for a number of other rare, familial idiopathic epilepsies.

Thus far nearly all the genes discovered to be involved in human epilepsies encode subunits of ion channels. Advances in the molecular biology of the rarer Mendelian-inherited idiopathic epilepsies are likely to radically alter our understanding of the pathophysiological basis of both acquired and inherited seizure disorders and facilitate the development of innovative new treatments for epilepsy.

Impact of Epilepsy
Hauser et al., Epilepsia (1980)

The attainment of a normal 'quality of life' for epilepsy patients is an important and almost universal aspiration. Arguably, however, the ultimate prognostic measure is the risk of premature death as a result of epilepsy.

The question of mortality in epilepsy was evaluated in the late 1970s by Hauser and colleagues. Residents of Rochester, Minnesota, with a diagnosis of epilepsy were identified using the Rochester Program Project. 618 residents were included in the prospective study, and observed for 8,233 person-years, with 475 followed up for at least

5 years or more. Forty-three patients were observed for over 30 years. The expected mortality was derived from yearly age and sex-specific person-years of follow-up determined from 1935–1974 life tables. The standardised mortality ratio (SMR) was calculated by comparing the observed and expected numbers of deaths in each cohort. In total there were 185 deaths through the 30 years of follow-up with 82 deaths expected. This results in an SMR of 2.3 which was statistically significant (95% confidence interval, 1.9–2.6). The SMR was particularly high (3.8) during the first 2 years after diagnosis. The early increased mortality rates were undoubtedly partly due to the underlying aetiology of the seizure disorder, such as cerebrovascular accidents, strokes and severe brain injury. Nevertheless, even in those patients with no clear underlying anatomical substrate, mortality rates remained elevated compared to the healthy population. As expected, there was an increased risk of death from cerebral tumours, cerebrovascular disease and accidents. Rather surprisingly, there was an increased number of deaths attributed to 'other diseases of the circulatory system' including noncerebral thromboembolism and aneurysms, the explanation of which remains elusive. Even patients with well-controlled epilepsy continued to have an increased SMR, particularly in the first 5 years following seizure remission, suggesting that the effects of seizures and epilepsy continue far beyond the point of diagnosis. Hauser and colleagues were thus the first to clearly demonstrate an increased mortality rate in patients with epilepsy, and on this basis it represents the seminal work in this field.

Rugg-Gunn et al., Lancet (2004)

Anatomical and functional connections between the brain and heart in both health and disease have long been established. Recently the interaction of the heart and brain in patients with epilepsy has been the subject of intense scrutiny. This has been driven by firstly, the publication of a number of important studies which have documented the frequent occurrence of cardiac rhythm changes during epileptic seizures and secondly, the lack of a clear pathophysiological mechanism for sudden unexpected death in epilepsy (SUDEP). SUDEP is defined as the sudden, unexpected, witnessed or unwitnessed, nontraumatic, and nondrowning death in patients with epilepsy with or without evidence for a seizure, and excluding documented status epilepticus, in which postmortem examination does not reveal a structural or toxicological cause for death. The incidence of sudden unexpected death is higher in epileptic patients compared to the normal population; up to 1,000/100,000 person-years in patients with pharmacoresistant epilepsy. This translates into a 1 in 100 chance of dying each year as a result of SUDEP.

Pathophysiological mechanisms of SUDEP are likely to be heterogeneous and multifactorial. Theories have focused on autonomic disturbance; particularly cardiac arrhythmias, central and obstructive apnoea and neurogenic pulmonary oedema. The possibility of structural or functional cardiac pathology predisposing patients with epilepsy to cardiac events has been proposed. There is extensive literature on the presence of ECG changes in patients with intracranial pathology despite normal cardiac examination at autopsy. Arrhythmias, conduction block and repolarisation ECG abnormalities have been reported in up to 56% of seizures[11].

In view of this we undertook a prospective long-term study of the incidence and nature of cerebrogenic cardiac arrhythmias in a small group of patients with pharmacoresistant focal epilepsy, a group with historically the highest risk of SUDEP. Twenty patients were implanted with an ECG loop recorder for up to 18 months. One patient was withdrawn due to a localised infection at the site of implantation. Over 220,000 patient hours of ECG recording were monitored, during which time 3377 seizures were reported by patients. Cardiac rhythm was captured on the implantable loop recorders in 377 seizures. Ictal bradycardia (less than 40 beats per minute) was seen in 0.24% of all seizures over the study period, and 2.1% of the recorded seizures. One patient developed supraventricular tachycardia lasting approximately 30 seconds. Seven of the 19 patients experienced ictal bradycardia at some point during the monitoring period. Four of these had severe bradycardia or periods of asystole which led to the insertion of a permanent pacemaker. There was no clear correlation between cardiac events and specific anti-epileptic drugs. Notably, only a small proportion of seizures for every patient were associated with significant cardiac events despite identical seizure characteristics presumably as a result of different patterns of cortical and subcortical propagation.

Clearly, the results do not yet prove that SUDEP is caused by ictal cardiac asystole although intuitively it remains a strong possibility. If this connection can be more firmly established the potential role of pacemaker insertion in preventing a proportion of SUDEP cases urgently needs to be evaluated.

Anti-Epileptic Drugs and the Foetus
Meador et al., New England Journal of Medicine (2009)
Reports of anti-epileptic drug-induced birth defects in humans date from the 1960s, and data continue to be collected in a number of epilepsy pregnancy registers[12]. Women with epilepsy who are taking an AED in monotherapy have at least a 2–3 times increased risk over the background population of having an infant with a major congenital malformation (4–9% chance for each pregnancy). However, uncontrolled epileptic seizures can lead to intrauterine growth retardation, injury, possible long-term cognitive delay and both maternal and foetal death. The management decisions are therefore complex and challenging.

There is emerging evidence that minor anomalies, learning difficulties and other problems may also be related to AED therapy. There are very few long-term follow-up studies of children exposed to AEDs *in utero*. Early observational studies suggested that mean IQ was significantly lower in children of women with epilepsy[13,14] and a growing number of retrospective and prospective studies have confirmed that developmental delay is more common in children born to mothers or fathers with epilepsy. It is challenging to disentangle the true effect of AED use from other interrelated and independent factors.

Most recently, an interim analysis of this large, prospective, observational, multi-centre study evaluating cognitive function in children exposed to AEDs *in utero* has been published. Between 1999 and 2004, Meador and colleagues enrolled pregnant women taking AEDs in monotherapy with the intention of evaluating cognitive performance of children at 3 and 6 years of age. Neuropsychometric data were available for 258 children at 3 years. Comprehensive maternal and child data were collected and analysed for associations. Significant independent predictors of child IQ included anti-epileptic drug, maternal IQ, maternal age, standardised dose of AED, gestational age at birth and prenatal use of folate. A striking dose-dependent association with child IQ and valproate use was seen, with children exposed to valproate *in utero* having an IQ on average 6–9 points lower than those exposed to other AEDs. This difference was most marked with higher doses and persisted despite adjustment for confounders. The strengths of this study include its prospective design, blinded cognitive assessments and detailed monitoring of multiple potential confounding variables. Conversely, it is a relatively small unrandomised study with no control group of unexposed children. Nevertheless, it is concordant with other data suggesting that valproate is associated with a higher rate of both major malformations and cognitive impairment and strongly suggests that valproate should not be used as a first-line anti-epileptic drug in pregnant women. Furthermore, there are concerns about its use in all women of child-bearing potential since approximately half of pregnancies are unplanned.

Summary and Conclusions

Epilepsy has challenged and frustrated us for almost 4000 years and although there have been important advances in the understanding of the pathophysiological basis, treatment and investigation of seizure disorders, many unanswered questions remain. Epidemiological studies have documented the natural history of this disorder and, following improvements in neuroimaging and therapeutics, we are now better equipped than ever to diagnose, classify, counsel and offer treatments on the basis of rigorous trial data. This does not always translate into a clinical benefit and, although most patients eventually enter long-term seizure remission, some continue to experience frequent seizures and too many patients die each year as a direct result of epilepsy. For the most part epilepsy is a treatable condition although medication at best suppresses rather than cures. Further drug development strategies and exploitation of the recent advances in the field of genomics may offer novel insights into seizure disorders and deliver more targeted and possibly neuroprotective therapies. Until then pharmacoresistant epilepsy will continue to have considerable physical, psychosocial and socioeconomic consequences for the individual and economic implications for the health and welfare services.

Key Outstanding Questions

1. What happens to the brain during the latent period between a cerebral injury and the later development of seizures?
2. Can we intervene during this period to prevent epileptogenesis?
3. Do seizures lead to other seizures, and do seizures harm the brain?
4. How can we develop more targeted drug therapies that will improvements in genomics facilitate this process?
5. How do we choose the best medication for an individual patient right from the start?
6. Will technologies such as deep brain stimulation, local drug delivery to the brain or targeted radiotherapy deliver more effective and better tolerated therapy?
7. Why do some patients die during seizures?
8. Why do patients have seizures?

References

Berkovic, S.F., *et al.* (2006) De-novo mutations of the sodium channel gene SCN1A in alleged vaccine encephalopathy: a retrospective study. *Lancet Neurology*, 5, 488–492. http://www.ncbi.nlm.nih.gov/pubmed/16713920

Hauptmann, A. (1912) *Luminal bei Epilepsie, 1907–1909.* http://jnnp.bmj.com/content/72/3/412.extract

Hauser, W.A., *et al.* (1980) Mortality in patients with epilepsy. *Epilepsia*, **21**, 399–412. http://onlinelibrary.wiley.com/doi/10.1111/j.1528-1157.1980.tb04088.x/abstract

Kwan, P., and Brodie, M.J. (2000) Early identification of refractory epilepsy. *New England Journal of Medicine*, **342**, 314–319. http://www.ncbi.nlm.nih.gov/pubmed/10660394

Leppert, M., *et al.* (1989) Benign familial neonatal convulsions linked to genetic markers on chromosome 20. *Nature* **337**, 647–648. http://www.nature.com/nature/journal/v337/n6208/abs/337647a0.html

Marson, A., *et al.* (2005) Immediate versus deferred antiepileptic drug treatment for early epilepsy and single seizures: a randomised controlled trial. *Lancet* **365**, 2007–2013. http://www.ncbi.nlm.nih.gov/pubmed/15950714

Marson, A.G., *et al.* (2007a) The SANAD study of effectiveness of carbamazepine, gabapentin, lamotrigine, oxcarbazepine, or topiramate for treatment of partial epilepsy: an unblinded randomised controlled trial. *Lancet*, **369**, 1000–1015. http://www.ncbi.nlm.nih.gov/pubmed/17382827

Marson, A.G., *et al.* (2007b) The SANAD study of effectiveness of valproate, lamotrigine, or topiramate for generalised and unclassifiable epilepsy: an unblinded randomised controlled trial. *Lancet*, **369**, 1016–1026. http://www.ncbi.nlm.nih.gov/pubmed/17382828

Meador, K.J., *et al.* (2009) Cognitive function at 3 years of age after fetal exposure to antiepileptic drugs. *New England Journal of Medicine*, **360**, 1597–1605. http://www.ncbi.nlm.nih.gov/pubmed/19369666

Medical Research Council Antiepileptic Drug Withdrawal Study Group. (1991) Randomised study of antiepileptic drug withdrawal in patients in remission. *Lancet*, **337**, 1175–1180. http://www.ncbi.nlm.nih.gov/pubmed/1673736

Rugg-Gunn, F.J., *et al.* (2004) Cardiac arrhythmias in focal epilepsy: a prospective long-term study. *Lancet*, **364**, 2212–2219. http://www.ncbi.nlm.nih.gov/pubmed/15610808

Steinlein, O.K., *et al.* (1995) A missense mutation in the neuronal nicotinic acetylcholine receptor alpha 4 subunit is associated with autosomal dominant nocturnal frontal lobe epilepsy. *Nature Genetics* **11**, 201–203. http://www.nature.com/ng/journal/v11/n2/abs/ng1095-201.html

Additional References

1. Berger, H. (1929) *Uber das Elektrenkephalogramm des Menchen.* 527–570.
2. Kwan, P., and Brodie, M.J. Phenobarbital for the treatment of epilepsy in the 21st century: a critical review. *Epilepsia* 2004;45:1141–1149.
3. Berg, A.T., and Shinnar, S. (1991) The risk of seizure recurrence following a first unprovoked seizure: a quantitative review. *Neurology*, **41**, 9659–9672.
4. Stokes, T., *et al.* (2004) Clinical guidelines and evidence review for the epilepsies: diagnosis and management in adults and children in primary and secondary care. Royal College of General Practitioners, London.
5. Luciano, A.L. and Shorvon, S.D. (2007) Results of treatment changes in patients with apparently drug-resistant chronic epilepsy. *Annals of Neurology*, **62**, 375–381.
6. Lossius, M.I., *et al.* (2008) Consequences of antiepileptic drug withdrawal: a randomized, double-blind study (Akershus Study). *Epilepsia*, **49**, 455–463.
7. Claes, L., *et al.* (2001) De novo mutations in the sodium-channel gene SCN1A cause severe myoclonic epilepsy of infancy. *American Journal of Human Genetics,* **68**, 1327–1332.
8. Tan, N.C., *et al.* (2004) Genetic association studies in epilepsy: 'the truth is out there'. *Epilepsia*, **45**, 1429–1442.

9. Singh, N.A., *et al.* (1998) A novel potassium channel gene, KCNQ2, is mutated in an inherited epilepsy of newborns. *Nature Genetics,* **18**, 25–29.

10. Phillips, H.A., *et al.* (1995) Localization of a gene for autosomal dominant nocturnal frontal lobe epilepsy to chromosome 20q 13.2. *Nature Genetics,* **10**, 117–118.

11. Opherk, C., *et al.* (2002) Heart rate and EKG changes in 102 seizures: analysis of influencing factors. *Epilepsy Research,* **52**, 117–127.

12. Harden, C.L., *et al.* (2009) Management issues for women with epilepsy – focus on pregnancy (an evidence-based review): II. Teratogenesis and perinatal outcomes: Report of the Quality Standards Subcommittee and Therapeutics and Technology Subcommittee of the American Academy of Neurology and the American Epilepsy Society. *Epilepsia,* **50**, 1237–1246.

13. Gaily, E., *et al.* (1988) Intelligence of children of epileptic mothers. *Journal of Pediatrics,* **113**, 677–684.

14. Scolnik, D., *et al.* (1994) Neurodevelopment of children exposed in utero to phenytoin and carbamazepine monotherapy. *Journal of the American Medical Association,* **271**, 767–770.

14 Motor Neuron Disease

Martin R. Turner and Kevin Talbot

Oxford Motor Neuron Disease Centre and Department of Clinical Neurology, University of Oxford, Oxford, UK

Introduction

The Oxford neurologist Professor Walter Bryan Matthews (1920–2001) commented in the second edition of his 1963 textbook *Practical Neurology* that:

> *The best test of a physician's suitability for the specialised practice of neurology is not his ability to memorise improbable syndromes but whether he can continue to support a case of motor neurone disease and keep the patient, his relatives and himself in a reasonably cheerful frame of mind.*

Motor neuron disease (MND), termed amyotrophic lateral sclerosis (ALS) in its commonest form and the terms being largely synonymous, is the condition that the neurologist dreads above all others. It is rare (incidence of 1–2/100,000/year) and there is ample justification for pessimism with relentless progression and death from respiratory failure within 3–4 years for 50% of patients. Over 100 drugs have been trialled without success. There are no consistent clues to aetiology from epidemiological study, and few from the small number of patients with familial forms of the disease.

The last 20 years has seen a vast improvement in the multidisciplinary palliative care of MND patients and despite the lack of major therapeutic advances there have been great strides in the understanding of motor neuron molecular biology and genetics. A quote from the godfather of MND, Jean-Martin Charcot, of over 120 years ago seems more likely to be realised than ever before:

> *Let us keep looking in spite of everything. Let us keep searching. It is indeed the best method of finding, and perhaps thanks to our efforts, the verdict we will give such a patient tomorrow will not be the same we must give this patient today.*

The Recognition of ALS as a Disease of Two Compartments
Charcot, Bureaux du Progrès Médical (1874)

The 19th century, the 'century of illumination', was a time when the physician had yet to specialise in the way characterised by modern healthcare delivery, and when an elite were able to devote their energies to rigorous clinico-pathological examination of patients. The French physician Jean-Martin Charcot (1825–1893) is renowned for insights far beyond MND. From his practice within the hallowed walls of the Paris Salpêtrière Hospital, the first published use of his term for the disease was in 1874 though Charcot had published the description of a case as early as 1865 in a female previously termed

Understanding Medical Research: The Studies that Shaped Medicine, First Edition. Edited by John A. Goodfellow. © 2012 John Wiley & Sons, Ltd. Published 2012 by John Wiley & Sons, Ltd.

a 'hysteric'[1]. In fact, an established pure lower motor neuron (LMN) syndrome termed 'progressive muscular atrophy' (PMA, now regarded as part of the spectrum of MND) can be credited to Cruvelhier, among others, some 20 years before Charcot's critical recognition of the involvement of an additional set of neurons beyond the LMNs. The UK physician Augustus Jacob Lockhart Clarke (1817–1880) appears to have made similar observations about upper motor neuron (UMN) involvement well before Charcot[2].

The most obvious sign of MND is muscle wasting, an indirect sign of lower motor neuron death. Akin to the leaves on a plant starved of their water supply, loss of LMNs leads to secondary muscle wasting, usually with visible coarse fasciculations. The primate motor system has a separate central compartment involving a descending corticospinal tract (CST) composed of upper motor neurons (UMNs) that form connections with multiple LMNs. These UMNs largely have their origins in the primary motor and premotor cortex. Charcot's great leap was to note the simultaneous involvement of the descending UMNs situated in the lateral parts of the spinal cord cross-sections he analysed, and which appeared pale and scarred. He observed that this 'sclerosis' appeared to be occurring simultaneously with the downstream muscle wasting (termed 'amyotrophy') caused by LMN loss at their origins in the spinal anterior horns. Thus emerged his concept of 'sclérose latérale amyotrophique'. The broader term MND emerged nearly a century later, coined by Lord Brain[3], although the two terms MND and ALS are largely used synonymously in modern parlance.

This simultaneous UMN and LMN involvement remains the cornerstone of the clinical diagnosis of MND to this day, particularly in the absence of any diagnostic test or biomarker. It is a highly unusual combination outside MND, and in the presence of progressive weakness without sensory involvement there are few true 'mimics' (though many textbooks continue to produce exhaustive lists of them). The site of onset (upper limb, lower limb and bulbar in equal proportions) and the spread of pathology in MND are very far from understood. For someone as masterful as Charcot, he seems in retrospect to have been a little hasty in his 1887 conclusions about the characterisation of his 'new' disease, a condition that has proved so resistant to therapeutic intervention and in which only recently is the complexity of pathophysiology emerging:

> *I do not think that elsewhere in medicine, in pulmonary or cardiac pathology, greater precision can be achieved. The diagnosis as well as the anatomy and physiology of the condition amyotrophic lateral sclerosis is one of the most completely understood conditions in the realm of clinical neurology.*

MND as a Cerebral as Well as a Spinal Disorder
Smith, Journal of Neurology, Neurosurgery & Psychiatry (1960)

In many of the earliest descriptions of MND, physicians noted the apparent sparing of the intellect in contrast to other progressive neurodegenerative disorders, here mentioned in an early (pre-Charcot) account of an MND patient 'Mr. P' by Dr Charles Bland Radcliffe and Augustus Jacob Lockhart Clarke[4]:

> *And Mrs. P, who was standing by the bedside at the time, removed all doubt upon this point by saying that her husband was 'too intelligent, if anything', and that he was never tired of hearing read books requiring attention and thought.*

However, in a largely neglected MND literature over the next century, that included Alzheimer[5], there emerged several reports of dementia in association with MND-like clinicopathological features. In 1960 Marion Smith, working at Queen Square in London, published a detailed neuropathological study of the brain in seven MND patients. She summarised her extensive 'extra-motor' findings in MND thus:

> *Degenerating myelinated nerve fibres are present from cortex throughout the brain-stem and cord in every case. The distribution of the degenerating fibres in the cortex is extensive. These fibres are present not only in the pre-central gyrus and paracentral lobule, but they are also abundant in the postcentral gyrus, and occur in considerable numbers in the adjacent parietal and frontal gyri . . . Numerous degenerating fibres are present in the corpus callosum. Degenerating fibres pass between the main group of degenerating fibres in the internal capsule and the lateral nucleus of the thalamus. Degenerating fibres are present in the basal ganglia, in particular in the ansa lenticularis and fasciculus lenticularis. Degenerating fibres are also present in the substantia nigra, the tegmentum and reticular formation of the brain-stem.*

In the subsequent half-century, a consistent syndrome of cognitive impairment as an inherent part of MND pathophysiology has been characterised. Although frank dementia remains rare, a more subtle 'dysexecutive' syndrome of impaired complex planning, and reduced verbal fluency is present in a significant proportion of MND patients[6].

Modern neuroimaging studies have supported all of Smith's findings[7–10]. The concept of MND as a 'multisystem' neurodegenerative disorder is now established and the older dogma of selective vulnerability of motor neurons less clear. Most recently the discovery of a common MND neuropathological hallmark in cases of fronto-temporal dementia has reinforced the concept of FTD and MND being two extremes of a continuum.

Identification of the Pathological Hallmarks of MND
Leigh et al., Neuroscience Letters (1988)

Ubiquitin recognises and binds to misfolded or damaged protein and targets it to chaperone proteins for export to the proteosome for degradation or sequestration and refolding. Neurons are post-mitotic cells with a low tolerance for misfolded or damaged protein, which is highly injurious. Prior to this 1988 study there was no clear pathological diagnostic hallmark which could be used to identify MND cases reliably. Leigh and colleagues developed an antibody against ubiquitin and studied post-mortem specimens of MND spinal cord, identifying a range of subcellular protein aggregates with characteristic morphologies which stained for ubiquitin and were unique to MND. Collectively these became known as ubiquitinated inclusions (UBIs) and became the focus of intense study to determine which proteins might be contained within.

There was vigorous debate at this time, some of which continues, whether ubiquitin accumulation in neurodegenerative disease was directly related to the neurodegenerative process, reflecting a failure of the proteosome system, or an epiphenomenon, or indeed a normal and appropriate cellular protective response to cell stress. Ubiquitin had already been identified in association with neurofilaments and tau in the brains of patients who had suffered in life from Alzheimer's or Parkinson's disease. However it was to be another 20 years before the identity of the major protein constituent of UBIs in the CNS of MND patients was identified.

The First Gene in Familial MND
Rosen et al., Nature (1993)

The concept that MND could be hereditary was denied by Charcot and given less attention than it deserved for much of the 20th century. However, to any neurologist seeing substantial numbers of MND patients, the occasional occurrence of individuals with a family history clearly indicating an autosomal dominant disorder was irrefutable and reports of such pedigrees began appearing in the 1950s. This led to the concept of familial ALS (fALS) and the systematic collection of DNA samples from affected families. In 1991 the first report of linkage of MND to a specific genetic region (the long arm of chromosome 21) appeared. In retrospect this seems to have been a stroke of luck as we now know that at least 80% of familial cases are not linked to this region.

In 1993 Rosen and colleagues published a paper in *Nature* which changed the landscape of MND research forever, bringing it into the molecular era. Using PCR and sequencing of individual exons they identified 11 different mutations in the gene for superoxide dismutase-1 (SOD1), which is in the middle of the chromosome 21 linkage region, in 13 families with fALS. Subsequent studies have shown that approximately 15–20% of fALS cases have mutations in SOD1, making this still by far the commonest genetic cause of MND.

SOD1 is a cytosolic enzyme which catalyses the conversion of toxic superoxide anion free radicals to harmless metabolites. Given the well-known harmful effect of free radicals on nerve cells and evidence that free radicals accumulate with aging, this immediately suggested that loss of dismutase activity was a plausible biological mechanism for motor neuron damage. The next 15 years was to be dominated by the search for a clear understanding of why mutations in SOD1, a ubiquitously expressed enzyme, should cause a disease with a high degree of specificity for motor neurons. If mutations induced a loss of the normal enzymatic function, other cell types in addition to motor neurons should be vulnerable. Interestingly the effect on the dismutase function of the resulting protein is highly variable with some mutations apparently even increasing free radical scavenging. There is now abundant evidence that mutations in SOD1 cause disease by leading to an acquired toxic property in the protein and not by inducing free radical mediated damage. However, almost two decades after the identification of the first gene for MND, the exact mechanism for motor neuron death is still uncertain.

An Animal Model
Gurney et al., Science (1994)

Within a year of the discovery of SOD1 as the first genetic cause of ALS, transgenic mice expressing mutant human SOD1 protein had been produced. Gurney's 1994 paper was the first report of such a mouse line and describes the model (SOD1 G93A) which, for better or for worse, has been the most commonly used tool in MND mouse model research to date. In total 12 different human SOD1 mutations have now been expressed in mice and these animals all demonstrate an isolated and ultimately fatal degeneration of motor neurons. That the mutant enzyme is expressed on a mouse background with a full complement of endogenous SOD1 enzyme function suggests that the disease is not caused by loss of the enzyme function and this has been formally proved by measuring the dismutase activity *in vivo* and by crossing the G93A model with a mouse expressing high levels of wild-type SOD1, which does not lead to rescue of the phenotype.

The model described in this much-quoted paper has led to a very large body of evidence that toxicity may involve mitochondrial damage, ER stress, axonal transport and a range of other pathways with potential for therapeutic targeting. Furthermore, as the technology for generating mouse models has advanced to allow selective expression of mutant protein in specific tissue such as neurons, glia and muscle, the important paradigm has emerged of MND as a disease in which the pathogenesis depends on non-neuronal cells.

However, the exact reason why these mice develop motor neuron disease has ultimately evaded researchers. Furthermore, of more than 100 drugs which have apparently shown effects in ameliorating the phenotype of the G93A mouse, not one has successfully translated into an effective new therapy for MND patients. These sobering facts require some careful re-evaluation of our whole approach to modelling neurodegeneration in rodents. Can an animal separated from humans by 50 million years of evolution, which lives for about 2.5 years and has considerably shorter motor neurons, really ever model a late-onset human disease which is in most cases sporadic? Has the technology for generating transgenic mice, in which a phenotype is 'forced' by massive over-expression of protein in a way which overrides physiological regulation, distorted the pathways to disease in a way which mask the key initiating steps of cell death most relevant to the human disease? Finally, we now know that SOD1-related ALS appears to have some distinct and important differences which single it out as separate pathological entity from most cases of ALS, a fact which may consign mouse models based on SOD1 mutations to obsolescence.

The First Disease-Modifying Treatment
Bensimon et al., New England Journal of Medicine (1994)

Randomised controlled trials have been performed in MND for nearly half a century. In 1956 Liversedge used a combination of glycocyamine and betaine therapy[11]. The rationale was their involvement in the biochemical pathway of creatine production, an important component of muscle metabolism. The author recorded that at that time the aetiology of MND remained elusive but was attributed to:

> A medley of factors, including chill, anxiety, toxicosis, injury and inevitably tobacco and alcohol.

Since then, a plethora of drugs have been tested in very variable circumstances, often with only small numbers of patients, and with tenuous rationale at times[12].

Excitotoxicity has been a lasting theme in MND pathophysiology for 20 years. It was recognised that, in culture, neuronal cell death could be induced by over-stimulation with naturally occurring excitatory amino acids such as glutamate. The findings of altered glutamate levels in the blood and CSF of ALS patients were supported by the report of reduced glutamate transport shortly afterwards[13]. This concept of over-stimulation of motor neurons as a key step in pathogenesis of MND has developed to some extent by inconsistent epidemiological links to physical exercise and athleticism[14], fuelled by high-profile sporting figures among the afflicted, including the legendary 1930s Yankees baseball player Lou Gehrig.

The benzothiazole riluzole found its original use as an ingredient of photographic developing solution and later in an industrial bleach. Legend has it that two scientists working in separate laboratories on the same floor accidentally swapped chemicals so that riluzole was screened in an *in-vitro* assay of glutamate inhibition and found to be effective[15]. It was then developed as a potential anticonvulsant but not achieve much success. Nonetheless, it was resurrected to assess its potential in the treatment of MND.

Gilbert Bensimon and colleagues wrote up the first multicentre randomised placebo-controlled trial of riluzole in 155 patients carried out over 21 months using death and tracheostomy as the primary outcome measures. Overall riluzole therapy was well tolerated and reduced mortality by a surprisingly high 39% at 12 months and by a more modest but still meaningful 19% at 21 months (p=0.046). A second larger study of 959 patients however showed only a "trend" to significant improvement in tracheostomy-free survival at 18 months (unadjusted p=0.08), equivalent to an estimated gain in survival of approximately 3 months at this time point[16].

The lack of subjective improvement, the inability to quantify individual slowing of progression, the misrepresentative distillation of the Lacomblez study in the statement "only worth an extra three months" and the lack of quality of life data in the trials are all cited as reasons for not prescribing or taking riluzole. The initially seismic reaction to the news in 1994, that after decades of unsuccessful trials one drug had at last been shown to make a difference to survival in MND, seems to have faded unduly fast.

Identification of Clinical Prognostic Factors
Haverkamp et al., Brain (1995)

Despite the uniformly median survival of 3–4 years from symptom onset, there is a large range of survival of the remaining 50%, with 5% of MND patients surviving beyond 10 years[17]. This heterogeneity, and how it relates to clinical features, has been a source of fascination since the earliest descriptions. Sir William Richard Gowers (1845–1915) noted:

> *When the progress at the commencement is rapid, it usually continues rapid, until the disease has attained a wide extent . . . . When it begins slowly it is usually slow throughout.*[18]

Prognostication is important in MND for care planning and decision making: the difference between an aggressive case of ALS running its course over 1 year and a 'flail arm' variant progressing over 8 years[19] is substantial. Natural history studies of clinic-based MND populations have identified three consistently adverse prognostic factors, namely:

- Bulbar-onset (affecting 25% of patients) rather than limb-onset (70%)
- Older age at symptom onset
- Rate of disease of progression (which generally does not change in an individual)

Even within bulbar-onset patients, longer surviving patients are recognised[20] and any robust prognostic model must consider multiple factors simultaneously. Haverkamp and colleagues used a clinic database to do exactly this in over 800 patients. This study also provided valuable descriptive data on interventions such as gastrostomy, comorbidities and immunological markers. They used the multivariate Cox proportional hazards model to generate a score composed of regression coefficients for several clinical attributes found to have independent prognostic value: age at symptom onset, slope of change of composite functional score, slope of change of respiratory sub-score, and the diagnostic latency. The model accurately predicted overall survival for 80% of patients, slightly under-estimating survival in those with "low-risk" and over-estimating it in those with "high-risk" profiles.

This pioneering model for accurately predicting survival using a handful of easily determined clinical features ultimately sets a very high benchmark for the emerging biofluid and neuroimaging biomarker candidates[21]. Therapeutic trials may be confounded by the enrolment of heterogeneous patients, and grouping patients of similar prognostic score at baseline may be a tool to help overcome this.

Standardised Measurement of Disease Progression and the Evolution of Clinical Trials
The ACTS Phase I-II Study Group, Archives of Neurology (1996)

Disease progression is a vital outcome measure in the context of MND therapeutic trials. In the absence of any precise way of measuring early pathological changes in the complex cortico-spinal and spinal-muscular motor unit, researchers have fallen back on clinical measures of disease progression.

These measures should be suitable for repetitive administration, demonstrate good interrater reliability and should measure something meaningful to the disease in question. The ALS Functional Rating Scale, based in part on the UDPDRS scale developed for Parkinson's disease, has been used as a standard measure in all ALS clinical treatment trials and studies of natural history since the original paper was published. One of the great strengths of this scale, which in its revised form (the ALSFRS-R) assesses 12 domains of function[22], is that it can be administered by patients themselves or their carers. It is now also frequently used in specialist clinic settings to assess disease progression and plan interventions. Although the rate of death is considered to be the most 'robust' measure of the effect of a drug in ALS trials, the ALSFRS-R will for the foreseeable future continue to be the best overall measure of disease progression.

The Discovery of TDP-43
Neumann et al., Science (2006)

For several decades after the characterisation of ubiquitinated inclusions as the pathological hallmark of MND, the identity of their constituents remained unknown. Purifying and analysing protein lysate from the tiny amounts available of affected neurons are challenging. Despite a number of attempts, this had proved intractable to standard biochemical techniques.

A major step forward came with the increasing recognition that MND and a subset of cases of frontotemporal dementia (FTD) share the same pathology. Neumann and colleagues took whole protein lysate from the cortex of patients with FTD and ubiquitin pathology and used the high molecular weight fractions to inject mice from which a panel of monoclonal antibodies were generated. These were in turn used to probe immunoblots of protein from FTD brains to identify an antibody which detected the major protein constituent of UBIs. This was then isolated from 2-D protein gels, sequenced by mass spectrometry and identified as the transactivation-responsive DNA-binding protein, TDP-43. Remarkably, anti-TDP-43 antibodies showed that TDP-43 is the major protein constituent of UBIs in MND, providing molecular confirmation of an overlap in pathology between MND and FTD. The translocation of TDP-43 to UBIs was associated with almost total depletion of the protein from its normal location in the nucleus. This suggested that the accumulation of TDP-43 in cytoplasmic aggregates was less likely to be a mere bystander effect than to have a direct role in the pathogenesis of motor neuron death. Further evidence of a direct role for altered TDP-43 in MND pathogenesis came from the identification of patients, both sporadic and familial ALS cases, carrying mutations in the TARDBP gene[23], which encodes TDP-43.

The identification of TDP-43 as an ALS-associated protein has had a major effect in shifting ALS research away from SOD1. It now seems clear that SOD1-associated familial ALS cases and transgenic mouse models do not demonstrate the same TDP-43 staining or nuclear-cytoplasmic translocation, suggesting that SOD1-associated ALS may not be the best model for the vast majority of cases. TDP-43 is known to modulate splicing of a subset of mRNA transcripts and may have other RNA modifying functions. The subsequent identification of mutations in the FUS/TLS gene[24] has focused attention on RNA processing as a common pathway in motor neuron vulnerability[25], representing a major paradigm shift. This also gives reason to hope that more relevant mouse models of MND can be developed for screening compounds with disease modifying potential.

Understanding Focality and Spread of Pathology
Ravits and La Spada, Neurology (2009)

Clinician scientists like John Ravits have only recently returned to the fundamental issues of focality and spread of pathology in MND, which have been debated since the time of Charcot and Gowers. Today this includes controversy about the 'dying back' of UMNs from diseased anterior horn cell LMNs versus distinct 'dying forward' of UMNs from their cerebral origins. Recognising (just as Gowers had eluded to) that the site of symptom onset, the rate of progression and the mixture of UMN versus LMN involvement are key variables in any equation that might explain the striking clinical heterogeneity seen in MND, Ravits studied 100 ALS patients clinically throughout their disease course and undertook detailed neuropathological analysis. The key findings can be summarised as follows:

- The site of onset is the most severely affected.
- Spread is outward along contiguous body regions.
- Upper and lower motor neuron signs are maximal at the same region.
- UMN and LMN loss is simultaneous but independent.
- Complexity arises because spread occurs within a complex 3D network of UMNs and LMNs, involving aspects of:
  - Convergence (one LMN receiving input from many UMNs)
  - Divergence (one UMN innervating many pools of LMNs)

This rigorous clinicopathological approach to MND is easy to demote in the face of enormous developments in molecular biology over the last half century, but may yet hold vital clues to the fundamental disease process in MND.

Summary and Conclusion

The modern concept of what defines MND reflects the rigorous clinico-pathological methods of Charcot and others, but 150 years on fundamental questions still remain

about the nature of variable upper motor neuron involvement and prognostic heterogeneity in MND. After the initial excitement about the discovery of SOD1 mutations,
only a handful of dominant genes have been found that account for only 3% of all cases,
and a growing realisation that this is a highly complex disorder involving polygenetic
factors and possibly subtle but catastrophic imbalances in motor and extra-motor
cerebral and spinal 'networks'. Close integration between the clinic and the laboratory
will be the key to any progress in developing effective disease modifying treatments that
have so far proved so frustratingly elusive for this devastating illness.

Key Outstanding Questions

1. What is the nature of the observed variation in focality and spread of pathology in
   MND? One disease or many?
2. Can we identify robust diagnostic, prognostic and therapeutic monitoring biomarkers from neuroimaging, neurophysiology, CSF or blood?
3. Can we identify those at risk of apparently sporadic MND in the general population
   before the earliest steps in the pathogenic pathway are taken?

Key Research Centres

1. Matthew Kiernan, Sydney, Australia
2. Wim Robberecht, Leuwen, Belgium
3. Vincent Meininger, Paris, France
4. Albert Ludolph, Ulm, Germany
5. Orla Hardiman, Dublin, Ireland
6. Vincenzo Silani, Milan, Italy
7. Leonard Van den Berg, Utrecht, Netherlands
8. Martin Turner and Kevin Talbot, Oxford, United Kingdom
9. Merit Cudkowicz, Cambridge, Massachusetts, United States

References

The ALS CNTF Treatment Study (ACTS) Phase I-II Study Group. The Amyotrophic Lateral
   Sclerosis Functional Rating Scale: Assessment of Activities of Daily Living in Patients with
   Amyotrophic Lateral Sclerosis. *Archives of Neurology* 1996;53(2):141–147. http://archneur.
   ama-assn.org/cgi/content/abstract/53/2/141

Bensimon G. *et al.* A controlled trial of riluzole in amyotrophic lateral sclerosis. ALS/Riluzole
   Study Group. *New England Journal of Medicine* 1994;330(9):585–591. http://www.ncbi.nlm.
   nih.gov/pubmed/8302340

Charcot J.-M. Amyotrophies spinales deuteropathiques sclérose latérale amyotrophique &
   Sclérose latérale amyotrophique. In: *Oeuvres complétes*. Bureaux du Progrès Médical, Paris,
   1874. http://www.archive.org/search.php?query=creator%3A%22Charcot%2C%20J.%20M.
   %20(Jean%20Martin)%2C%201825-1893%22

Gurney M.E. *et al.* Motor neuron degeneration in mice that express a human Cu, Zn superoxide
   dismutase mutation. *Science* 1994;264(5166):1772–1775. http://www.ncbi.nlm.nih.gov/
   pubmed/8209258

Haverkamp L.J. *et al.* Natural history of amyotrophic lateral sclerosis in a database population. Validation of a scoring system and a model for survival prediction. *Brain* 1995;118(3): 707–719. http://brain.oxfordjournals.org/content/118/3/707.abstract

Leigh P.N. *et al.* Ubiquitin deposits in anterior horn cells in motor neurone disease. *Neuroscience Letters* 1988; 93(2–3):197–203. http://www.sciencedirect.com/science/article/pii/030439408890081X

Matthews W.B. *Practical neurology.* Blackwell, Oxford, 1963.

Neumann M. *et al.* Ubiquitinated TDP-43 in frontotemporal lobar degeneration and amyotrophic lateral sclerosis. *Science* 2006;316(5796):130–133. http://www.ncbi.nlm.nih.gov/pubmed/17023659

Ravits J.M. and La Spada A.R. ALS motor phenotype heterogeneity, focality, and spread: deconstructing motor neuron degeneration. *Neurology* 2009;73(10):805–811. http://www.ncbi.nlm.nih.gov/pmc/articles/PMC2739608/?tool=pubmed

D.R. *et al.* Mutations in Cu/Zn superoxide dismutase gene are associated with familial amyotrophic lateral sclerosis. *Nature* 1993;362(6415):59–62. http://www.nature.com/nature/journal/v362/n6415/abs/362059a0.html

Smith M.C. Nerve fibre degeneration in the brain in amyotrophic lateral sclerosis. *Journal of Neurology, Neurosurgery & Psychiatry* 1960;23(4):269–282. http://www.ncbi.nlm.nih.gov/pmc/articles/PMC497425/?tool=pubmed

Additional References

1. Charcot J.-M. Sclérose des cordons latéraux de la moelle épinière chez une femme hystérique atteinte de contracture permanente des quatre membres. *Bull de la Société Méd. des Hôpit. de Paris* 1865:24–35.

2. Turner MR, *et al.* Lockhart Clarke's contribution to the description of amyotrophic lateral sclerosis. *Brain.* 2010 epub Jun 30.

3. Brain W.R. *Motor neurone disease: diseases of the nervous system.* 6th ed. Oxford University Press; London, 1962. p. 531–543.

4. Radcliffe CB and Lockhart Clarke J. An important case of paralysis and muscular atrophy with disease of the nervous centres. *British and Foreign Medico-Chirurgical Review* 1862:30.

5. Alzheimer A. On a case of spinal progressive muscle atrophy with accessory disease of bulbar nuclei and the cortex. *Archiv. fur Psychiatrie* 1891;23:459–485.

6. Phukan J, *et al.* Cognitive impairment in amyotrophic lateral sclerosis. *Lancet Neurology* 2007 Nov;6(11):994–1003.

7. Ludolph AC, *et al.* Frontal lobe function in amyotrophic lateral sclerosis: a neuropsychologic and positron emission tomography study. *Acta Neurol. Scand.* 1992;85(2):81–89.

8. Abrahams S, *et al.* Word retrieval in amyotrophic lateral sclerosis: a functional magnetic resonance imaging study. *Brain* 2004;127(Pt 7):1507–1517.

9. Turner MR, *et al.* Evidence of widespread cerebral microglial activation in amyotrophic lateral sclerosis: an [(11)C](R)-PK11195 positron emission tomography study. *Neurobiology of Disease* 2004;15(3):601–609.

10. Filippini N, *et al.* Corpus callosum involvement is a consistent feature of amyotrophic lateral sclerosis. *Neurology* 2010 in press.

11. Liversedge LA. Glycocyamine and Betaine in Motor-Neurone Disease. *Lancet* 1956: 1136–1138.

12. Turner MR, *et al.* Clinical trials in ALS: an overview. *Semin. Neurol.* 2001;21(2):167–175.

13. Rothstein JD, *et al.* Decreased glutamate transport by the brain and spinal cord in amyotrophic lateral sclerosis. *New England Journal of Medicine* 1992;326(22):1464–1468.

14. Harwood CA, *et al.* Physical activity as an exogenous risk factor in motor neuron disease (MND): a review of the evidence. *Amyotroph. Lateral. Scler.* 2009;10(4):191–204.
15. Turner MR, *et al.* Riluzole and motor neuron disease. *Practical Neurology* 2003;3 (3):160–170.
16. Lacomblez L, *et al.* Dose-ranging study of riluzole in amyotrophic lateral sclerosis. Amyotrophic Lateral Sclerosis/Riluzole Study Group II. *Lancet* 1996;347(9013):1425–1431.
17. Turner MR, *et al.* Prolonged survival in motor neuron disease: a descriptive study of the King's database 1990-2002. *Journal of Neurology, Neurosurgery & Psychiatry* 2003;74 (7):995–997.
18. Gowers WR. Chronic spinal muscular atrophy. In: A manual of diseases of the nervous system. P. Blakiston, Philadelphia, 1893:471–498.
19. Hu MT, *et al.* Flail arm syndrome: a distinctive variant of amyotrophic lateral sclerosis. *Journal of Neurology, Neurosurgery & Psychiatry* 1998;65(6):950–951.
20. Turner MR, *et al.* The diagnostic pathway and prognosis in bulbar-onset amyotrophic lateral sclerosis. *Journal of the Neurological Sciences* 2010;294(1-2):81–85.
21. Turner MR, *et al.* Biomarkers in amyotrophic lateral sclerosis. *Lancet Neurology* 2009; 8(1):94–109.
22. Cedarbaum JM, *et al.* The ALSFRS-R: a revised ALS functional rating scale that incorporates assessments of respiratory function. BDNF ALS Study Group (Phase III). *Journal of the Neurological Sciences* 1999;169(1–2):13–21.
23. Sreedharan J, *et al.* TDP-43 mutations in familial and sporadic amyotrophic lateral sclerosis. *Science* 2008;319(5870):1668–1672.
24. Vance C, *et al.* Mutations in FUS, an RNA processing protein, cause familial amyotrophic lateral sclerosis type 6. *Science* 2009;323(5918):1208–1211.
25. Bäumer D, *et al.* The role of RNA processing in the pathogenesis of motor neuron degeneration. *Expert Rev. Mol. Med.* 2010 in press;12:e21–doi:10.1017/S1462399410001523.

15 Migraine

Mark W. Weatherall

Princess Margaret Migraine Clinic, Department of Clinical Neurology, Charing Cross Hospital, London, UK

Headache roameth over the desert, blowing like the wind, Flashing like lightening, it is loosed above and below.

Sumerian verses, 7th century BC

The immediate antecedent of an attack is a condition of unstable equilibrium and gradually accumulating tension in parts of the nervous system more immediately concerned, while the paroxysm itself may be likened to a storm, by which this condition is dispersed and equilibrium for the time being restored.

Edward Living, *On Megrim* (1873)

The world shouts at the person with migraine.

Peter Goadsby (2008)

Introduction

What is migraine? For something so universal, so long recognised as a common part of human experience, to continue to defy incontrovertible and final definition seems extraordinary, until one understands the complexity of this often debilitating neurological condition. Migraine, as the clinicians and scientists whose work is recorded in this article understood it, is a disorder characterised by a tendency to recurrent moderate or severe headaches, often associated with nausea and sensitivity to lights, noise and movement.

Headaches readily recognisable as migraine can be found in the medical and lay literature throughout recorded history: in the ancient Egyptian papyri and the works of Hippocrates and Galen; through to the detailed clinical and anatomical descriptions of Thomas Willis. Theories of headache causation in this literature mirror the prevailing worldview, for the most part deriving explanation from Aristotelian humoural theory, as refined by Galen, and the Arabic medical encyclopaedists such as Ibn'Sena (Avicenna).

The high watermark of the premodern literature is the monograph *On Megrim*, published in 1873 by the English physician Edward Liveing. Originally constructed as an MD thesis, Liveing's monograph contains extensive clinical descriptions of migraine auras, headache and associated features, as well as reviews of prevailing theories of causation, and Liveing's own theory of 'nerve-storms'. Liveing's work was regarded by no less a luminary than William Gowers as just about the only thing worth reading on migraine, and in recent decades, through the advocacy of Oliver Sacks and John Pearce, it

Understanding Medical Research: The Studies that Shaped Medicine, First Edition. Edited by John A. Goodfellow. © 2012 John Wiley & Sons, Ltd. Published 2012 by John Wiley & Sons, Ltd.

has become regarded as a masterpiece of the genre. It did not, however, lead to changes in the understanding or treatment of migraine at the time. It was instead the vascular theories of migraine put forward by du Bois Reymond, Mollendorf and Peter Wallwork Latham that provided the background for most of the research on migraine in the first eight decades of the 20th century. The reason for this was the discovery of an efficacious antimigraine drug with undoubted vascular effects: ergotamine.

Migraine and Ergotamine
Graham and Wolff, Archives of Neurology and Psychiatry (1938)
Ray and Wolff, Archives of Surgery (1940)

The first report of the efficacy of ergot of rye in the suppression of head pain appears in the *British Medical Journal* in 1868. Various groups were involved in unpicking the complex pharmacology of ergot in the following decades, but it was Stoll at Sandoz Pharmaceuticals in Basel, Switzerland, who isolated ergotamine in the second decade of the 20th century. Reports in the 1920s and 1930s attested to its effectiveness in migraine headache. In parallel with this work, advances in neurosurgical technique allowed increasingly sophisticated attempts to localise brain function, including pain. These strands of work were brought together in the 1930s by Harold Wolff, a neurologist now widely regarded as a pioneer of experimental studies of migraine pathophysiology. The above papers are absolutely fundamental to what came after.

In their 1938 paper, Graham and Wolff recorded changes in the amplitude of the pulsations in the extra-cranial arteries during attacks of migraine and observed the effects of ergotamine upon this. They showed that pulse amplitudes increased during migraine, and that both pressure on the carotid artery ipsilateral to the headache, and the administration of ergotamine tartrate, reduced pulse amplitudes and diminished the intensity of the headache.

Ray and Wolff's intraoperative experiments on 45 patients (selected from a 'large group' by virtue of being 'intelligent and co-operative', 'relatively free of apprehension and of preoccupation with pain', and of undergoing operative procedures such that they were 'not too prostrated or inarticulate to describe their sensations') showed that pain, but not other sensations, could be evoked by electrical, mechanical, thermal or chemical stimulation of dural blood vessels and sinuses and of the large intracerebral arteries. These painful sensations were localised predominantly to the ophthalmic branch of the trigeminal nerve, where primary headaches typically manifest. This provided a theoretical basis for observations of pain in conditions in which pain-sensitive structures became inflamed, displaced or distended.

These observations also formed the basis of much of Wolff's landmark monograph *Headache and Other Head Pain*, which immediately became the standard work on the subject, and is now in its eighth edition. Wolff himself was cautious about extrapolating his findings in the extra-cranial arteries to those of the intracranial arteries, pointing out that if dilatation of the dural and cerebral arteries was responsible for migraine, one would expect this to be prevented in cases of raised intracranial pressure; this appeared to be true for headaches induced by vasodilators, such as histamine, but not for migraine itself. Nonetheless, a simplistic vascular theory (aura caused by vasoconstriction, and headache by vasodilatation) was distilled from his monograph into countless student lectures and textbooks, and is still believed by many otherwise well-informed doctors to this day.

It is important to understand that Wolff's conception of migraine involved not only the vasodilatation of blood vessels, blocked by ergotamine, but also the existence of perivascular nociceptive factors that damaged local tissues and increased sensitivity to pain in migraine attacks. This was thought possibly to have an allergic basis. Various candidate substances were studied during the 1940s and 1950s, including histamine, acetylcholine, bradykinin and serotonin. The most powerful known serotonin antagonist, lysergic acid (LSD), was not clinically useful because of its hallucinogenic effects. In 1959, however, the Italian neurologist Federigo Sicuteri published a study demonstrating that 1-methyl-D-lysergic acid butanolamide (methysergide), a more powerful serotonin antagonist than LSD but not a vasodilator, was a safe and effective prophylactic treatment for headache.

Introduction of the Serotonin Antagonists
Sicuteri, International Archives of Allergy (1959)

Sicuteri treated 18 patients with migraine, 11 of whom were pretreated with placebo in an embryonic type of cross-over study. Improvements were noted in all cases over the follow-up period of 15–60 days; 50% of the patients were rendered free of attacks. An indication of the importance of the change in attitude towards to migraine when methysergide was introduced into clinical practice may be gathered from the recollections of the American neurologist Neil Raskin, who in 2008 recalled that 'I was still in training when methysergide was introduced in 1960. It was quite astonishing how this drug changed physicians' thinking about the nature of migraine. Prior to that time, and all through the 40s and 50s, migraine was thought to be predominantly psychosomatic. I think back to all those patients that I had sent to psychiatric consultants who came back to me with "no psychopathology"; the common response was that the psychiatrists were not sophisticated enough. Suddenly, patients could take a few tablets of methysergide and within a week they were headache-free. No change in their internal milieu. Cured. Unfortunately, there were some problems with methysergide, but this drug's ability to antagonize certain actions of serotonin peripherally abruptly transformed migraine from a psychosocial problem into a scientific one'[1].

A spate of further studies followed, including the first well-conducted randomised controlled trial in headache[2]. Sicuteri showed that increased levels of 5-HIAA (the main metabolite of serotonin) could be found in the urine during migraine attacks, and a series of papers from Jim Lance's group in Sydney began to delineate the role of platelet dysfunction in migraine (platelets being the main repository of serotonin in the body). A second serotonin antagonist, pizotifen, was developed as a migraine prophylactic by Sandoz in the 1960s, appearing at around the time that reports of methysergide-induced retroperitoneal, cardiac and pulmonary fibrosis began to appear. The fortuitous observation that patients in trials of beta-blockers for hypertension reported decreased migraine frequency opened up a new avenue of prophylactic treatment in the 1970s.

Contemporary readers may be surprised that Sicuteri's study included patients with both migraine and cluster headache, now universally regarded as distinctive conditions. The question of how one should differentiate between different headache disorders was at this time an active one. In 1962 an Ad Hoc Committee (of the recently formed American Headache Society) on the Classification of Headache (with Harold Wolff serving on it until his death from a stroke that year at the age of 63) produced a diagnostic classification that remained influential throughout the 1960s and 1970s. The basis of this classification was clinical, heavily influenced by extensive patient case series such as that published by Selby and Lance in 1960[3].

By the early 1980s, the limitations of the Ad Hoc Committee's classification had become clear, particularly in regard to achieving homogeneous patient populations for research studies. New primary headache disorders such as paroxysmal hemicrania and hemicrania continua had been described by Otto Sjaasted's group. A committee (and subsequently 12 subcommittees) of the International Headache Society was formed to produce a more definitive replacement.

Headache Classification
Headache Classification Committee of the International Headache Society, Cephalalgia (1988)

The *International Classification of Headache Disorders* was not light reading, extending to 54 pages of tightly drawn operational definitions for 70 types and 90 subtypes of primary and secondary headaches, not to mention 16 pages of references and two pages of definitions. The authors recognised the potential for its users to be daunted, exhorting them from the outset, 'please do not be overwhelmed. It is big, complicated, but not supposed to be learned by heart.' It is perhaps the only document of its type and importance to apologise in the introduction that 'however tedious and irritating it may be, operational diagnostic criteria must be introduced, if headache research is to accomplish significant advance in the future'. The authors were correct in their assumption that its importance would lie in providing international consensus on what types of patients should be included in the research trials, as well as in reinforcing the distinctions between migraine and the growing list of other primary headache disorders. Like all documents drawn up by committees, it had its limitations and omissions, chronic headache disorders being particularly poorly served. Some of those limitations and omissions have been corrected in the second edition of the *Classification*, published in 2004, and subsequent appendices and revisions. Healthy debate still ensues whenever the subject of headache classification comes up at international headache meetings, but now, even if we still cannot answer the question 'What is headache?', it is easier to answer the question 'Which headache is this?'

By the time of the publication of the ICHD-I, the vascular theories of migraine pathophysiology that had held the ascendancy over the previous decades had started to come under sustained challenge. The basis of this challenge was both clinical and experimental. The clinical challenge was to explain the vascular basis of migraine aura, a spreading or evolving combination of positive and negative neurological features experienced by about 20% of migraine sufferers, usually immediately prior to the headache phase of their attack. Beautiful images of visual aura had been produced by the astronomer Hubert Airy in the 19th century, and reproduced in (amongst other places) Liveing's monograph *On Megrim*. The gold standard clinical description of visual aura, however, was that published by the visual physiologist Karl Laishley in 1940.

An Account of Auras
Lashley, Archives of Neurology and Psychiatry (1941)

Lashley's work was classic psychophysics. He studied his own visual auras meticulously, noting that they always started at or near the centre of fixation, spreading laterally and never impinging upon the midline. Some of his auras had scintillating zigzag edges;

others were exclusively negative. Lashley mapped these phenomena onto the known anatomy of the occipital cortex, postulating that a wave of inhibition (sometimes preceded by intense excitation) must propagate away from the occipital pole at a speed of approximately 3 mm/min.

Lashley's concept was difficult to reconcile with the prevailing idea that aura was due to constriction of cerebral vessels, then followed by headache-inducing vasodilatation, a theory dating back to the 1870s and seemingly reinforced by the work coming out of Wolff's group. In 1958 the Canadian neurologist PM Milner pointed out that a potential alternative physiological mechanism could be found in the work of the Brazilian physiologist Aristedes Leão, undertaken while studying for a doctorate in physiology at Harvard Medical School, and published in the *Journal of Neurophysiology* in 1944. Leão was studying experimental models of epilepsy; when he tried to induce seizures by electrical stimulation of the cortex of rabbits, he instead found an orderly and progressive flattening of cortical electrical activity, spreading away from the point of stimulation, followed some time afterwards by recovery of function in the same pattern. The speed at which this wave of cortical spreading depression (CSD) crossed the cortex was approximately 3 mm/min[4].

Neither Leão's work nor Milner's insight led immediately to further studies on the neural basis of aura. CSD is very difficult to demonstrate neurophysiologically in humans, except in extreme situations such as the aftermath of subarachnoid haemorrhage. Nonetheless, this appealing hypothesis gained increasing credence in the early 1980s, when Martin Lauritzen and Jes Olesen of the Danish headache group published a series of experimental studies definitively favouring CSD over more straightforward cerebral vasoconstriction as the cause of aura.

Olesen, Annals of Neurology (1981)

The Danish group studied blood flow in aura by means of [133]Xenon single-photon emission computed tomography (^{133}Xe-SPECT). This isotope, given by carotid injection (which induced attacks in some patients), was cleared more quickly in areas of the brain with high regional cerebral blood flow (rCBF), allowing rCBF to be estimated. During aura, transient oligaemia was seen to spread anteriorly from the occipital pole in a pattern that did not respect the territorial distributions of the major cerebral arteries. Intriguingly, oligaemia lingered into the headache phase, persisting well beyond the resolution of clinical symptoms. Refinements in functional neuroimaging in the intervening decades, including the introduction of positron emission tomography (PET) and functional magnetic resonance imaging (fMRI), have allowed increasingly detailed spatial and temporal localisation of changes in cerebral blood flow, all supporting the hypothesis that CSD is the biological substrate of migraine aura.

Functional imaging seemed to have provided an answer to the question of where aura originates. Could it also provide clues as to the location of the processes that generate headache? The answer to this seemed to be answered in the affirmative in 1995.

Weiller et al., Nature Medicine (1995)

This PET study included nine patients studied during spontaneous attacks of migraine without aura, before and after treatment and in the headache-free interval. Significantly higher rCBF was found in median brainstem structures, contralateral to the side of the pain, persisting beyond the resolution of the headache. Spatial resolution was not precise; the area involved included the periaqueductal gray, the midbrain reticular formation and the locus coeruleus. This area had already been implicated in migraine generation by observations that patients who had undergone electrode implantation in the midbrain to treat chronic pain had, on occasion, developed new-onset unilateral migraines. More recently cases have appeared of patients with new onset migraines triggered by brainstem inflammation or haemorrhage from a brainstem cavernoma.

Further imaging work with PET and fMRI has since replicated and extended these findings. The idea that CSD is the physiological substrate of aura has been further supported by studies showing that many effective migraine prophylactics inhibit CSD *in vivo*, and more recently that tonebersat, a specific CSD-blocker, whilst not a useful drug for the acute or prophylactic treatment of migraine as a whole, may have some useful effects in migraine with aura. CSD has been found to be remarkably widespread in nature, even occurring in locusts, thus suggesting an important evolutionary role for this process, the nature of which remains as yet obscure. Similarly obscure are the answers to questions such as how CSD might trigger headache mechanisms in the brain, and what triggers such mechanisms in people who do not experience aura.

The Development of Triptans

Answers to these questions depend on increased understanding of exactly how and where headache-generating processes take place. Once again, one of the major driving forces behind advances in the understanding of migraine physiology came from the generation of new drugs to treat the condition. The pathophysiological advances of the 1930s and 1940s followed the introduction of ergotamine, and derived in no small part from attempts to understand how it worked. Similarly, the introduction in the 1980s of a new class of drugs, the $5\text{-HT}_{1B/1D}$ agonists ('triptans'), provided a huge stimulus to the advances in the understanding of the neural basis of migraine in the 1990s. Ironically the stimulus to this work originated in studies of the serotonin antagonist methysergide. In 1974 the Rotterdam physiologist Pramod Saxena showed that methysergide casued selective vasoconstriction in the cephalic arteriovenous anastomoses of the carotid bed. A decade later Saxena demonstrated the existence of an 'atypical' serotonin receptor, at which methysergide appeared to exert a partial agonist effect. This was later isolated and christened the 5-HT_{1B} receptor. Around this time his laboratory was visited by a team from Glaxo led by the British pharmacologist Patrick Humphry, who brought with him some novel compounds in development which were believed to be selective serotonin, or serotonin subtype, agonists.

Humphry et al., British Journal of Pharmacology (1988)

The choice of this paper may be surprising. It is a closely argued piece of clinical pharmacology designed to show that GR43175 was a highly selective agonist for the 5-HT1-like receptor. It does not mention migraine, except in the title of one of the references; this was a study published by Humphry the previous year in which another 5-HT in development had been given intravenously to migraine sufferers with some success. The compound used in 1987 (AH25085) was not commercially viable as its oral bioavailability was very poor. GR43175, on the other hand, was a different matter, and within 3 years its effectiveness as an injectable, and then an oral migraine treatment was established beyond doubt. The triptans (and there are now seven commercially available varieties, each with its own idiosyncrasies) are now the mainstay of acute migraine treatment, a multibillion-dollar industry, and the clearest demonstration yet of the benefits that basic neuropharmacology can bring to the relief of the suffering of patients with migraine.

But how do these drugs work? Whilst not downplaying the importance of events occurring in and around the pain-sensitive structures of the head, interest in the late 1980s and early 1990s started to switch towards the brain structures involved in processing painful stimuli from these areas. These studies were made possible by advances in microiontophoresis and techniques for studying neurotransmitter and gene expression (such as c-fos staining). Out of these studies emerged the central concept of the trigeminovascular system.

The Trigeminovascular System and Migraine
Goadsby and Edvinsson, Annals of Neurology (1993)

Goadsby and Edvinsson's paper brings basic science directly to the bedside. Using the electrical stimulation of the trigeminal ganglion in anaesthetized cats as an animal model, they showed that this caused the release of calcitonin-gene related peptide (CGRP) into the cerebral vasculature. CGRP was believed to be a potent vasodilator, and indeed laser Doppler flowmetry showed significant increases in cerebral blood flow associated with this. Both changes were antagonised by the administration of sumatriptan or dihydroergotamine. In human volunteers, elevations of CGRP levels were seen during attacks, levels being normalised by the administration of sumatriptan. Parallel changes were not seen in the levels of other vasoactive neuropeptides such as neuropeptide Y (NPY) or substance P (SP). Elevated vasoactive intestinal peptide (VIP) levels were seen in patients with parasympathetic-associated symptoms such as nasal congestion or rhinorrhoea.

Throughout the late 1990s and early 2000s, the role of CGRP was elucidated in numerous studies. Demonstrating the relevance of these studies *in vivo* has been helped by the development of a human experimental model through which some migraineurs develop a delayed headache after the administration of glyceryl trinitrite (GTN) that is indistinguishable clinically from their usual migraine. Arguments have raged over exactly where the triptans exert their effects, not least because several members of the class are thought not to cross a normally functioning blood–brain barrier. One intriguing insight arises from the work on Rami Burstein and colleagues on cutaneous allodynia in migraine. This symptom is common in migraine, and extends beyond the immediate area in which the pain is felt, suggesting that it arises from central rather than peripheral sensitisation. The clinical relevance of this observation is that, as they put it memorably in the title of one of their papers, treatment with triptans appears to be a race against the development of allodynia[5]. This, in combination with recent trials confirming the consensus view that triptans work best when given early in the attack, suggests that they exert their major effect on the release of CGRP around peripheral blood vessels.

In another example of the oscillation between the laboratory and clinical advances in headache medicine, the discovery that CGRP is involved in migraine pathophysiology has led to the development of a new class of migraine treatments, CGRP antagonists, that have shown real promise in Phase II and Phase III clinical trials in the first decade of the

21st century. Another area in which the links between clinicians and basic scientists have borne fruit in the last two decades has been in the genetics of migraine. The first fruit of this collaboration came with the discovery by Dutch workers of the first gene for familial hemiplegic migraine (FHM), a rare form of the condition first described in a family from Bristol in the *British Medical Journal* in 1910[6].

Migraine Genetics
Ophoff et al., Cell (1996)
Since the publication of this paper, a further two FHM genes have been isolated, both of which code for cell membrane ion channels (the Na^+/K^+-ATPase gene ATP1A2, and the sodium channel α-subunit encoding gene SCNA1). None of these genes seem to be more widely implicated in the commoner forms of migraine however. Modern techniques of genome-wide analysis have been brought to bear on this issue, and several candidate areas have been identified that may contain genes involved in various aspects of migraine pathophysiology. In future, the work of Aarno Palotie and colleagues on the complex genetic basis of migraine may well press hard for inclusion[7]. Alongside this new emphasis on the genetics of migraine, there has been a resurgence in interest in its epidemiology, particularly in the links between migraine and vascular disorders such as stroke, patent foramen ovale, and rare vasculopathies such as CADASIL, including longitudinal studies of the MRI abnormalities not infrequently found in the brains of migraineurs.

So, to return to where we started, what is migraine? What can we now say with any certitude about this most common of neurological disorders? We can say that the cause is genetic, that we are either migraineurs or we are not, even if we cannot say why so many us seem to be; we can say that the dichotomy between the vascular and neural theories of migraine is a false one; that migraine truly is a neurovascular disorder; and finally we can tell our patients that we have effective treatments for them, with scientific research holding out the promise of more to come in the not-too-distant future.

Key Outstanding Questions
1. Is CSD definitely the biological substrate of migraine aura?
2. How does CSD trigger headache in migraine?
3. Does 'silent' CSD occur in people who suffer from migraine without aura?
4. Where and how exactly do triptans and CGRP antagonists work?
5. What is the role of vascular factors (such as PFOs) in triggering migraine?
6. Is migraine a progressive disorder in some people?

Key Research Groups
1. Peter Goadsby, United States and United Kingdom
2. Jes Olesen, Denmark
3. Steven Silberstein, United States
4. Hans-Christopher Diener, Germany
5. Richard Lipton, United States
6. Michel Ferrari, Netherlands
7. David Dodick, United States

References

Goadsby, P.J., and Edvinsson, L. (1993) The trigeminovascular system and migraine: studies characterizing cerebrovascular and neuropeptide changes seen in humans and cats. *Annals of Neurology*, **33**, 48–56. http://onlinelibrary.wiley.com/doi/10.1002/ana.410330109/abstract

Graham, J.R., and Wolff, H.G. (1938) Mechanism of migraine headache and action of ergotamine tartrate. *Archives of Neurology and Psychiatry*, **39**, 737–763. http://archneurpsyc.ama-assn.org/cgi/content/summary/39/4/737

Headache Classification Committee of the International Headache Society (1988) Classification and diagnostic criteria for headache disorders, cranial neuralgias, and facial pain. *Cephalalgia*, **8**(Suppl. 7), 1–96. http://onlinelibrary.wiley.com/doi/10.1111/cha.1988.8.issue-s7/issuetoc

Humphry, P.P.A., *et al.* (1988) GR43175, a selective agonist for the 5-HT1-like receptor in dog isolated saphenous vein. *British Journal of Pharmacology*, **94**, 1123–1132. http://www.ncbi.nlm.nih.gov/pmc/articles/PMC1854075/?tool$^1/_4$pubmed

Kernick, D., and Goadsby, P. (2008) *Headache: a practical manual*. Oxford University Press, Oxford.

Lashley, K.S. (1941) Patterns of cerebral integration indicated by the scotoma of migraine. *Archives of Neurology and Psychiatry*, **42**, 259–264. http://archneurpsyc.ama-assn.org/cgi/content/summary/46/2/331

Liveing, E. (1873) *On megrim, sick headache*. Arts and Boeve Publishers, Nijmegen.

Olesen, J., *et al.* (1981) Focal hyperaemia following by spreading oligaemia and impaired activation of rCBF in classical migraine. *Annals of Neurology*, **9**, 344–352. http://onlinelibrary.wiley.com/doi/10.1002/ana.410090406/abstract

Ophoff, R.A., *et al.* (1996) Familial hemiplegic migraine and episodic ataxia type-2 are caused by mutations in the Ca2þ channel gene CACNL1A4. *Cell*, **87**, 543–552. http://www.cell.com/retrieve/pii/S0092867400813732

Ray, B.S., and Wolff, H.G. (1940) Experimental studies on headache: pain sensitive structures of the head and their significance in headache. *Archives of Surgery*, **41**, 813–856. http://archsurg.ama-assn.org/cgi/content/summary/41/4/813

Sicuteri, F. (1959) Prophylactic and therapeutic properties of 1-methyllysergic acid butanolamide in migraine. *International Archives of Allergy*, **15**, 300–307. http://www.ncbi.nlm.nih.gov/pubmed/14446408

Weiller, C., *et al.* (1995) Brain stem activation in spontaneous human migraine attacks. *Nature Medicine*, **1**, 658–660. http://www.nature.com/nm/journal/v1/n7/pdf/nm0795-658.pdfv

Wolff, H.G. (1948) *Headache and other head pain*. Oxford University Press, New York.

Additional References

1. Solomon, S., *et al.* (2008) American headache through the decades: 1950 to 2008. *Headache*, **48**, 671–677.

2. Southwell, N., *et al.* (1964) Methysergide in the prophylaxis of migraine. *Lancet*, **1**(7332), 523–524.

3. Selby, G., and Lance, J.W. (1960) Observations on 500 cases of migraine and allied vascular headache. *Journal of Neurology, Neurosurgery & Psychiatry*, **23**, 23–32.

4. Leão, A.A.P. (1944) Spreading depression of activity in the cerebral cortex. J. Neurophysiol., **7**, 359–390.

5. Burstein, R., *et al.* (2004) Defeating migraine pain with triptans: a race against the development of cutaneous allodynia. Ann. Neurol., **55**(1), 19–26.

6. Clarke, J.M. (1910) On recurrent motor paralysis in migraine, with report of a family on which recurrent hemiplegia accompanied the attacks. *British Medical Journal*, **1**, 1534–1538.

7. Wessman, M., *et al.* (2004) The molecular genetics of migraine. Ann. Med, **36**(6), 462–473.

16   Multiple Sclerosis

Alasdair Coles and Alastair Compston

Department of Clinical Neurosciences, University of Cambridge, Cambridge, UK

Introduction

Having been recognised only since the late 19th century, there has been just over 100 years of research on multiple sclerosis. A picture has emerged of this disease as an inflammatory disorder of the central nervous system, caused by a complex interplay of multiple genetic susceptibility alleles and unknown environmental triggers. We have tried to illustrate this in our choice of landmark papers, at the same time being aware that strong cases could be pressed for other studies. Many lines of scientific attack on the disease have benefited from increasingly potent weapons, and in many cases our papers reflect the application of the very latest technology of the day. Finally we note that three of our 'top ten' were authored by Ian McDonald (1933–2006), testimony to his extraordinary contribution to understanding multiple sclerosis[1].

1916: The Pathological Anatomy of the Lesion in Multiple Sclerosis
Dawson, Transactions of the Royal Society of Edinburgh (1916)

James Dawson (1870–1927) left the greatest pathological account of multiple sclerosis (MS) in the English language. At that time there was much debate as to whether the disease was 'inflammatory' or 'developmental' (degenerative). Some promoted a theory of a primary vascular, inflammatory, aetiology[2], suggesting that infections initiate the changes in blood vessels. Others explained the aetiology with reference to direct damage to nerve fibres, an 'intrinsically weakened' system or a developmental disturbance. Müller, the most articulate teacher from the developmental school, proposed that any participation of the blood vessels within the lesion is secondary[3] and his concept of 'multiple gliosis' as the essential process rehearses the final position taken by Charcot[4] and most of his school. Others proposed a toxin- or microorganism-induced primary degeneration of the myelin sheath with secondary inflammation and blood vessel changes[5]. But, as often is the case, the best account was the first: Rindfleisch[6] assigned priority to the blood vessels, proposing a sequence in which a chronic irritative condition of the vessel wall alters the nutrition of nerve elements, leading to atrophy and monster glia (Deiters or Rindfleisch cells).

Reviewing the histology of nine personal cases, Dawson devotes the majority of his text to one patient, L.W. She was admitted to hospital in Edinburgh on 4 April 1910 with a 2-year history of weakness and tremor in all four limbs, dysarthria and sphincter disturbance. In May she had an episode of brainstem demyelination, in August she lost

Understanding Medical Research: The Studies that Shaped Medicine, First Edition. Edited by John A. Goodfellow. © 2012 John Wiley & Sons, Ltd. Published 2012 by John Wiley & Sons, Ltd.

vision in both eyes, developed increasing bulbar failure and died from septicaemia in September. After listing the tragic accumulation of lesions throughout the brain and spinal cord of the unfortunate L.W., Dawson attempts a clinicopathophysiological correlation. Weakness in the legs is consistent with the extensive spinal cord gliosis, intention tremor with lesions in the superior cerebellar peduncles and red nuclei, disordered eye movements with the periaqueductal plaques and the several cranial nerve palsies with involvement of the pons and medulla. Dawson shows that old lesions are characterised by complete absence of myelin, dense fibrillary tissue, persistence of axis cylinders, numerous blood vessels, no active myelin degeneration and an abrupt transition to normal tissue. In acute lesions, the differences are infiltrated blood vessels, active demyelination with fat granule cells and transitional zones shading into normal tissue. He illustrates the text with 22 colour and 434 black-and-white figures in 78 plates.

Dawson summarises his ideas to include a sequence of events that produces recognisable clinical characteristics when directed at glia, leading to degeneration of the myelin sheath with fat granule cell formation, and a reactive change in glia involving cell proliferation with fibril formation culminating in sclerosis. The whole process is triggered and modified by fluctuating exogenous factors, causing the characteristic relapses.

1960: Evidence for an Immune Response within the Central Nervous System
Lowenthal et al., Journal of Neurochemistry (1960)

The most consistent laboratory abnormality in MS is the finding of a restricted number of 'oligoclonal' immunoglobulins within the cerebrospinal fluid (CSF). These are produced by B cells in the parenchyma of the central nervous system (CNS) and drift into CSF like oil in the sump. However any role in the pathogenesis of MS remains completely unknown. Their everyday importance is as a biomarker supporting the diagnosis of MS, being found in 90–95% of people with the disease; but also in conditions having an inflammatory basis and, rarely, apparently by chance. The history of their discovery is intimately tied to technological advances.

In their 1942 paper, Kabat and Landlow showed that the ratio of gamma-globulin to albumin in CSF is normally identical to serum, except in patients with neurosyphillis[7]. They concluded that 'the data would suggest that some formation of gamma globulin could take place within the tissues of the CNS and be poured into CSF', a novel concept.

Lowenthal and colleagues, at the Neurochemical Research Laboratory, Antwerp, pioneered the application of agar electrophoresis to CSF proteins. They saw for the first time multiple sharp gamma-globulin bands in CSF of patients with MS, which were not present in normal individuals, and they distinguished these from the increased bands seen in subacute sclerosis panencephalitis. CSF electrophoresis was now being promoted as a diagnostic aid for MS in clinical practice.

The next innovation was isoelectric focusing of agarose-gel electrophoresis, which improved sensitivity. Hans Link and colleagues improved the definition of the 'oligoclonal bands' (a term he coined), and showed that these were largely due to the presence of IgG antibodies[8].

The scientific dividend from the discovery of CSF oligoclonal bands has been frustratingly small; with no consistent antigenic target and being unaffected by most effective therapies. The recent discovery of meningeal B cell lymphoid follicles, and the moderate efficacy of B-cell depleting antibodies, has reawakened interest in the role of B cells and antibodies[9].

1970: An Exemplary Trial of Steroid Treatment of the Acute Relapse
Rose et al., Neurology (1970)

> *In 1960, at a symposium concerned with the evaluation of drug therapy in neurologic and sensory diseases, the many particular difficulties involved in the clinical trials of therapy in multiple sclerosis were recognized, including those pertaining to the conduct of cooperative studies.*

So opens this 59-page report on a trial of ACTH as a treatment of MS relapse. By 1965 there was agreement that ACTH did not influence MS in the long term, but conflicting small-scale reports on its short-term effect on relapses. Rose and colleagues suspected that ACTH might have a small effect, which would require careful trial design to reveal. So they insisted on a placebo control and on the use of ten neurology centres to maximise recruitment of the required number of patients. They described as a particular strength: 'a statistical centre office and staff, backed by computer facilities, ensured randomization, diminished bias in data review, and provided opportunity for the multiple analyses that were required for the extensive clinical observations'.

Each patient was in hospital for 2 weeks, receiving twice-daily injections of diminishing doses of ACTH or placebo. They were assessed each week for 4 weeks on several scales. 52 pages of charts, tables and text describe the results. The conclusion, confirmed many times since, was 'the Disability Status Scale, together with the Functional Systems, comprises an adequate system of evaluating change in a therapeutic trial of MS and, of all the measures used in this study, apparently is the most consistent indicator of change'.

The primary outcome measure was comparison of patients' disability at baseline with 4 weeks after starting treatment. There was a significant difference in favour of ACTH, but the authors were not impressed; with the size of benefit falling between week 3 and 4, suggesting that it might disappear on extended follow-up. Secondly, they questioned whether the statistically significant difference was clinically significant.

Soon clinicians moved to using synthetic corticosteroids rather than using ACTH. The lack of extended follow-up in the Rose study was corrected by a study in Wales of 50 people with MS treated with placebo or intravenous methylprednisolone[10] and more still was learnt from the effect of steroids on optic neuritis[11]. The conclusion of all of these was that steroids reduce the duration of a relapse, but have no impact on the extent of residual disability or subsequent disease course.

1972: The First Clinical Demonstration of Demyelination
Halliday et al., Lancet (1972)

Ian McDonald and Martin Halliday showed that visual evoked potentials (VEPs) can detect past episodes of optic neuritis, and so introduced a non-invasive test to assist in the diagnosis of suspected MS.

Martin Halliday demonstrated in 1963 that people with MS have delayed somatosensory evoked potentials[12], but the changes were not robust and he soon turned his attention to VEPs. Meanwhile Tom Sears and Ian McDonald had demonstrated the electrical consequences of CNS demyelination[13]. They showed that direct microinjection of diphtheria toxin into the spinal cord of the cat produces a highly circumscribed demyelinating lesion which leads to conduction block, or prolongation of the refractory period for transmission and an impaired ability to transmit high-frequency trains of impulses.

Ian McDonald then studied 19 patients with unilateral optic neuritis, 17 in the acute phase, with flash VEPs and a new technique, 'pattern' VEPs (an alternating black-and-white checkerboard). In optic neuritis the mean latency of VEPs in the affected eye was 155 msec, an increase of 30%; and the peak amplitude was halved at 3.68 microV. In the five patients seen acutely with visual acuities of 6/60 or less, there was no evoked response at all; but as their vision recovered over weeks so their VERs reappeared, although much delayed and remained so, even when visual acuities had recovered to normal, for up to 5 years. Pattern-evoked responses elicited more reproducible and sensitive responses than a flash response. The authors concluded: 'since a persistently increased latency may be present with normal optic discs, fields, and fundi, the technique described here provides a useful objective test for previous damage to the optic nerve. Its potential usefulness in the diagnosis of multiple sclerosis when patients present with clinical evidence of only a single lesion not involving the visual system is obvious'.

They went on to show that abnormal VEPs were sensitive markers of previous optic neuritis, including subclinical optic neuritis[25] and to propose diagnostic criteria incorporating VEPs[15]. To date, the only clinical diagnostic test that can demonstrate that a central neurological lesion is *demyelinating* is the cortical evoked potential, of which the pattern-evoked visual potential is by far the most sensitive and robust.

1972: Identifying the Primary Genetic Association for Multiple Sclerosis
Naito et al., Tissue Antigens (1972)

The most important association of MS with alleles of the human leukocyte antigen (HLA) system, began to be uncovered in the early 1970s. HLAs were first identified as serum factors in transplant recipients that reacted against a third-party 'tissue', and which were associated with transplant rejection. A key figure was Paul Terasaki at UCLA who developed the microcytotoxicity test; a tissue typing test for organ transplant donors and recipients that required only 1 microliter each of antisera[16].

In 1972 Terasaki's group concluded from 94 patients and 871 controls that HL-A3 was overrepresented in MS patients. Furthermore they demonstrated that the geographical variation in prevalence of MS paralleled the prevalence of HL-A3. They summarised some of the epidemiology suggesting an environmental cause and concluded that 'the evidence to date on MS, however, is still consistent with the idea that a genetic difference in susceptibility underlies some environmental influence'.

Soon after this paper, Casper Jersild and colleagues from Copenhagen wrote a brief letter to the *Lancet* to make some generic points around HLA genetics. They described correction for multiple testing, the need for replication datasets and the usefulness of meta-analyses. Illustrating their argument, they announced the results of HLA serotyping in 36 Danish patients with multiple sclerosis followed by a replication set in 71 other patients. From these analyses, HL-A7 emerged as most associated with multiple sclerosis. However, when the Danes merged their data with that from the Terasaki study, and corrected for multiple testing, only HL-A3 retained significance. This set the tone for the years to follow of underpowered studies leading to false positive results and real associations revealed by combining datasets[17].

In 1976 Terasaki and one of the authors of this chapter discovered the association with the class II allele HLA-*DR15*[18,19] which remains the best characterised candidate susceptibility gene for MS. Only in the last few years has there been sufficient power in the techniques and cohorts to uncover small individual genetic contributions of a host of other alleles[20].

The finding that MS is associated with the HLA system implicates the immune system in its pathogenesis, explains some of the geographical variation of the disease, provides a molecular substrate for the interaction of genetics and environment and suggests treatment directed at the T-lymphocyte, the T cell receptor and the class II molecule.

1973: Remyelination Is Possible in the CNS
Gledhill et al., Nature (1973)

A principal hope of people affected by MS is reversal of damage already accrued, and trials of potential remyelinating therapies are being conducted. Key steps that made such therapies possible were the demonstrations that remyelination was possible in the CNS, that this was mediated by the oligodendrocyte precursor and that it was accompanied by functional improvement. We have chosen the paper which definitively demonstrated remyelination in the adult mammalian CNS and showed how to identity demyelinated fibres.

Previous authors had shown that remyelinating cells differed from the mature oligodendrocyte[21] and that, at the level of electron microscopy, axons were surrounded by thin myelin lamellae, which they considered to be evidence for remyelination[22].

In 1973 Richard Gledhill, Barry Harrison and Ian McDonald compressed the spinal cord of three adult cats. This caused early demyelination with retained axons, and remyelination beginning 3 weeks later. Their main discovery, under the electron microscope, was that the remyelinated sheath is abnormally thin with a reduced internodal distance. Under the light microscope, they found no evidence for the presence of Schwann cells, so concluded that oligodendrocytes had been responsible for the remyelination. These ultrastructural characteristics have become the defining features used to recognise remyelinated axons in experimental and human pathological studies.

The next important step was the demonstration that such remyelinated axons could restore function. This work was also supervised by Ian McDonald working with the electrophysiologist Ken Smith[23].

1977: Plotting the Epidemiology of MS
Kurtzke, Journal of Neurology (1977)

John Kurtzke saw action in World War II as a pharmacist's mate. On discharge, he went to medical school and spent most of his professional life as a neurologist in the Veteran's Administration service. He wrote his first paper on MS in 1953[24] and is still publishing[25].

He is responsible for the industry-standard 'Kurtzke Scale' of disability[26] and he organised the first placebo-controlled clinical trial in MS[27]. But, his principal contribution has been the careful documentation and analysis of the varying prevalence of MS around the world and especially within the cohorts of US military personnel. Characteristic of his papers are a distrust of complex statistics and meticulously presented hand-drawn charts.

Kurtzke laid out the big picture of MS epidemiology and pointed out that the assertion of the day, that latitude determined MS prevalence, is incorrect. In Asia and the Pacific, latitude seemed not a factor at all and 'at 40° north, for example, MS is high in America, medium in Europe, and low in Asia'. In Europe and North America, there are zones of high frequency of MS between 65° and 45° north latitude. Neighbouring these (in Europe to the north, east and south; in the United States' southern region; and the remainder of Australia) are zones of medium frequency; everywhere else as of low frequency.

Measured serially in the same small region, Kurtzke asserted that the prevalence appears stable over time although our experience in East Anglia, United Kingdom, is different[28]. One area stands out as having a high prevalence of MS; this Fennoscandian focus: 'This clustering, as well as the broader geographic distributions already considered, mean to me that the occurrence of MS is intrinsically related to geography, and therefore that MS is an acquired, exogenous, environmental disease'. By comparing the age at which migration alters the risk of acquiring MS, he concluded that the key exposure occurs between the ages of 10 and 15 years, and that there is an 'incubation' period of some 20 years before the disease manifests. He then presented new data on the risk in veterans by race and gender, showing that it is greatest in white women. Thus, he concludes 'MS is the white man's burden spread from western Europe'. Kurtzke argued that if MS is due to an infectious agent, rather than a toxin, transmissibility should be evident. This is why he was so keen to discuss possible 'epidemics'. In 1977, he had just returned from a second visit to the Faroe Islands, where there seemed to be a cluster of new cases following the stationing of British troops. He was to visit the Faroes many more times, and has just recently advanced the idea that gastrointestinal infections mediated the transmission between British troops and Faroese[29], although this is a debated interpretation[30,31].

1981: The First Evidence Showing That MS Is Treatable: The End of the Beginning?
Jacobs et al., Science (1981)
'There is evidence that multiple sclerosis is caused (at least partially) by a viral infection of the central nervous system that acts as a 'trigger' for repeated exacerbations of neurologic symptoms characteristic of the disease. Interferon is a naturally occurring biologic product with potent antiviral activities. It does not cross the blood–brain barrier in significant quantity when administered systemically, but can be safely administered intrathecally'. So opens Larry Jacobs' landmark paper on the use of interferon in MS.

There are many problems with this paper. Its premise, that viral infections are the remedial cause, is probably incorrect; its analysis is flawed; and, rightly, it met with considerable controversy. However, it deserves selection because it introduced an intervention that does, to a degree, suppress disease activity; and, in Larry Jacobs, it introduced one pioneer of the disease modifying therapies, or 'DMTs'.

From the Roswell Park Memorial Institute (now Roswell Park Cancer Institute) in Buffalo, New York came the first evidence that interferons can ameliorate chronic active hepatitis and kill tumour cells *in vitro*[32]. At around that time, Larry Jacobs arrived as a young neurologist and with colleagues contemplated using interferon to treat amyotrophic lateral sclerosis, but soon turned to MS.

Verveken suggested that interferon had failed in previous studies[33,34] because it does not cross the blood–brain barrier, and suggested that administration should be intrathecal. Jacobs took up this suggestion, with a study group of 20 patients, four with relapsing-remitting disease, four with relapsing-progressive disease and 12 who were 'stable with residua'. Ten received natural interferon-beta by lumbar puncture, twice a week for 4 weeks, then monthly for 5 months. Ten patients were used as unblinded controls. Patients were followed up for over a year. At the end of the study, two of the interferon-treated patients had experienced four relapses, compared to ten relapses from six controls: for the first time, there was a hint that relapse rate in MS might be modified.

Jacobs' paper deserved some of the criticism that followed[35]. There are simple arithmetical errors in the tables and the primary outcome is not statistically significant, as was erroneously claimed. Jacobs' reliance on a change in relapse rate before and after treatment is potentially distorted by regression to mean.

However, the data were encouraging and more studies followed. He went on to produce a much more rigorous trial and did show a definite effect[36]. However, another trial had to be stopped early because it exacerbated rather than ameliorated disease activity[37]. Thereafter, interferons derived from recombinant technology were given systemically. Still there were problems. Recombinant interferon-alpha was shown to have no efficacy in 1986[38], and recombinant interferon-gamma (Immuneron, Biogen) provoked relapses[39]. However Ken Johnson, another key figure in the interferon story, managed to get interferon-beta 1b (Betaseron), licensed in 1993 following further positive studies[40].

1983: A Step towards Increased Diagnostic Accuracy
Poser et al., Annals of Neurology (1983)

Charles Poser wrote in 1965, 'many clinicians thus insist that there is, . . . in diagnosing MS, an . . . almost mystic diagnostic item frequently referred to as the "feel" or the "smell" of the patient, and which can best be characterized by the almost classical, pontifical pronouncement: 'Don't ask me why I think that this patient has MS, I just know!"'.[41]

Poser's motivation to introduce diagnostic criteria for MS was to improve the quality of epidemiological studies. In a classic paper in 1965[41] he asked 190 neurologists in 53 countries to read 30 case records and decide if they had 'probable', 'possible' or 'unlikely' MS. There was a consistent two-thirds diagnostic accuracy across the board of geography and experience. Somewhat embarrassingly, people regarded as MS experts performed rather worse than general neurologists and between individual diagnosticians there was a great deal of variety. He analysed symptoms and signs helpful in making the diagnosis from which he derived a rather complex scoring system to refine the clinician's suspicion of MS. Ultimately, Poser's scoring system was just too complex and it never took off.

In the United States, neurologists continued to use the Schumacher 1965 criteria; however, this focused just on the 'probable' group and did not incorporate the growing literature on paraclinical tests or imaging[42]. In the United Kingdom, the McDonald and Halliday criteria[30] gained favour, as they recognised the value of evoked potentials. Poser was not satisfied, so he set out in 1982 to come up with comprehensive diagnostic criteria for research. He gathered at Washington the luminaries of MS, including George Ebers, Ian MacDonald and Donald Paty. They proposed four categories of MS: 'clinically definite, laboratory-supported definite, clinically probable and laboratory-supported probable'. At last 'paraclinical' evidence of a lesion could be substituted for clinical evidence.

Poser's criteria lasted nearly two decades until replaced by the 2001 McDonald criteria[43], which were themselves modified in 2005 and, most recently, in 2010[44]. Much of Poser's thinking remains, but he did not agree with the elevation in importance of MRI; 'one of the big problems I see now is the numbers of patients who have minimal symptoms, and maybe some abnormal MRI findings, who have been treated for MS for years and who have never had it. I see people like this every week in my office'[45]. Of critical importance for the writers of the new McDonald is the ability to make the diagnosis as early as possible, to allow the introduction of therapies. So the absolute requirement for a second clinical attack has been dropped; instead, any new MRI disease activity after a clinically isolated syndrome now fulfils the criteria to diagnose MS. This process has reached its apotheosis under the 2010, where it is proposed that evidence of dissemination *in time* can be derived from a single MRI scan *during* a clinically isolated syndrome, if it shows the simultaneous presence of asymptomatic gadolinium-enhancing lesions and non-enhancing lesions at any time.

1988: Surrogate Markers in Life for Disease Activity in MS
Miller et al., Brain (1988)

Magnetic resonance imaging (MRI) of the brain has become an invaluable technique for the diagnosis and management of people with MS, as well as into research of its pathogenesis and treatment. The paper we have selected is not the first study of MS using MRI. But it is, in our view, the first to bring new understanding of the pathogenesis.

The importance of this study lies in the insights it gave to the natural history of MS, particularly to the realisation that there is continued disease activity even during periods of clinical stability. David Miller and colleagues sought to determine how to judge the age of an individual MRI lesion in order to help in two contexts: firstly, in the assessment of the patient with a clinically isolated syndrome (where lesions of different age would suggest dissemination in time and hence the probability of MS); and, secondly, in therapeutic trials. They turned to the recently developed paramagnetic agent, gadolinium DTPA.

Ten patients with MS were scanned initially, eight of whom were experiencing a relapse at the time. Fifty-six contrast enhancing lesions were observed in total compared to none in the two nonrelapsing patients. In six of eight patients, an enhancing lesion was seen which was anatomically congruent with the relapse phenotype. A second scan was performed between 3 and 5 weeks later in nine of these patients. Of the previous 54 enhancing lesions, only 12 persisted. But 12 new lesions had appeared. Six months later, eight patients were rescanned and 15 new lesions seen, of which eight showed enhancement. In passing, the authors note that some enhancing lesions were seen in the cortex, and one enhancing spinal cord lesion is shown.

For the first time the dynamics of plaque formation could be studied and some of the controversies arising from static pathological studies resolved. The observation that enhancement was seen as the first abnormality in every new lesion which appeared on interval scans placed breakdown of the blood–brain barrier as an initiating event. They suggested that the elevated T1/T2 ratio of enhancing lesions reflected the increased intracellular water associated with acute inflammation; and the low T1/2 ratio of old non-enhancing lesions might reflect increased extracellular water from leakage of an incompletely repaired blood–brain barrier. Cortical plaques, which were known from pathological studies but had not been seen on unenhanced scans could now be visualised.

For most contemporary readers, the big news was the revelations on the frequency of new lesions in people apparently with stable MS. This had several implications. For research, MRI provided a sensitive measure of brain inflammation. Another advance was that gadolinium-enhancing lesions could be used to reduce the duration and cohort sizes of clinical trials.

The findings of this paper were soon ratified. Henry McFarland at the National Institutes of Health (Bethesda) produced a study of six patients with 'early, mild, relapsing-remitting multiple sclerosis' scanned monthly for 8–11 months and showed that 'numerous enhancing lesions were observed irrespective of clinical activity'; and, again, suggested that these lesions be used as an outcome measure in clinical trials[46].

Conclusion

Forty years ago, multiple sclerosis was regarded by the average neurologist as uninteresting and untreatable, and those affected by the disease were left with little hope of cure or relief. Now, through work such as that we have mentioned here, we have: effective immunotherapies; agents which can promote remyelination in animals; a treasure trove of genetic associations and clues to environmental triggers to plunder for novel tractable pathways; and hope for neurologist and patient alike.

Key Outstanding Questions

1. Do the >50 established genetic associations identify a treatable pathological pathway?
2. What are the environmental triggers of multiple sclerosis (current candidates are low vitamin D, lack of sunshine, viral infections, and smoking)?
3. Is early and powerful suppression of inflammation in relapsing-remitting multiple sclerosis sufficient to prevent the progressive phase of the disease?
4. Why does remyelination fail in multiple sclerosis, and can this failure be prevented?

Key Research Centres

1. Institute of Neurology, London, United Kingdom
2. University of California San Francisco, United States
3. University of Cambridge, Cambridge, United Kingdom
4. Max Planck Institute of Neurobiology, Martinsried, Germany
5. University of Vienna, Vienna, Austria

References

Dawson, J.D. (1916) *The histology of disseminated sclerosis*. Trans. R. S. Edin. http://www.einstein.yu.edu/uploadedFiles/EJBM/21Maglione73.pdf

Gledhill, R.F., *et al.* (1973) Pattern of remyelination in the CNS. *Nature*, **244**(5416), 443–444. http://www.nature.com/nature/journal/v244/n5416/abs/244443a0.html

Halliday, A.M., *et al.* (1972) Delayed visual evoked response in optic neuritis. *Lancet*, **i**, 982–985. http://www.thelancet.com/journals/lancet/article/PIIS0140-6736 (72)91155-5/abstract

Jacobs, L., *et al.* (1981) Intrathecal interferon reduces exacerbations of multiple sclerosis. *Science*, **214**, 1026–1028. http://www.sciencemag.org/content/214/4524/1026.abstract

Kurtzke, J.F. (1977) Geography in multiple sclerosis. *Journal of Neurology*, **215**(1), 1–26. http://www.springerlink.com/content/n3022326nq5616u1/

Lowenthal, A., *et al.* (1960) The differential diagnosis of neurological diseases by fractionating electrophoretically the CSF proteins. *Journal of Neurochemistry*, **6**, 51–60. http://onlinelibrary.wiley.com/doi/10.1111/j.1471-4159.1960.tb13448.x/abstract

Miller, D.H., *et al.* (1988) Serial gadolinium enhanced magnetic resonance imaging in multiple sclerosis. *Brain*, **111**, 927–939. http://brain.oxfordjournals.org/content/111/4/927.abstract

Naito, S., *et al.* (1972) Multiple sclerosis: association with HL-A3. *Tissue Antigens*, **2**, 1–4. http://onlinelibrary.wiley.com/doi/10.1111/j.1399-0039.1972.tb00111.x/abstract

Poser, C.M., *et al.* (1983) New diagnostic criteria for multiple sclerosis: guidelines for research protocols. *Annals of Neurology*, **13**(3), 227–231. http://onlinelibrary.wiley.com/doi/10.1002/ana.410130302/abstract

Rose, A.S., *et al.* (1970) Cooperative study in the evaluation of therapy in multiple sclerosis: ACTH vs placebo: final report. *Neurology*, **20**, 1–59. http://www.neurology.org/content/20/5_Part_2.toc

Additional References

1. McDonald, W.I. (1999) Chance and design. *Journal of Neurology*, **246**(8), 654–660.
2. Williamson, R.T. (1894) The early pathological changes in disseminated sclerosis. *Medical Chronicle (Manchester)*, **19**, 373–379.
3. Muller, E. (1910) Über sensible Reizerscheinungen bei beginnender multipler sklerose. *NeurolischCentralblatt*, **29**, 17–20.
4. Charcot, J.-M. (1868) Histologie de la scl_erose en plaques. *Gazett Hôpitaux*, **41**, 554–558.
5. Huber, O. (1895) Zur patholüsschen Anatomie der multiplen Sklerose der Ruckenmarks. *Archiv für pathologïsche Anatomie*, **140**, 396–410.
6. Rindfleisch, E. (1863) Histologisches Detail zur grauen Degeneration von Gehirn und Rückenmark. *Archiv für pathologïsche Anatomie Physiol. Klin. Med.* (Virchow), **26**, 474–483.
7. Kabat, E.A., *et al.* (1942) An electrophoretic study of the protein components in cerebro-spinal fluid and their relationship to the serum proteins. *Journal of Clinical Investigation*, **21**(5), 571–577.
8. Link, H. (1972) Oligoclonal immunoglobulin G in multiple sclerosis brains. *Journal of the Neurological Sciences*, **16**(1), 103–114.
9. Cross, A.H., and Wu, G.F. (2010) Multiple sclerosis: oligoclonal bands still yield clues about multiple sclerosis. *Nature Reviews Neurology*, **6**(11), 588–589.
10. Milligan, N.M., *et al.* (1987) A double-blind controlled trial of high dose methylprednisolone in patients with multiple sclerosis: 1. Clinical effects. *Journal of Neurology, Neurosurgery & Psychiatry*, **50**(5), 511–516.
11. Beck, R.W., *et al.* (1992) A randomized, controlled trial of corticosteroids in the treatment of acute optic neuritis. The Optic Neuritis Study Group. *New England Journal of Medicine*, **326**(9), 581–588.

12. Halliday, A.M., and Wakefield, G.S. (1963) Cerebral evoked potentials in patients with dissociated sensory loss. *Journal of Neurology, Neurosurgery & Psychiatry*, **26**, 211–219.

13. McDonald, W.I., and Sears, T.A. (1970) Focal experimental demyelination in the central nervous system. *Brain*, **93**(3), 575–582.

14. Halliday, A.M., *et al.* (1973) Visual evoked response in diagnosis of multiple sclerosis. *British Medical Journal*, **4**(5893), 661–664.

15. McDonald, W.I., and Halliday, A.M. (1977) Diagnosis and classification of multiple sclerosis. *British Medical Bulletin*, **33**(1), 4–9.

16. Terasaki, P.I., and McClelland, J.D. (1964) Microdroplet assay of human serum cytotoxins. *Nature*, **204**, 998–1000.

17. Jersild, C., *et al.* (1972) HL-A antigens and multiple sclerosis. *Lancet*, **1**(7762), 1240–1241.

18. Compston, D.A., *et al.* (1976) B-lymphocyte alloantigens associated with multiple sclerosis. *Lancet*, **2**(7998), 1261–1265.

19. Terasaki, P.I., *et al.* (1976) Multiple sclerosis and high incidence of a B lymphocyte antigen. *Science*, **193**(4259), 1245–1247.

20. De Jager, P.L., *et al.* (2009) Meta-analysis of genome scans and replication identify CD6, IRF8 and TNFRSF1A as new multiple sclerosis susceptibility loci. *Nature Genetics*, **41**(7), 776–782.

21. Bunge, M.B., *et al.* (1961) Ultrastructural study of remyelination in an experimental lesion in adult cat spinal cord. *Journal of Biophysical and Biochemical Cytology*, **10**, 67–94.

22. Perier, O., and Gregoire, A. (1965) Electron microscopic features of multiple sclerosis lesions. *Brain*, **88**(5), 937–952.

23. Smith, E.J., *et al.* (1979) Central remyelination restores secure conduction. *Nature*, **280**(5721), 395–396.

24. Berlin, L., *et al.* (1953) Acute respiratory failure in multiple sclerosis and its management. *Journal of Nervous and Mental Disease*, **117**(2), 160–161.

25. McLeod, J.G., *et al.* (2011) Migration and multiple sclerosis in immigrants to Australia from United Kingdom and Ireland: a reassessment. I. Risk of MS by age at immigration. *Journal of Neurology*, 25 January.

26. Kurtzke, J.F. (1983) Rating neurologic impairment in multiple sclerosis: an expanded disability status scale (EDSS). *Neurology*, **33**(11), 1444–1452.

27. Berlin, L., and Kurtzke, J.F. (1957) Isoniazid in treatment of multiple sclerosis. *Journal of the American Medical Association*, **163**(3), 172–174.

28. Robertson, N., *et al.* (1996) Multiple sclerosis in south Cambridgeshire: incidence and prevalence based on a district register. *Journal of Epidemiology and Community Health*, **50**(3), 274–279.

29. Wallin, M.T., *et al.* (2010) Multiple sclerosis in the Faroe Islands. 8. Notifiable diseases. *Acta Neurologica Scandinavica*, **122**(2), 102–109.

30. Poser, C.M., and Hibberd, P.L. (1988) Analysis of the 'epidemic' of multiple sclerosis in the Faroe Islands. II. Biostatistical aspects. *Neuroepidemiology*, **7**(4), 181–189.

31. Poser, C.M., *et al.* (1988) Analysis of the 'epidemic' of multiple sclerosis in the Faroe Islands. I. Clinical and epidemiological aspects. *Neuroepidemiology*, **7**(4), 168–180.

32. Horoszewicz, J.S., *et al.* (1979) Noncycling tumor cells are sensitive targets for the antiproliferative activity of human interferon. *Science*, **206**(4422), 1091–1093.

33. Ververken, D., and Billiau, C.H. (1979) Intrathecal administration of interferon in MS patients. In: *Humoral immunology in neurological disease*. Ed. L.A. Karcher and A.D. Strosberg. Plenum, New York, 625–627.

34. Fog, T. (1980) Interferon treatment of multiple sclerosis patients: a pilot study. In: *Search for the cause of multiple sclerosis and other chronic disease of the nervous system*, 491–493. Verlag Chemie, Weinheim.

35. Berry, C.C. (1982) Intrathecal interferon for multiple sclerosis. *Science,* **217**(4556), 269–270.
36. Jacobs, L., *et al.* (1986) Multicentre double-blind study of effect of intrathecally administered natural human fibroblast interferon on exacerbations of multiple sclerosis. *Lancet,* **2** (8521–8522), 1411–1413.
37. Milanese, C., *et al.* (1990) Double blind study of intrathecal beta-interferon in multiple sclerosis: clinical and laboratory results. *Journal of Neurology, Neurosurgery & Psychiatry,* **53**(7), 554–557.
38. Camenga, D.L., *et al.* (1986) Systemic recombinant alpha-2 interferon therapy in relapsing multiple sclerosis. *Archives of Neurology,* **43**(12), 1239–1246.
39. Panitch, H.S., *et al.* (1987) Exacerbations of multiple sclerosis in patients treated with gamma interferon. *Lancet,* **1**(8538), 893–895.
40. IFNB Multiple Sclerosis Study Group (1993) Interferon beta-1b is effective in relapsing remitting multiple sclerosis. I. Clinical results of a multicenter, randomized, double-blind, placebo-controlled trial. IFNB Multiple Sclerosis Study Group. *Neurology,* **43**(4), 655–661.
41. Poser, C.M. (1965) Clinical diagnostic criteria in epidemiological studies of multiple sclerosis. *Annals of the New York Academy of Science,* **122**, 506–519.
42. Schumacher, G.A., *et al.* (1965) Problems of experimental trials of therapy in multiple sclerosis: report by the Panel on the Evaluation of Experimental Trials of Therapy in Multiple Sclerosis. *Annals of the New York Academy of Science,* **122**, 552–568.
43. McDonald, W.I., *et al.* (2001) Recommended diagnostic criteria for multiple sclerosis: guidelines from the International Panel on the diagnosis of multiple sclerosis. *Annals of Neurology,* **50**(1), 121–127.
44. Polman, C.H., *et al.* (2011) Diagnostic criteria for multiple sclerosis: 2010 revisions to the McDonald criteria. *Annals of Neurology,* **69**(2), 292–302.
45. Poser, C.M. (2006) Revisions to the 2001 McDonald diagnostic criteria. *Annals of Neurology,* **59**(4), 727–728.
46. Harris, J.O., *et al.* (1991) Serial gadolinium-enhanced magnetic resonance imaging scans in patients with early, relapsing-remitting multiple sclerosis: implications for clinical trials and natural history. *Annals of Neurology,* **29**(5), 548–555.

17 The Autoimmune Basis for Guillain-Barré Syndrome

John A. Goodfellow and Hugh J. Willison

Neuroimmunology Group, Division of Clinical Neuroscience, University of Glasgow, Glasgow, UK

Introduction

Guillain-Barré syndrome (GBS) is the most common cause of acute flaccid paralysis and affects approximately 1–2 per 100,000 population per year. The clinical presentation is very varied, but generally consists of an acute, symmetrical, ascending weakness of the limbs which can vary from mild to complete tetraplegia with respiratory failure. There are usually paraesthesias, pain and numbness. It is one of the few putative autoimmune diseases for which there is strong, comprehensive evidence of the auto-immune process. Here we will discuss the historically important studies that have led to the view that GBS consists of a number of distinct pathological subtypes with an autoimmune basis, and leave the reader with a larger conceptual framework with which to form and evaluate current and future research and clinical questions.

What Is Guillain-Barré Syndrome?

GBS is a clinical syndrome classically presenting as an acute flaccid ascending weakness with some sensory disturbance. Loss of tendon reflexes is the norm and there is a characteristically elevated CSF protein without a rise in white cells. Although the early descriptions refer to 'ascending paralysis', the distribution and progression of weakness is very variable; however, there is usually a general symmetry of weakness in legs and arms. There are numerous 'regional variants' where the weakness appears more focal, such as an oropharyngeal form or Miller Fisher syndrome (MFS) where the weakness is restricted to the extra-ocular muscles. There is often a history of a recent upper respiratory tract illness or diarrhoeal gastroenteritis within the previous month. Complications such as infections associated with respiratory and bulbar failure, auto-nomic instability and pulmonary emboli contribute to a mortality of around 5–10%, but around 80% of patients will have made an almost complete recovery at 12 months.

Describing the Syndrome
Guillain, Barré and Strohl, Bull. Soc. Méd. Hôp. Paris (1916)

In 1916 Georges Guillain, Jean Alexander Barré and Andre Strohl described a syndrome of acute ascending flaccid weakness in two French soldiers in the trenches of World War I. Although similar descriptions existed at the time, such as that of fellow

Understanding Medical Research: The Studies that Shaped Medicine, First Edition. Edited by John A. Goodfellow. © 2012 John Wiley & Sons, Ltd. Published 2012 by John Wiley & Sons, Ltd.

Frenchman Jean Landry, the important contribution they made was to take the recently developed technique of the lumbar puncture and describe a high level of CSF protein in the absence of a raised white cell count. This effectively excluded polio which at the time was a devastating and far more common cause of acute flaccid weakness. In true French fashion, they prescribed lamb chops and Bordeaux wine as therapy and both patients made a full recovery.

Defining the Pathology
Haymaker and Kernohan, Medicine (1949)

In 1949 Haymaker and Kernohan published a large 'clinic-pathological report' of 50 fatal cases of GBS. This was, and perhaps remains, one of the largest and most extensive studies on the pathology of GBS in humans. It solidified the concept that clinically variable subjects all had a similar underlying pathological process affecting the peripheral nerves and should be considered part of a spectrum. This turned contemporary debate away from discussing the minutiae of inclusion and exclusion criteria of distinct clinical subtypes and instead focused attention on understanding the disease process of clinically variable neuropathies. They proposed a pathological process whose earliest stages involved oedema and damage to peripheral nerves and nerve roots. Following this was an inflammatory infiltrate of lymphocytes and phagocytes that the authors suggested may have been secondary to the initial damage. Demyelination was observed and proposed to precede axonal degeneration which was also a prominent feature in these cases. A natural hypothesis that followed from this proposed schema was that there may be an infectious, immune or toxic factor that led to the initial oedema and nerve damage. By furthering the probability that GBS was an inflammatory disease of the peripheral nerves, this study brought the idea that it may be an infectious or post-infectious autoimmune phenomenon to the fore. As we shall see below, this notion has remained useful and in many ways was the conceptual ancestor of the modern theory that molecular mimicry with microbial antigens and the production auto-antibodies are major contributors to GBS pathology.

Waksman and Adams, Journal of Experimental Medicine (1955)

Six years later, Waksman and Adams described experimental allergic neuritis (EAN) for the first time in their mammoth 40-plus-page report published in the *Journal of Experimental Medicine*. A testimony to a time when medical journals were able to devote much space to baroque language and discussion, this carefully described animal model closely mirrored the clinical features of human GBS. Inspired by the existing model of experimental allergic encephalitis (still widely used for multiple sclerosis), the authors extracted various components of peripheral nerve myelin and immunised rabbits. The result was a dramatic and convincing post-immunisation, symmetrical, ascending paralysis. In their own words, it was 'one of the first laboratory models of non-infectious inflammatory disease of peripheral nerves' and bore 'certain resemblances to . . . Guillain-Barré syndrome'. The research community were similarly convinced, and it quickly became a model which would dominate research focus for over 40 years. EAN was, and remains, an attractive model of GBS for several reasons. Firstly it is difficult to dispute the similarity of clinical disease in the animal model with the human disease, even including the hallmark high CSF protein and low white cell counts. However, Waksman and Adams themselves cautioned that it is 'highly speculative that a disease of the PNS of a rabbit may be the same as a well known human disease merely because of a certain similarity of pathologic findings'. Secondly it was a relatively easily produced model that offered opportunity to scientifically investigate the disease process. Thirdly the inflammatory nature of the condition was broadly consistent with existing notions of the underlying pathological process in humans. It was *broadly* consistent in that Waksman and Adams clearly showed that their model was an inflammatory disease. However it was largely a T-cell mediated process and the cellular infiltration was seen at the earliest stages of the disease. This was slightly at odds with the scheme proposed by Haymaker and Kernohan who had envisioned the cellular response as being secondary. Nonetheless, an inflammatory disease of the peripheral nerves is what the research community had developed and they rightly began to explore it and its implications for human disease.

Asbury et al., Medicine (1969)

Following the widespread acceptance of the importance of T cells in mediating the primary damage in EAN, Adams went on to carry out a pathological study on humans in 1969. The authors were particularly interested in the role of T cells in human GBS. They were not disappointed by their findings from autopsies of 19 fatal cases. They found a prominent inflammatory infiltrate present at all stages of the disease, including in four patients who died within 7 days of disease onset. Asbury and colleagues proposed their own pathological sequence which differed in some important ways from that of the 1949 study. They suggested that there was no nerve damage until activated lymphocytes infiltrated nerve fibres and phagocytosed Schwann cells or excreted mediators of tissue damage. Severe demyelination led to axonal injury with distal denervation and possibly proximal cell body death. This sequence was based on their autopsy findings and would prove to be consistent with the major findings of studies on the neuroimmunology of EAN where the nerve damage is mediated by a T cell-dependent cellular immune response. It was later established that T cells activate macrophages which then phagocytose Schwann cells and secrete chemokines and nitric oxide which contribute to nerve damage.

This study brought about an overall shift in thinking about GBS. The humoral or toxic circulating factors suggested by Haymaker and Kernohan faded to the background as T cells became favoured and seen as the central pathological feature of the human disease and the driver of injury in the animal model. However, the basic idea of GBS as an autoimmune disease remained and the search began for auto-reactive T cells and a plausible trigger in human GBS. Over the next 30 years, this would be the dominant theory of the pathogenesis of GBS and today remains a very useful model of inflammatory demyelination of the peripheral nerves.

Saida et al., American Journal of Pathology (1979) and Science (1979)

Despite the dominance of the T cell hypothesis a number of groups continued to investigate the possibility that noncellular elements within the immune system were key factors in pathogenesis. Two studies published in 1979 can be seen as landmarks in establishing a theory of auto-antibody mediated peripheral nerve injury that was distinct from the recognised T cell mechanisms. In April Saida and Saida published a study in The

American Journal of Pathology in which they showed that intraneural injection of anti-GalC serum in Wistar rat sciatic nerve produced focal demyelination and 'an acute inflammatory reaction consisting of endoneurial oedema, polymorphonuclear cell infiltration and fibrin extravasation'. Later that year Saida and Saida reported in *Science* their version of EAN which was produced with immunisation with GalC. This model involved injecting bovine brain gangliosides repeatedly into rabbits, of which a proportion would then go on to develop a flaccid paralysis within months. The authors acknowledged that 'the possible role of cell-mediated immunity cannot be excluded' but emphasised that 'the absence of perivenular cuffing of small lymphocytes in early lesions in this study also support the concept that GalC-induced EAN may be primarily antibody-dependent rather than the result of tuberculin-like delayed hypersensitivity'.

Together these studies provided experimental grounds for arguing for a primary pathogenic role of antineuronal or antimyelin antibodies in inflammatory neuropathy. Although published in widely read journals, this particular model did not capture the imagination of the research community in the same way that the traditional EAN model did, and the T cell theory was still the dominant mode of thinking about human GBS. This was probably at least in part due to the uncertain existence or relevance of anti-GalC antibodies in human disease. Indeed it is generally thought that these particular antibodies may be a secondary epiphenomenon. Despite such concerns the basic idea of an antibody-mediated pathology remained attractive to some and most researchers now acknowledged the need to investigate this arm of the immune system in more detail.

Assessing Treatment
The Guillain-Barré Syndrome Study Group, Neurology (1985)
While debate continued as to the pathogenesis, efforts were also ongoing into establishing an effective treatment for GBS. In the early 1980s, a large multicentre randomised controlled trail comparing plasma exchange (PEx) and conservative treatment in GBS patients was carried out across several centres in the United States. The group reported their results in 1985, and the results established PEx as a valid and effective treatment as well as providing additional support to the notion that the humoral immune system was involved in pathogenesis. The study was prompted by three lines of circumstantial evidence: anecdotal reports of PEx being effective in GBS patients; the responsiveness of some patients with chronic inflammatory peripheral nerve disorders to PEx; and evidence of 'circulating factors in serum of GBS patients that impede peripheral nerve function in experimental studies'. Thus it was designed primarily to determine the effectiveness of a specific therapy but also to potentially address the longstanding question as to whether the humoral arm of the immune system is involved in the pathogenesis. The PEx group improved quicker and had better functional outcomes at 4 weeks and 6 months. Patients who required mechanical ventilation and those who received PEx within 7 days of onset particularly benefited from the treatment. PEx was also shown to be as safe as conventional treatment. It is thus widely accepted to have answered both research questions to some extent and certainly persuaded the authors of an editorial in the same issue to say that they would offer PEx to their patients in a similar clinical context.

The main criticism of the study is that it was not blinded. The authors understandably considered it unethical to perform sham PEx on critically ill patients so the study design was open to both placebo and unblinding biases. For example the clinical grading system that was used to rate patient improvement could have been affected by a placebo effect and unblinding. There were no electrophysiological tests carried out which might have offered an opportunity for blinding and a more objective assessment of outcome. However, electrophysiological assessment in GBS is often very variable and improvements or deterioration in these parameters do not always correlate with clinically important improvements. The lack of blinding remains a valid criticism of the study, and so the results were overall interpreted cautiously.

In addition, not all patients receiving PEx had the same replacement regime, and this was not taken into consideration in analysis of the results: some patients were reconstituted with plasma, some with reconstituted albumin solution. This led some to question whether PEx was beneficial because it *added* some factor to the patient rather than *removing* a putative pathogenic one. Again, this was probably a valid observation and the question of the pathogenesis of GBS remained unresolved. Subsequent large controlled trials would further demonstrate the effectiveness of both PEx and also that intravenous immune globulin (IVIg) is as effective but that there is no benefit from combining therapies[1]. Since IVIg is cheaper and more straightforward to administer than PEx it is now generally the first line treatment in GBS but remains a 'nonspecific' therapy.

Clinical Variants and Neuroimmunology
Feasby et al., Brain (1986)
In 1986 a Canadian group reported their findings from a combined clinical electrophysiological and autopsy study on five GBS patients. These five patients had clinically defined GBS with inexcitable nerve conduction, instead of the more commonly seen pattern of slowed conduction velocity consistent with widespread demyelination. One of these patients died in the acute phase of the illness and the autopsy was to reveal some findings that would radically change the way we understood GBS. Rather than finding the expected demyelination and florid inflammatory cell infiltration of peripheral nerves that had been the pathological hallmark of the disease since Kernohan and Haymaker in the 1940s and Asbury, Arnason and Adams in the 1960s, the investigators found severe axonal degeneration without inflammation or demyelination. They went on to argue whether that 'was a single clinical entity or multiple', whether there were any clinical criteria that would delineate subtypes and whether the pathogenesis was the same in different types. Some argued that the electrophysiological findings could be accounted for by an extensive distal demyelination and that there was only really one disease process and one type of GBS. Although the autopsy findings were difficult to place into this view the pathology was based on only one patient. Thus acute motor axonal neuropathy (AMAN) was born as a conceptual entity. This remained fairly speculative in the eyes of some, but this would soon change with a series of reports that both established AMAN as a real occurrence and direct attention to its autoimmune basis.

Chiba et al., Annals of Neurology (1992)
Another rare clinical variant of GBS, Miller Fisher syndrome (MFS), soon came to the forefront of research in the early 1990s. In 1992 Chiba and colleagues at the University of Tokyo in Japan reported the presence an antiganglioside antibody in six patients

with MFS. Antiganglioside antibodies had been described previously in GBS, but they were found only in a minority of patients and the association with disease was unclear. This report identified anti-GQ1b antibodies as the serological hallmark of this rare form of GBS, being present in all patients. In 1956 the famous stroke physician Miller Fisher described the triad of ataxia, areflexia and ophthalmoplegia in a case report in the *New England Journal of Medicine*[2]. He postulated that it was of the same aetiology of GBS except that the nerve damage was restricted to the extra-ocular motor nerves. In clinical practice there is considerable of overlap between classical GBS and patients with ocular, bulbar and generalised weakness and so the description of a highly specific and sensitive serological marker in what was seen as a regional variant of GBS was hugely significant. In this 1992 report, Chiba demonstrated an increase in serum anti-GQ1b antibody in the early phase which reduced with time. The authors proposed it as a diagnostic marker (and it remains a useful diagnostic test in MFS) and argued that it could be pathogenic. Although MFS is rare and makes up less than 10% of GBS cases, this connection with anti-GQ1b antibodies (later shown to be present in over 95% of cases) and subsequent studies on this syndrome have yielded many insights into the pathogenesis of GBS. It led the way to the discovery that there is a regional variation in the expression of gangliosides within the peripheral nervous system, with GQ1b being enriched in the extra-ocular nerves and muscle spindles and sparse in other nerves. This beautifully explains the correlation between antibody specificity and clinical symptoms in MFS. Further studies explored the distribution of other gangliosides and found that GM1 and GD1a are more highly expressed in motor than in sensory nerves and roots and GD1b more highly expressed in sensory than in motor. Much of the clinical heterogeneity of human GBS is now ascribed to regional and individual differences in ganglioside expression levels and fine specificity of antibodies, a concept first developed from observations on this rare clinical variant (Figure 17.1).

Yuki et al., Journal of Experimental Medicine (1993)

Shortly after the Chiba's report of anti-GQ1b antibodies in MFS, another Japanese group reported a case of GBS in which they detected elevated levels of anti-GM1 antibodies and for the first time directly linked this to a preceding infection. Their patient had had watery diarrhoea for 4 days, and then 6 days after this resolved he developed the cardinal features of GBS: ascending flaccid weakness, areflexia and high CSF protein with normal cellularity. Electrophysiological tests revealed a predominantly motor axonal neuropathy, thus confirming a diagnosis of AMAN. They then confirmed *C. jejuni* infection by showing a fourfold rise in level of anti-*C. jejuni* antibody and by culturing it from a stool sample. This culture was identified as being Penner type O:19, a relatively rarer strain which subsequent studies would show is more common as a preceding agent in patients who develop GBS. This was grown and the lipopolysaccharide (LPS) was purified and, using a combination of mass spectrometry and NMR spectroscopy, its structure was shown to contain a terminal tetrasaccharide identical to the human ganglioside GM1. The authors then went on to 'speculate that infection by C. jejuni (PEN 19) induces high production of anti-GM1 antibody in patients with an immunogenetic background, thereby leading to the abolishment of tolerance, and that the anti-GM1 antibody binds to motor nerve terminals causing motoneuron inexcitability and the eventual development of muscular weakness' and that their results 'should be of use in establishing the mechanism of the pathogenesis of GBS after infection as well as the mechanisms of other

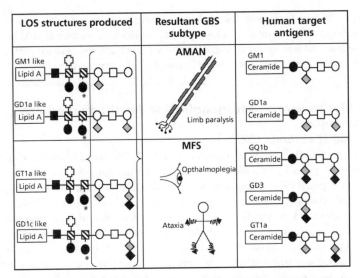

Figure 17.1 Lipo-oligosaccharides (LOS) produced by GBS-associated strains of *C. jejuni*, resultant GBS subtypes and human target antigens. *C. jejuni* strains produce LOS with ganglioside-like moieties attached to a lipid A core. The clinical subtype of GBS depends upon which ganglioside-like moiety is present and on the anatomical distribution of gangliosides. Adapted with permission from Rinaldi and Willison, *Current Opinion in Neurology*, 2008, **21**, 540–546.

autoimmune diseases'. Although Campylobacter-asscociated GBS had been previously reported by Tattersfield[3] and other infections were known to precede GBS, the development of the concepts of AMAN, *C. jejuni* infection, and pathogenic antiganglioside antibodies thus paved the way for this first clear demonstration of how molecular mimicry could underlie human GBS. It was a tantalising case report which highlights how single cases can still have a significant contribution to medical research as it opened the gate to a flood of larger studies which would further link infectious agents, antiganglioside antibodies and clinical subtypes.

Hafer-Macko et al., Annals of Neurology (1996)

Ten years after Feasby introduced the controversial concept of AMAN, a group at Johns Hopkins produced a detailed pathological study on seven fatal cases arsing in relation to an extensive studied cohort of paediatric GBS cases in Hebei Province, China. This Hopkins–Hebei partnership has provided us with many remarkable insights into GBS pathogenesis. By this time the existence of the subtype was more firmly established and the link with preceding *C. jejuni* infection and the production of antiganglioside antibodies was surfacing as an attractive autoimmune mechanism. In their analysis of the autopsy tissue, the authors found IgG and complement deposition along the axolemma of motor fibres, particularly at the nodes of Ranvier, prior to the development of Wallerian-like degeneration. Myelin remained intact as macrophages 'were recruited into the affected nodes' where they 'dissected into the internodal periaxonal space'. In an important step in the development of the B-cell theory of GBS, the investigators argued that 'simple binding of antibody, alone or with subsequent activation of complement at the nodes of motor fibres, can be sufficient to impair conduction'. The thinking on human GBS had thus come full circle and resounded with the 1949 hypothesis of Haymaker and Kernohan: at least a proportion of GBS patients were seen as having a primarily axonal neuropathy mediated by soluble factors (antibody and complement) in which cellular infiltration was scant or a secondary phenomenon.

The Mechanism of Antiganglioside Antibody-mediated Nerve Injury
Halstead et al., Brain (2008)

The most clinically relevant animal model of AMAN is probably one developed by Japanese groups led by Yuki and Kusunoki. This depends upon chronic administration of purified gangliosides to Japanese white rabbits to produce a flaccid monophasic weakness[4] or an ataxic syndrome[5]. In these models sensitised animals developed high titres of anti-GM1 or anti-GD1b IgG antibodies, acute flaccid limb weakness, IgG deposition on motor axons and Wallerian-like degeneration of peripheral nerves without prominent demyelination or inflammation. Although a persuasive replication of the clinical and pathological entity, this model does not strictly speaking directly demonstrate or explore the pathogenic action antiganglioside antibodies. It provides a fairly comprehensive account of the pathogenesis of GBS, but there are two important areas in which it is somewhat limited. The trigger in the animal model is the administration of purified ganglioside, which obviously is not a part of the human condition and it therefore does not address the crucial initiating events in GBS. Secondly, it has not been extensively used to uncover the precise pathogenic actions of antiganglioside antibodies.

Another model developed largely in the United Kingdom and the Netherlands has been used to describe the mechanisms of antiganglioside antibody-mediated nerve injury.

In this model Hugh Willison, Jaap Plomp and colleagues used certain relatively rare serotypes of *C. jejuni* more commonly found in patients with GBS that had lipopolysaccharides structures with epitopes identical to various gangliosides to produce antiganglioside antibodies in mice. Over several studies they went on to show that the antibodies damaged nerve terminals by binding and activating the complement cascade. Their 2001 publication in Brain is an important landmark in establishing the pathogenic action of anti-GQ1b antibodies[6] and a 2005 paper established that anti-GD1a antibodies, the serological hallmark of AMAN, have a similar pathogenic potential[7]. This model employed *ex vivo* neuromuscular preparations to demonstrate nerve injury and so there was no robust clinical phenotype. Nonetheless, it remained a powerful proof-of-principle for the pathological potential of antiganglioside antibodies and complements Yuki's rabbit model.

The natural next step was to develop novel strategies for treatment of the autoantibody-mediated injury and in 2008 Halstead and colleagues published such a study. In this study, Halstead produced an *in vivo* model in the mouse using monoclonal anti-GQ1b antibodies derived from mice immunised with LPS from *C. jejuni* strains associated with MFS. As in the *ex vivo* model, Halstead again demonstrated that this *in vivo* injury was dependent upon antibody binding and activation of the terminal complement complex and, significantly, also showed that use of the therapeutic compound eculizumab (a humanised mouse monoclonal antibody which prevents the formation of the terminal complement complex) prevented the electrophysiological and morphological injury to motor nerves and stopped the development of respiratory paralysis. The editors highlighted it as a milestone in the study of autoimmune neuropathy that has now set the stage for the first clinical trials for a specific therapy every bit as inventive as Guillain, Barré and Strohl's prescription of lamb chops and Bordeaux.

Summary and Conclusions

Our understanding of human Guillain-Barré syndrome has advanced considerably since 1916 when Guillain, Barré and Strohl described their two patients with the condition that now bears their name. Debate from autopsy and electrophysiological studies has led us to understand it as having an underlying spectrum of pathological changes and that different subtypes correlate well with different auto-antibodies. The establishment of EAN as an animal model in the 1950s led to a wealth of information on the molecular pathogenesis of inflammatory neuropathies and it continues to be widely used today. The early hypothesis of a circulating, soluble immune factor that may contribute to injury initially did not lead to much fruitful research. However, combined with the increasing evidence for a post-infectious trigger from *C.jejuni* and the various lines of evidence for an underlying autoimmune basis for the axonal form of GBS, the antiganglioside antibody-mediated model of nerve injury has begun to be more widely accepted and has now been used to test putative novel therapies. We now await human clinical trials of rational, specific immunotherapy in Guillain-Barré syndrome.

Key Outstanding Questions

1. Is there a specific auto-antibody that is associated with AIDP, the main form of GBS?
2. Why do some individuals produce antiganglioside antibodies in response to *C. jejuni* infection while others do not? Why does their immune system still have these self-reactive antibodies?
3. To what extent is the cellular arm of the immune system responsible for the demyelination and axonal injury seen in human GBS?
4. Are there any specific immunotherapeutic strategies available for patients with GBS that are more effective than, or avoid the adverse risks of, IVIg or plasma exchange?

Key Research Centres

1. Prof Willison, Neuroimmunology Research Group, Division of Clinical Neurosciences, University of Glasgow, Glasgow, United Kingdom
2. GBS Research Group, Department of Neurology, Academic Hospital Rotterdam, Rotterdam, Netherlands
3. Kusunoki Reaseach Group, Kinki University School of Medicine, Osaka, Japan
4. Peripheral Nerve Centre, Johns Hopkins School of Medicine, Baltimore, Maryland, United States

References

Asbury, A.K., *et al.* (1969) The inflammatory lesion in idiopathic polyneuritis: its role in pathogenesis. *Medicine (Baltimore)*, **48**(3), 173–215. http://journals.lww.com/md-journal/Citation/1969/05000/The_Inflammatory_Lesion_in_Idiopathic_Polyneuritis.1.aspx

Chiba, A., *et al.* (1992) Serum IgG antibody to ganglioside GQ1b is a possible marker of Miller Fisher syndrome. *Annals of Neurology*, **31**(6), 677–679. http://onlinelibrary.wiley.com/doi/ 10.1002/ana.410310619/abstract

Feasby, T.E., *et al.* (1986) An acute axonal form of Guillain-Barre polyneuropathy. *Brain*, **109**(6), 1115–1126. http://brain.oxfordjournals.org/content/109/6/1115.abstract

Guillain, G., *et al.* (1916) Sur un syndrome de radiculo-nérvrite avec hyperalbuminose du liquid céphalorachidien sans réaction cellulaire. Remarques sur les caractères cliniques et graphiques des réflexes tendineux. *Bulletin de la Société Médicale des Hôpitaux de Paris*, **40**, 1462–1470.

The Guillain-Barré Syndrome Study Group (1985) Plasmapheresis and acute Guillain-Barre syndrome. The Guillain-Barre Syndrome Study Group. *Neurology*, **35**(8), 1096–1104. http:// www.neurology.org/content/35/8/1096.abstract

Hafer-Macko, C., *et al.* (1996) Acute motor axonal neuropathy: an antibody-mediated attack on axolemma. *Annals of Neurology*, **40**(4), 635–644. http://onlinelibrary.wiley.com/doi/10.1002/ ana.410400414/abstract

Halstead, S.K., *et al.* (2008) Eculizumab prevents anti-ganglioside antibody-mediated neuropathy in a murine model. *Brain*, **131**(5), 1197–1208. http://www.ncbi.nlm.nih.gov/pubmed/18184663

Haymaker, W.E., and Kernohan, J.W. (1949) The Landry-Guillain-Barré syndrome; a clinico-pathologic report of 50 fatal cases and a critique of the literature. *Medicine (Baltimore)*, **28**(1), 59–141. http://journals.lww.com/md-journal/Citation/1949/02000/The_Landry_Guillain_ Barre_Syndrome__A.3.aspx

Saida, T., *et al.* (1979) Experimental allergic neuritis induced by sensitisation with galactocerebro-side. *Science*, **204**(4397), 1103–1106. http://www.sciencemag.org/content/204/4397/1103.abstract

Saida, K., *et al.* (1979) In vivo demyelination induced by intraneural injection of anti-galactocerebroside serum: a morphologic study. *American Journal of Pathology*, **95**(1), 99–116. http://www.ncbi.nlm.nih.gov/pmc/articles/PMC2042286/?tool=pubmed

Waksman, B.H., and Adams, R.D. (1955) Allergic neuritis: an experimental disease of rabbits indu-ced by the injection of peripheral nervous tissue and adjuvants. *Journal of Experimental Medicine*, **102**(2), 213–236. http://www.ncbi.nlm.nih.gov/pmc/articles/PMC2136504/?tool=pubmed

Yuki, N., *et al.* (1993) A bacterium lipopolysaccharide that elicits Guillain-Barre syndrome has a GM1 ganglioside-like structure. *Journal of Experimental Medicine*, **178**, 1771–1775. http:// www.ncbi.nlm.nih.gov/pmc/articles/PMC2191246/?tool=pubmed

Additional References

1. Hughes, R.A., *et al.* (2007) Immunotherapy for Guillain-Barré syndrome: a systematic review. *Brain*, **130**(9), 2245–2257.

2. Fisher, M. (1956) An unusual variant of acute idiopathic polyneuritis (syndrome of ophthalmoplegia, ataxia and areflexia). *New England Journal of Medicine*, **255**(2), 57–65.

3. Rhodes, K.M., and Tattersfield, A.E. (1982) Guillain-Barré syndrome associated with Campylobacter infection. *British Medical Journal*, **285**(6336), 173–174.

4. Yuki, N., *et al.* (2001) Animal model of axonal Guillain-Barré syndrome induced by sensitization with GM1 ganglioside. *Annals of Neurology*, **49**(6), 712–720.

5. Kusunoki, S., *et al.* (1996) Experimental sensory neuropathy induced by sensitisation with ganglioside GD1b. *Annals of Neurology*, **39**(4), 424–431.

6. O'Hanlon, G.M., *et al.* (2001) Anti-GQ1b ganglioside antibodies mediate complement-dependent destruction of the motor nerve terminal. *Brain*, **124**(5), 893–906.

7. Goodfellow, J.A., *et al.* (2005) Overexpression of GD1a ganglioside sensitizes motor nerve terminals to anti-GD1a antibody-mediated injury in a model of acute motor axonal neuropathy. *Journal of Neuroscience*, **25**(7), 1620–1628.

18 Helicobacter pylori, Peptic Ulcers and Gastric Cancer

Anahita Dua[1] and Emad M. El-Omar[2]

[1]Department of General Surgery, Medical College of Wisconsin, Milwaukee, USA
[2]Gastrointestinal Group, Institute of Medical Sciences, School of Medicine & Dentistry, Aberdeen University, Aberdeen, UK

Introduction

Dyspeptic disorders probably date back to the dawn of time, but actual gastric and duodenal ulcers were first demonstrated on autopsy in the late 17th and early 18th centuries respectively. With industrialisation in the early 20th century, peptic ulcers, and their serious complications of bleeding, perforation and gastric outlet obstruction, became a scourge of modern life. Ulcers were synonymous with a stressful life characterised by excessive smoking, hard work and near mental breakdown. The assumption since the beginning of the 20th century was that ulcers were caused by excessive gastric acid and the famous Schwartz dogma of 'no acid no ulcer', that dated back to 1910, was the accepted wisdom. This 'physiological' explanation of peptic ulcers made sense and fitted the established new discoveries related to control of gastric acid secretion. Many academic chairs in many distinguished universities were established on the back of work delineating the pathophysiology of peptic ulcers.

The obsession with acid initially led to a surgical revolution that saw millions of desperate patients undergo major surgical procedures such as partial gastrectomy, vagotomy with drainage and later highly selective vagotomy. Such procedures were designed to corrupt the acid secretory capacity of the stomach but with side effects that left many patients with worse problems. In the early seventies a pharmacological revolution took over the management of this disease. The discovery of histamine-2 (H_2) receptors and how to antagonise them by the late Sir James Black was a defining moment. Several pharmacological companies soon invested heavily in this advance and the world was introduced to H_2 antagonists and later proton pump inhibitors (PPIs). These drugs profoundly inhibit acid secretion and heal ulcers effectively. However, upon cessation of treatment, ulcers quickly recurred and patients were essentially sentenced to a lifetime of dependence on medication or the threat of major surgery. The economic cost of managing such patients was phenomenal.

In the early 1980s, an unknown registrar in gastroenterology (Barry Marshall) working in Perth, Western Australia was looking for a research project to complement his clinical training. He was given a choice of working with an unknown but astute pathologist (Robin Warren). Warren had been claiming that he could see bacteria in biopsies of patients with gastritis and peptic ulcers. At the time this was considered a scientific heresy and this pathologist kept his thoughts to himself. Marshall was quite intrigued by this

Understanding Medical Research: The Studies that Shaped Medicine, First Edition. Edited by John A. Goodfellow. © 2012 John Wiley & Sons, Ltd. Published 2012 by John Wiley & Sons, Ltd.

observation and decided, thankfully, to take on this project. The rest as they say was history. Little did these two 'unknown' doctors know at the time, but the story of *Helicobacter pylori* was born and culminated in the award of the Nobel Prize for Medicine to these two pioneers. The choice of our first paper therefore must acknowledge this momentous development.

An Infectious Theory
Marshall and Warren, Lancet (1984)

In 1984 Marshall and Warren described 'unidentified curved bacilli in the stomach of patients with gastritis and peptic ulceration'. They designed a small pilot study of 20 patients in order to support their hypothesis that there was an association between antral gastritis and bacteria. They found that over half their biopsy specimens contained this unnamed curved bacilli and there seemed to be an association between the number of bacilli and severity of the gastritis. This was enough to convince Marshall and Warren who then set out to 'confirm the association between antral gastritis and the bacteria, to discover associated gastrointestinal diseases, to culture and identify the bacteria, and to find factors predisposing to infection'. Biopsy specimens were taken from 100 consecutive patients who presented for gastroscopy. Patients filled out a questionnaire relating to gastritis symptoms, which showed that the only symptom that correlated with gastritis was 'burping'. The real excitement came from the biopsy specimens which demonstrated spiral or curved bacilli in 58 patients. The bacilli cultured from 11 of those biopsies were Gram-negative, flagellate, microaerophilic and related to the genus Campylobacter. It was notable that the bacilli were present in 38 of the 40 patients with active chronic gastritis, DU or gastric ulcer. However, the bacteria were detected in only 2 of 31 patients with no inflammation. The authors were surprised to find that peptic ulcer was the only endoscopic finding associated with histological gastritis and what they termed 'pyloric campylobacter'. They concluded that this Campylobacter bacillus (which they incorrectly named as *Campylobacter pyloridis*) was an important factor in the aetiology of these gastrointestinal diseases but were clear in stating their uncertainty as to the role in pathophysiology.

There were many critics of this work and the majority remained sceptical. The main criticism was that it was purely descriptive, lacked insight into pathogenesis and did not fulfil Koch's postulates for causation. Frustrated by the lack of acceptance, which in all honesty was justified at that time, Marshall embarked on a remarkable experiment.

The Human Guinea Pig and Koch's Postulates
Marshall et al., Medical Journal of Australia (1985)

Marshall argued that the only way he could convince sceptics that his discovery was genuine was if a human ingested the bacterium and could show that it induced gastritis in a previously normal stomach. There was ever going to be one volunteer for this landmark experiment: Marshall himself. Unbeknown to his wife, he had decided to act as his own guinea pig. Crucially, he had established prior to ingesting the culture medium that his stomach was histologically normal. He then simply walked into the microbiology lab, obtained the pure bacterial culture and gulped it! A mild illness developed, which lasted

14 days. On the tenth day after the ingestion of bacteria, histologically proven gastritis was present, by the second week 'several colleagues observed that he developed "putrid" breath' and by day 14 this had largely resolved. The paper describes nicely the syndrome of acute pyloric campylobacter gastritis. For the first time ingestion of a pure bacterial culture could be shown to cause gastric inflammation. He proposed that this disorder may progress to a chronic infection predisposing to peptic ulceration.

Many papers started to appear looking at the prevalence of this organism in different upper gastrointestinal diseases and in healthy populations. It was estimated that half the world's population was colonised by these organisms. It also became clear that duodenal and gastric ulcers that were not caused by aspirin or nonsteroidal anti-inflammatory drugs (NSAIDs) were invariably associated with this infection. In other words, while half the world had the infection, all ulcer patients were essentially colonised. By that stage, the original *Campylobacter pyloridis* had undergone two name changes. Initially it was changed to *Campylobacter pylori*, but it was soon realised that it was not in fact a *Campylobacter* and justified classification into a new genus as *Helicobacter pylori* (*H.pylori*). We will hereafter refer to the infection by its ultimate and correct name. The crucial question now was to explain how this gastric disease can cause ulceration in the upper gastrointestinal tract.

How Does an Infection in the Antrum Cause Ulcers in the Duodenum? The Gastrin Link
Levi et al., Lancet (1989)

It was known that duodenal ulcer patients produce excessive amounts of gastric acid due to a large parietal cell mass. Parietal cells are present in the corpus of the stomach and secrete gastric acid in response to the hormone gastrin released from the G cells residing in the antrum. Gastrin is a meal-stimulated hormone that drives the major part of gastric acid secretion. In this paper John Calam and his group at the Hammersmith, London, demonstrated that antral colonisation by *H. pylori* causes a significant rise in basal and meal-stimulated gastrin secretion. This gastrin link was crucial and paved the way for discovering the full pathophysiology of *H. pylori*-induced peptic ulcer disease. They studied 31 DU patients and determined *H. pylori* status, plasma gastrin levels and gastric acid secretion. Of the 31 patients, 25 were colonised with *H. pylori* and had a higher basal and meal-stimulated plasma gastrin concentration along with a higher peak acid output as compared to the 6 patients who were not colonised. They proposed that *H. pylori* infection in the gastric antrum increased antral gastrin release and hypothesised that *H. pylori* organisms use their urease enzyme to split urea and generate alkaline ammonia. The alkaline cloud surrounding the organism protects it from the acidic environment but also has a profound physiological effect: normally gastrin release is inhibited by a fall in gastric pH, which prevents excessive acid from being secreted. If the pH of the gastric mucus layer is increased by the ammonia generated by *Helicobacter*'s urease enzyme the stomach would consequently secrete more acid. While this hypothesis turned out to be somewhat inaccurate, it stimulated several key studies that finally outlined the key pathophysiology of ulcers.

For a start, the level of hypergastrinaemia induced by *H. pylori* infection was the same in ulcer patients compared to infected healthy volunteers. Why then were ulcer patients producing so much acid in response to the same degree of hypergastrinaemia? Equally, what would happen if the infection was eradicated? Would the hypergastrinaemia normalise, and would that have an effect on gastric acid secretion? These questions were essential for understanding the pathophysiology of ulcers and for offering a permanent cure for the disease. The next paper perhaps contributed the most to understanding these basic pathophysiological events.

What Is the Effect of *Helicobacter pylori* on Gastric Physiology?
El-Omar et al., Gastroenterology (1995)

A sizeable part of the work on the effect of *H. pylori* on gastric physiology was uncovered by Professor McColl's team in Glasgow, United Kingdom. They had been engaged in some friendly competition with the Calam group at the Hammersmith and this was an exciting period that contributed some valuable insight. McColl's team studied *H. pylori* infected DU patients and infected and uninfected healthy volunteers. They also studied infected subjects (DU and healthy) before and after eradication. A major obstacle was the lack of an easy and reproducible test of meal-stimulated acid secretion. Available tests were cumbersome and lacked the sensitivity to detect subtle changes in acid secretion that may result from eradication. El-Omar and colleagues developed an alternative test that relied on intravenous administration of gastrin releasing peptide (GRP). GRP is naturally produced by the stomach in response to the presence of food and in turn causes the release of gastrin. By giving this intravenously, one could mimic the effects of a meal without the disadvantage of the presence of food within the stomach and hence have an easier and more reliable ability to measure the stimulated acid secretion. This GRP test allowed the team to answer the above questions. When compared to the *H. pylori*-negative healthy subjects, patients who had both DU and *H. pylori* infection demonstrated the following abnormalities: (1) threefold increase in basal acid output, (2) sixfold increase in acid response to GRP, (3) increased maximal acid response to exogenous gastrin, (4) increased ratio of basal acid output to maximal gastrin-stimulated output and (5) increased ratio of maximal GRP-stimulated acid output to maximal gastrin-stimulated output. All of these abnormalities resolved completely following successful eradication of *H. pylori*, except for the increased maximal acid output to gastrin which was unchanged. The authors concluded that these infection-induced acid secretory disturbances were consistent with impaired inhibitory control and the basis of the mechanism by which *H. pylori* predisposes to DU.

The full story is now generally accepted as the following: *H. pylori* infection causes inflammation in the antrum with release of proinflammatory cytokines causing an increase in gastrin release and a reduction in its antagonist and inhibitor somatostatin. The net effect is that acid secretion in subjects with a large parietal cell mass is markedly increased and bicarbonate secretion is reduced. The delivery of large amounts of acid into the unprotected duodenum is harmful and can lead to inflammation and damage. In response to this constant injury the duodenum undergoes a protective metaplasia with development of several patches of gastric type mucosa. Gastric metaplasia within the duodenum leads to further colonisation by *H. pylori* organisms from the adjacent antrum, leading to inflammation in these metaplastic patches and a weakening of the defences. Peptic ulcers invariably form in such patches. Thus we finally have an explanation as to why ulcers form in areas that appear well away from the site of original infection.

Crucially, eradication of the infection leads to normalisation of the physiological abnormalities and a return to normal acid secretion. This explains why eradicating the infection offers a permanent cure compared to the near inevitable recurrence seen with the use of anti-secretory drugs. At the end of all of this we have gone a full circle! First it was thought that acid caused ulcers (Schwarz dogma), then an infection caused ulcers (the pylorites) and finally we have an infection that causes increased acid as the most likely scenario! The race was now on to see if (1) antibiotics could kill the bacterium and (2) whether this would help ulcer patients.

A Simple Treatment That Cures Ulcers?
Hentschel et al., New England Journal of Medicine (1993)

By 1993 a few eradication regimens had been tried with variable success. There was a raging debate about the best choice of treatment for *H. pylori* infection. Marshall and others had advocated the choice of bismuth, which had established anti-ulcer effects and was also antimicrobial. Thus, although bismuth was certainly effective in reducing the rate of recurrence of DUs, it was unclear whether this was due to its antimicrobial effects or to its direct cytoprotective effects on the gastroduodenal mucosa. This was an important question because, left unanswered, it meant one could not say with certainty that *H. pylori* eradication *per se* was a necessary part in curing the diathesis. Equally, everyone knew that DUs had a high recurrence rate, and it was essential to prove that recurrence was no longer a problem after eradication. Hentschel and colleagues addressed these questions in this landmark paper. They randomised 104 *H. pylori* infected patients with recurrent DUs to either a treatment group of amoxicillin plus metronidazole or placebos taken orally over a 12-day period. All patients were given ranitidine cover for 6 or 10 weeks. Patients underwent endoscopy once prior to treatment and then periodically during the 12 month follow-up. This was a double-blind, randomised controlled trial and the results were staggering. Of the 52 patients randomised to the antibiotic arm, 46 had successful eradication of the infection compared with only 1 of the 52 who received the placebo. Ulcers were healed in 6 weeks in 92% of patients on the antibiotics arm of the study versus 75% on the placebo arm. At 12 months of follow-up, DUs recurred in only 4 of the 50 patients given antibiotics and in 42 of the 49 given placebo. Ulcers recurred in 1 of 46 patients in whom *H. pylori* had been eradicated, and in 45 of 53 in whom *H. pylori* persisted. The authors concluded that 'In patients with recurrent duodenal ulcer, eradication of *H. pylori* by a regimen that does not have any direct action on the mucosa is followed by a marked reduction in the rate of recurrence, suggesting a causal role for *H. pylori* in recurrent duodenal ulcer'.

The clinical and economic impact of this paper was phenomenal. By today's standards perhaps the power of the study was rather modest, but very few treatments that are so simple and cheap have been shown to be so effective at curing a major human disease. The pharmaceutical companies that had made billions from anti-secretory medications were rightly worried! Peptic ulcer disease, for so long a scourge of modern life, is an infectious disease that *can be cured* by simple and cheap antibiotics. Marshall and Warren were vindicated, and their hands were firmly heading for the Nobel Prize.

The Power of the NIH Consensus Statements
'Helicobacter pylori in Peptic Ulcer Disease', NIH Consensus Statement (1994)

After a decade of hard work since the 1984 *Lancet* paper, there was a need for leadership to bring about a wide-scale change in medical practice in relation to PUD. In 1994 the National Institute of Health (NIH) commissioned a consensus development conference on the role of *H. pylori* in PUD which brought together gastroenterologists, surgeons, infectious disease specialists, epidemiologists, pathologists and even members of the public to address six fundamental questions, as detailed below. The resulting statement was very cautious, was evidence based and provided for the first time clear management guidance.

1. What is the causal relationship of *H. pylori* to upper gastrointestinal disease?

The panel concluded that a causal relationship was hard to establish between *H. pylori* and PUD, due to the lack of animal model and because only a small portion of patients colonised by the bacteria develop ulceration. These doubts were answered by the development of several animal models that reproduced the disease. There is now no reasonable doubt that *H. pylori* infection causes peptic ulcers.

2. How does one diagnose and eradicate *H. pylori* infection?

They concluded that invasive tests including endoscopy with a gastric biopsy, biopsy with direct detection of urease activity in the tissue specimen, and biopsy with a culture of the *H. pylori* organism were all suitable. However, non-invasive tests that are highly sensitive and specific, namely serology for immunoglobulin G antibodies to *H. pylori* antigens and breath tests of urease activity using orally administered C14- or C13-labeled urea, should also be considered. In current practice, we rely on the urea breath tests, which are the most sensitive and specific and also on serology.

3. Does eradication of *H. pylori* infection benefit the patient with PUD?

The statement concluded that eradication of *H. pylori* has been shown to enhance the healing of ulcers and modestly decrease the amount of time it takes to heal. Further evidence soon followed that eradication not only prevents recurrence of simple chronic ulcers but also complicated ones that had bled previously.

4. What is the relationship between *H. pylori* infection and gastric malignancy?

Reports at that time were suggesting that *H. pylori* infection was also associated with gastric cancer. This was proven beyond doubt in subsequent years, but at the time of the NIH consensus meeting only epidemiological evidence was available. The NIH statement was therefore rather cautious in its conclusions but left the door open for further progress on this front.

5. Which *H. pylori* infected patients should be treated?

'All patients with peptic ulcers who are infected with *H. pylori* should be treated with antimicrobials regardless of whether they are suffering from the initial presentation of the disease or from a recurrence'. This statement led, almost overnight, to a massive change of practice. Every patient with ulcers now demanded the new treatment, and every health care provider was obliged to consider it. There was no stopping the *Helicobacter* juggernaut now.

6. What are the most important questions that must be addressed by future research in *H. pylori* infections?

The statement highlighted a few key areas, including the following:

a. Population pockets specifically children, patients with gastric ulcers, and patients with duodenal or gastric ulcers with complications need to be further studied.

b. How should patients with initial dyspepsia symptoms be treated? Subsequent work has shown that eradication of the infection in patients with non-ulcer dyspepsia probably cures a small but significant proportion. Current clinical practice therefore dictates that dyspeptic patients who have no alarm symptoms may be tested for the infection and treated if found positive.

c. Further research revolving around virulence factors, bacterial genetics, mechanisms of immunity, animal models, antibiotic resistance and modes of transmission needs to be conducted.

The *H. pylori* Genome
Tomb et al., Nature (1997)

By 1997 reports were appearing of complete microbial genome sequences. *H. pylori*'s genome was amongst the first to be published. This offered a tremendous opportunity to quiz the organism and its associated diseases. As early as 1991 certain strains of *H. pylori* were recognised as more virulent than others. Some were found to produce a virulence factor called cytotoxin associated gene A (CagA), which increases the risk of PUD and gastric cancer. This was the product of a gene that resided in an island of genes (named the cag pathogenicity island) that became the major focus of research in the 1990s and beyond. CagA protein is now regarded as an oncoprotein whose introduction into host cells can trigger pathways that lead to gastric carcinogenesis. When the genome was published it offered a chance to discover other virulence factors and targets for bactericidal attack. Tomb and colleagues sequenced *H. pylori* strain 26695. They showed that it had a circular genome of 1,667,867 base pairs and 1590 predicted coding sequences. Using sequence analysis they determined that the bacteria had a system allowing motility, iron scavenging, and the restriction and modification of DNA; explaining its potential role in neoplasia. Adhesins, lipoproteins and other outer membrane proteins were identified and testified to the complex interactions that take place between the host and pathogen. The authors determined, based on the presence of homopolymeric tracts, dinucleotide repeats in coding sequences, and the many sequence-related genes encoding outer membrane proteins, that *H. pylori* probably uses recombination and slipped-strand mispairing within repeats as mechanisms for antigenic variation and adaptive evolution.

One of the most important findings was that the survival of *H. pylori* in acidic conditions depends partly on its ability to establish a positive inside-membrane potential in low pH. Understanding the mechanism by which *H. pylori* maintains its survival in the inhospitable gastric niche presents another target for future treatment options, perhaps even a vaccine. The long-term benefits of this work will continue to be reaped for many years.

H. pylori and Gastric Cancer
Parsonnet et al., New England Journal of Medicine (1991)

Gastric cancer is the second most common cause of cancer-related death and the predicted incidence for 2010 is 1.1 million with the majority of this health burden being borne by economically lesser-developed countries. Long before H. pylori was discovered, we had a working model for the pathogenesis of gastric cancer proposed by an outstanding pathologist, Pelayo Correa, who had spent a lifetime studying it. The Correa model established that gastric cancer starts with a chronic superficial gastritis with the potential to progress through atrophic gastritis, intestinal metaplasia, dysplasia and finally gastric adenocarcinoma[1]. When Correa proposed his model there was no explanation for the initial chronic superficial gastritis. It was thought that some luminal factor must be responsible (e.g. high salt, alcohol, smoking, dietary components and carcinogens). The answer of course was very simple: most cases of chronic superficial gastritis are caused by H. pylori infection. By the early 1990s, several key epidemiological studies were published that shed considerable light on the relationship between gastric cancer and H. pylori.

This paper by Parsonnet and colleagues addressed the question of seemingly negative H. pylori serology at the time of diagnosis of the cancer. They obtained stored sera from healthy individuals decades previously and followed them up to determine if having prior infection with H. pylori increased the risk of subsequent development of gastric cancer. They had access to a cohort of 128,992 subjects followed up since the mid-1960s at a health maintenance organisation. From this cohort they selected 186 cases that developed gastric cancer and 186 controls matched for age, sex and race. The mean time between collection of the serum and the diagnosis of gastric cancer was 14.2 years. 84% of the gastric cancer patients compared to 61% of the controls were seropositive for H. pylori infection (odds ratio, 3.6; 95% confidence interval 1.8–7.3). Interestingly, past history of peptic ulcer disease was protective against gastric cancer (odds ratio 0.2). The authors concluded that infection with H. pylori was associated with an increased risk of gastric cancer and suggested that it may be a cofactor in its pathogenesis.

In the same issue of the *New England Journal of Medicine*, another study reported similar findings[2]. In this case, the cohort was that of Japanese American men living in Hawaii. H. pylori was found to increase the odds ratio for gastric cancer to 6.0 (95% confidence interval 2.1–17.3). By 1994, there was enough evidence to prompt the International Agency for Research on Cancer (IARC) to declare H. pylori a Group I (definite) carcinogen, a scientific equivalent to being inducted into the carcinogenesis hall of fame! The IARC statement was very bold and was met with considerable scepticism, but in the ensuing 16 years evidence from epidemiological and interventional studies in humans as well as rodent and cell biological studies have convinced many that this bacterial infection is indeed the key factor in the initiation of the neoplastic process in the stomach.

H. pylori and the Gastric Cancer versus Duodenal Ulcer Phenotype
Uemura et al., New England Journal of Medicine (2001)

In the late 1990s, the paradox of having an infectious agent that causes two conditions (peptic ulcers and gastric cancer) that are somewhat mutually exclusive became apparent. Uemura and colleagues in Japan prospectively studied 1526 Japanese patients who had duodenal ulcers, gastric ulcers, gastric hyperplasia, or non-ulcer dyspepsia at the time of enrolment. 1246 of these patients had *H. pylori* infection, and 280 were negative. The mean follow-up was 7.8 years, and the patients underwent endoscopy with biopsy at baseline and then between 1 and 3 years after enrolment. Gastric cancers developed in 36 (2.9%) of the infected and none of the uninfected patients. The authors identified corpus predominant gastritis as the most serious gastric phenotype giving a relative risk for cancer of 34.5 (95% CI 7.1–166.7). Presence of severe gastric atrophy and intestinal metaplasia were also distinct risk factors. Interestingly, none of the 275 patients with duodenal ulcers (DU) developed gastric cancer, confirming previous studies that DU disease protects from this malignancy.

Thus we have a clear picture emerging of an infection that causes a variable pattern of gastritis in different people. There are three main gastric phenotypes that result from chronic *H. pylori* infection: (1) the commonest by far is a mild pangastritis that does not affect gastric physiology and is not associated with significant human disease, (2) a corpus-predominant gastritis associated with gastric atrophy, hypochlorhydria and increased risk of gastric cancer (the gastric cancer phenotype) and (3) an antral-predominant gastritis associated with high gastric acid secretion and increased risk of duodenal ulcer disease (the DU phenotype).

The Role of Host Genetics in Outcome of *H. pylori* Infection
El-Omar et al., Nature (2000)

H. pylori causes damage by initiating chronic inflammation in the gastric mucosa mediated by an array of cytokines. Genetic polymorphisms directly influence inter-individual variation in the magnitude of cytokine response contributing to the clinical outcome. El-Omar and colleagues speculated that the most relevant genes would be those whose products were involved in handling the *H. pylori* attack and those mediating the resulting inflammation. The initial search, reported in this *Nature* paper, focused on genes that were most relevant to gastric physiology, particularly gastric acid secretion. It was hypothesised that an endogenous agent that was up-regulated in the presence of *H. pylori*, has a profound pro-inflammatory effect and was also an acid inhibitor would be the most relevant host genetic factor to be studied. Interleukin 1 beta (IL-1β) fitted this profile perfectly. It was shown that pro-inflammatory *IL-1* gene cluster polymorphisms (*IL-1B* encoding IL-1β and *IL-1RN* encoding its naturally occurring receptor antagonist) increase the risk of gastric cancer and its precursors in the presence of *H. pylori*. Individuals with the pro-inflammatory *IL-1* genotypes are at increased risk of developing hypochlorhydria and gastric atrophy in response to the infection. This risk also extends to gastric cancer itself with a two- to threefold increased risk of malignancy compared to subjects who have the less pro-inflammatory genotypes.

The association has been confirmed independently by other groups covering Caucasian populations but with no apparent association in Asians. Several other host genetic factors have been uncovered, and there seems little doubt that host genetics play an important role in determining who develops an ulcer or a cancer and who escapes major damage (Figure 18.1). This *Nature* paper opened up a new avenue for research, an avenue that will lead in due course to definition of a gastric cancer genetic risk profile[3]. Such a

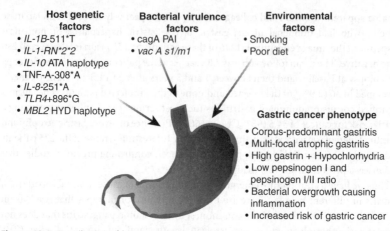

Host genetic factors
- *IL-1B*-511*T
- *IL-1-RN**2*2
- *IL-10* ATA haplotype
- TNF-A-308*A
- *IL-8*-251*A
- *TLR4*+896*G
- *MBL2* HYD haplotype

Bacterial virulence factors
- cagA PAI
- *vac A s1/m1*

Environmental factors
- Smoking
- Poor diet

Gastric cancer phenotype
- Corpus-predominant gastritis
- Multi-focal atrophic gastritis
- High gastrin + Hypochlorhydria
- Low pepsinogen I and pepsinogen I/II ratio
- Bacterial overgrowth causing inflammation
- Increased risk of gastric cancer

Figure 18.1 Contribution of host genetic, bacterial virulence and environmental factors in pathogenesis of *H.pylori*-induced gastric cancer. Reproduced with permission from Amieva and El-Omar, *Gastroenterology* 2008.

profile could be used in conjunction with testing for *H. pylori* infection and will refine the search for those who might benefit from eradication therapy.

Summary and Conclusion

The discovery of *H. pylori* infection was a highlight of 20th-century medicine. It is very rare that one can claim that a serious human disease has virtually disappeared in one's lifetime, but this is true of peptic ulcer disease. Equally our understanding of gastric cancer is perhaps the best of any solid malignancy and victory against it is in sight. A Nobel Prize for Medicine was awarded to Marshall and Warren in recognition of their work on *H. pylori* and peptic ulcer disease. Another legacy will likely come with eradication of gastric cancer, perhaps in two decades or so. In our choices for these ten papers, we strived for those that introduced novel ideas and propelled the field forward. There are clearly many more worthy papers that are equally important and their omission is in no way a reflection of their reduced priority, merely a reflection of our bias and ignorance.

Key Outstanding Questions

1. Will eradication of *H. pylori* infection prevent the development of gastric cancer?
2. If the above is true, at what stage should the infection be sought out and eradicated?
3. Is there a 'point of no return' beyond which cancer will develop regardless of eradication of the infection?
4. Will mass eradication of infection bring its own problems such as gastro-oesophageal reflux disease and oesophageal adenocarcinoma?
5. Can we develop a single highly effective antibiotic against *H. pylori*?
6. Will a vaccine ever succeed, and if it does, can we use it safely on a mass scale?

Key Research Centres

1. Timothy C Wang, PI, Division of Digestive and Liver Diseases, Columbia University Medical Center, New York, United States
2. Martin J Blaser, PI, Department of Microbiology, Department of Medicine, New York University School of Medicine, New York, United States
3. David Y Graham, PI, Section of Gastroenterology and Hepatology, Baylor College of Medicine, Houston, United States
4. Francis Megraud, PI, Laboratoire de Bactériologie-Enfants Hopital Pellegrin, Bordeaux, France
5. Peter Malfertheiner, PI, Otto-von-Guericke-Universität Magedeburg Medizinische Fakultät Zentrum für Innere Medizin Klinik für Gastroenterologie, Hepatologie und Infektiologie, Magdeburg, Germany
6. Emad El-Omar, PI, Gastrointestinal Group, Immunology and Inflammation Theme, Institute of Medical Sciences, School of Medicine & Dentistry, Aberdeen University, Aberdeen, United Kingdom

References

El-Omar, E.M., et al.(1995) Helicobacter pylori infection and abnormalities of acid secretion in patients with duodenal ulcer disease. *Gastroenterology*, **109**(3), 681–691. http://www.ncbi.nlm.nih.gov/pubmed/7657096

El-Omar, E.M., et al.(2000) Interleukin-1 polymorphisms associated with increased risk of gastric cancer. *Nature*, **404**, 398–402. http://www.nature.com/nature/journal/v404/n6776/full/404398a0.html

Helicobacter pylori in peptic ulcer disease (1994) *NIH Consensus Statement*, **12**(1), 1–23. http://consensus.nih.gov/1994/1994HelicobacterPyloriUlcer094html.htm

Hentschel, E., et al.(1993) Effect of ranitidine and amoxicillin plus metronidazole on the eradication of Helicobacter pylori and the recurrence of duodenal ulcer. *New England Journal of Medicine*, **328**(5), 308–312. http://www.ncbi.nlm.nih.gov/pubmed/8419816

Levi. S., et al. (1989) Campylobacter pylori and duodenal ulcers: the gastrin link. *Lancet*, **1**(8648), 1167–1668. http://www.ncbi.nlm.nih.gov/pubmed/2566737

Marshall, B.J., and Warren, J.R. (1984) Unidentified curved bacilli in the stomach of patients with gastritis and peptic ulceration. *Lancet*, **1**, 1311–1315. http://www.thelancet.com/journals/lancet/article/PIIS0140-6736(84)91816-6/Abstract

Marshall, B.J., et al. (1985) Attempt to fulfil Kochs postulates for pyloric Campylobacter. *Medical Journal of Australia*, **142**(8), 436–439. http://www.ncbi.nlm.nih.gov/pubmed/3982345

Tomb, J.F., et al. (1997) The complete genome sequence of the gastric pathogen Helicobacter pylori. *Nature*, **388**, 539–547. http://www.ncbi.nlm.nih.gov/pubmed/9252185

Parsonnet, J., et al. (1991) Helicobacter pylori infection and the risk of gastric carcinoma. *New England Journal of Medicine*, **325**, 1127–1131. http://www.ncbi.nlm.nih.gov/pubmed/1891020

Uemura, N., et al. (2001) Helicobacter pylori infection and the development of gastric cancer. *New England Journal of Medicine*, **345**, 784–789. http://www.ncbi.nlm.nih.gov/pubmed/11556297

Additional References

1. Correa, P., et al. (1975) A model for gastric cancer epidemiology. *Lancet*, **2**(7924), 58–60.
2. Nomura, A., et al. Helicobacter pylori infection and gastric carcinoma among Japanese Americans in Hawaii. *New England Journal of Medicine*, **325**(16), 1132–1136.
3. Amieva, M.R., and El-Omar, E.M. (2008) Host-bacterial interactions in Helicobacter pylori infection. *Gastroenterology*, **134**(1), 306–323.

19   Acute Liver Failure

James O'Beirne and Andrew K. Burroughs

Royal Free Sheila Sherlock Liver Centre, Royal Free Hospital, London, UK

Introduction

Liver failure is defined as the loss of the normal synthetic and metabolic capacity of the liver. Two forms are recognised depending on the presence or absence of underlying chronic liver disease. Chronic liver failure (CLF) is the loss of liver function associated with underlying cirrhosis, commonly over months or years, and may be associated with complications such as variceal bleeding, ascites, hepatorenal syndrome and hepatic encephalopathy. Acute liver failure (ALF) is the abrupt loss of liver function over days or weeks on the background of a normal liver. ALF is a potentially recoverable condition due to the ability of the liver to regenerate whereas chronic liver failure is generally irreversible because the cirrhotic liver cannot regenerate. More recently the term 'acute on chronic liver failure' (ACLF) has entered into the literature. ACLF is an abrupt reduction in liver function in a patient with underlying chronic liver disease secondary to a precipitating insult such as sepsis or bleeding. In ACLF resolution of the acute insult may result in improvement of liver function.

Prior to the 1960s, liver failure was known by numerous nonspecific terms such as massive hepatic necrosis, acute yellow atrophy and acute hepatic coma[1-3]. It was not until the advent of needle liver biopsy that the distinction between acute and chronic liver failure could be readily made. The current specialty of hepatology reflects the importance of the distinction of the different types of liver failure. ALF is generally managed in dedicated intensive care units (ICU) in liver transplant centres where patients can be supported until hepatic recovery occurs or transplantation is required. CLF is generally managed in primary and secondary care where the care of the patient is optimised by applying evidence from large randomised controlled trials in areas of the complications of cirrhosis.

In this chapter, we illustrate how the modern management of acute liver failure has been informed by key studies in these different areas.

Definitions of Acute Liver Failure
Lucké and Mallory, American Journal of Pathology (1946)
O'Grady et al., Lancet (1993)

As early as 1946 it was appreciated that there were distinct patterns of progression amongst patients with acute hepatitis who developed encephalopathy. Lucké and Mallory described a very rapidly progressive, and a less rapid form of the illness in a small cohort of patients. The terms 'fulminant liver failure' and 'subacute liver failure'

Understanding Medical Research: The Studies that Shaped Medicine, First Edition. Edited by John A. Goodfellow. © 2012 John Wiley & Sons, Ltd. Published 2012 by John Wiley & Sons, Ltd.

emerged and were refined in 1970 when Trey and Davidson published their definition of fulminant hepatic failure.[4] They defined fulminant hepatic failure as a 'potentially reversible condition, the consequence of severe liver injury, with an onset of encephalopathy within 8 weeks of the appearance of the first symptoms and in the absence of pre-existing liver disease'. This was a useful definition but did not include a subgroup of patients with a slower progression and a much worse prognosis. This subgroup was further characterised by the Kings College group in 1986 in a paper describing 47 patients with an evolution of jaundice to encephalopathy of between 8 and 26 weeks. These patients were described as having *late onset hepatic failure* and had a mortality rate of over 80%.[5] It was very clear from these two descriptions that subsets of patients with liver failure existed and that the tempo of the onset of the illness could inform clinicians as to the aetiology and likely prognosis.

ALF is a rare disease with an estimated incidence of 1 to 6 cases per million/year[6]. The development of dedicated liver units like that at Kings College was instrumental in allowing the study of patients in larger numbers and led to the publication of O'Grady and colleagues seminal paper in 1993. This is a landmark paper in ALF for a number of reasons. Firstly, the findings were derived from the largest cohort of patients ever described and was before the widespread application of emergency liver transplantation for this indication (1972–1985). This allowed the true natural history to be studied and set the foundation for the use of the definitions in liver transplantation. Secondly, the standardised definitions allowed outcome to be compared between units even in different countries where the dominant aetiologies may be different.

The paper proposed a new standardised definition of ALF based on the time interval between the onset of jaundice and the development of hepatic encephalopathy. Biochemical and clinical data, including the presence of cerebral oedema, and outcome were collected on the 635 patient cohort and analysed in relation to the time interval between the onset of jaundice and encephalopathy. The onset of jaundice rather than the onset of symptoms (as used in the Trey and Davidson definition) was chosen to reduce the bias of the subjective interpretation of mild symptoms early in the disease and also because an earlier study had identified jaundice as an independent risk factor for a poorer outcome. The most common aetiology of liver failure was poisoning with paracetamol (310 cases). Of the nonparacetamol cases the cause of liver failure was hepatitis B virus (37%), hepatitis A virus (20%), sero-negative or indeterminate (36%) or drug reaction in the remainder. A simple analysis of survival compared to the interval between jaundice and encephalopathy revealed some rather interesting findings.

When the paracetamol cases were excluded most survivors were clustered in the group who had developed encephalopathy within 7 days of jaundice. The incidence of cerebral oedema in this group was very high at 69% but paradoxically the survival of this group of patients was better than the rest of the cohort at 36%. All the patients with paracetamol poisoning developed encephalopathy with 7 days from jaundice, and the survival in this group was also good at 34.4%. It therefore appeared that despite having a higher incidence of cerebral oedema and a more acute presentation those patients who developed encephalopathy with 7 days of jaundice had a relatively good prognosis and the authors described this group as having 'hyperacute liver failure'.

In patients where the interval between jaundice and encephalopathy was greater than 4 weeks the survival was extremely low at 14%. These patients had a low incidence of

Table 19.1 Classification of acute liver failure according to O'Grady et al., Lancet (1993)

	Hyperacute liver failure	Acute liver failure	Sub-acute liver failure
Encephalopathy	Yes	Yes	Yes
Duration of jaundice before encephalopathy (days)	0–7	8–28	29–72
Cerebral oedema	Frequent	Common	Rare
Prothrombin time	+++	++/+++	+
Bilirubin	+	+++	+++
Prognosis (% survival)	40%	20%	10%
Typical Example	Paracetamol	Hepatitis B	Sero-negative

Note: The presentation of liver failure can give an indication as to the likely prognosis, aetiology and presence of complications.

cerebral oedema (14%) and a modest degree of coagulopathy (median prothrombin time 34 seconds). The dominant aetiology was sero-negative or indeterminate liver failure (83%). These patients therefore seemed to be prognostically and aetiologically distinct from the rest of the cohort and the authors defined them as suffering from 'subacute liver failure'.

The remaining patients who developed encephalopathy greater than 7 days but less than 4 weeks following the onset of jaundice were termed as suffering from 'acute liver failure'. They had a high incidence of cerebral oedema (56%) but unlike the hyperacute group had a very poor prognosis with a survival of 7%. The severity of coagulopathy was greater than the subacute group and similar to the hyperacute group. A high proportion was suffering from sero-negative or indeterminate liver failure in addition to other aetiologies except paracetamol.

The major conclusion of this study was that the definition of ALF could be refined based upon readily available clinical and biochemical data. The proposed classification imparted information about likely prognosis and the likely aetiology: most patients with hyperacute liver failure had paracetamol as the likely cause whereas in subacute liver failure the cause was almost always sero-negative or indeterminate. Conversely, if the aetiology was known, the likely clinical course could be predicted (Table 19.1).

Thus patients with a hyperacute presentation (likely paracetamol) are predicted to have a rapid clinical course (either deterioration or improvement) and are rapidly transferred to the ICU where management to prevent or treat cerebral oedema is easily applicable. In contrast, patients with sero-negative or indeterminate liver failure are managed less often in the ICU, have a much worse prognosis and are considered for liver transplantation at a much earlier stage of encephalopathy.

Prognostication in Acute Liver Failure
O'Grady et al., Gastroenterology (1988, 1989)

In the early 1980s, liver transplantation for ALF was not widely applied and there were no criteria to guide clinicians as to which patients may benefit from the procedure. Often liver transplantation was applied too late when complications such as cerebral oedema, coagulopathy and refractory hypotension contributed to a poor outcome. Some advocated that all patients with ALF should be offered liver transplantation given that the overall outcome was so poor. This did not take into account the small but significant proportion who might survive with intensive medical management alone. There was a need for prognostic indicators that could be applied early in the illness when a transplantation organ could be identified and a transplant could occur if needed. Likewise, patients with a predicted good prognosis could safely avoid transplantation and its attendant complications.

In 1989 O'Grady and colleagues outlined criteria for the selection of patients for liver transplantation in ALF. The fact that these have stood the test of time is a reflection of the size of the original data set and the careful analysis performed using a set of parameters that had already shown prognostic importance in the experience of the authors and previous publications. They used 588 patients to develop a prognostic model which was then tested in a further cohort of 175 patients to ascertain the sensitivity and specificity.

They studied a series of static (aetiology, age and jaundice to encephalopathy time) and dynamic variables (prothrombin time, pH, creatinine, liver function tests and haematological parameters) in a stepwise logistic regression model. For each dynamic variable they measured the value at admission and the peak value.

Of the static variables, aetiology was the most important. Hepatitis A and paracetamol had the best prognosis whereas drug reactions and sero-negative had low survival (13.6% and 9% respectively). The second most important static variable was age. In patients with paracetamol aetiology the age effect was not very pronounced. However, in drug reaction or viral hepatitis patient's survival was noted to be very poor in those aged less than 10 years or greater than 40.

Jaundice to encephalopathy time was only assessed in patients with a non-paracetamol aetiology on the basis that paracetamol poisoning follows a predictable course with the peak of encephalopathy occurring in the first week. There was a highly significant difference between survival in patients who developed encephalopathy within 7 days and those who developed hepatic encephalopathy later (34.0% vs. 6.7%).

Of the dynamic variables assessed the strongest predictor of outcome was arterial pH (reflecting the severity of liver failure and the degree of associated multiple organ failure): a pH less than 7.3 was associated with only a 15% survival rate. A peak bilirubin level greater than 300 μmol/L conferred a very poor prognosis with over 70% of patients. Prothrombin time had previously been shown to be an important determinant of survival in ALF[7]. In O'Grady's study a prothrombin time greater than 100 seconds was associated with a survival rate of less than 20% independent of the aetiology.

Certain variables appeared to show important differences between the paracetamol and non-paracetamol groups so the authors constructed separate models for paracetamol and non-paracetamol cases then tested in a further cohort of 121 patients admitted to the liver failure unit.

An arterial pH of less than 7.3 was able to predict 97% of the deaths in the validation group, but this finding was only present in less than half the admitted patients. A peak prothrombin time of greater than 100 seconds was able to predict 79% of the 43 deaths. After excluding patients with a pH less than 7.3 the best predictor of death was a combination of a prothrombin time of greater than 100 seconds and a creatinine greater than 300 μmol/L in the presence of at least grade 3 encephalopathy. In the validation cohort this combination predicted 67% of the deaths, and when used in combination

Table 19.2 Kings College Hospital Criteria for the selection of patients for emergency liver transplantation

Paracetamol-induced	Non-paracetamol-induced
pH < 7.3 (irrespective of grade of encephalopathy)	Prothrombin time > 100 secs (irrespective of grade of encephalopathy)
Or all three of the following:	Or three of the following:
Prothrombin time > 100 secs	Age < 10 or > 40 years old
Serum creatinine > 300 μmol/L	Adverse aetiology (sero-negative or drug reaction)
Grade 3 encephalopathy or above	Jaundice to encephalopathy time greater than 7 days
	Prothrombin time > 50 secs
	Serum bilirubin > 300 μmol/L

Source: Adapted from O'Grady et al., *Gastroenterology* (1989).

with arterial ph < 7.3, 77% of the deaths were correctly predicted giving a specificity of 0.94 with a sensitivity of 0.45 and a predictive accuracy of 0.83.

For non-paracetamol-induced cases the mixture of 3 static and 2 dynamic variables were assessed in a validation of cohort of 54 patients admitted over 1 year again using the same cut offs. All the patients with a prothrombin time of greater than 100 seconds died regardless of other parameters. If any three of prothrombin time > 50 seconds, bilirubin > 300 μmol/L, age <10 or > 40, jaundice to encephalopathy time >7 days or adverse aetiology were present, regardless of the grade of encephalopathy, then 96.4% of patients died.

The criteria based on this paper (Table 19.2) continue to remain in clinical use today for the selection of patients for liver transplantation. In a recent meta-analysis of 18 studies comprising over 1000 patients examining the accuracy of the 'Kings College Criteria' for nonparacetamol aetiologies, the criteria still had excellent predictive ability especially when applied dynamically[8]. For paracetamol-induced liver failure, the criteria are still robust and indeed are a prerequisite for registration for emergency liver transplantation in the United Kingdom but sensitivity is rather low meaning that some patients still die despite never fulfilling the criteria.

Pathophysiology of ALF: Multiple Organ Failure and Covert Tissue Hypoxia
Bihari et al., Journal of Hepatology (1985)

The commonest mode of death in ALF remains either multiple organ failure or cerebral herniation (CH) from intracranial hypertension (ICH). The pathophysiology leading to these is incompletely understood but seminal studies done in the 1980s have shaped the critical care management of ALF. One of the key observations was the importance of the arterial pH in determining the prognosis of patients with ALF. The metabolic acidosis seen in ALF is secondary to hyperlactataemia in part from the over-production of lactate due to anaerobic respiration but also due to inadequate clearance of lactate by the failing liver.

Bihari and colleagues investigated 32 patients with ALF during the first 48 hours of grade 4 hepatic encephalopathy[9]. Based on measurements of oxygen extraction, the authors proposed that in ALF there was a greater systemic availability of oxygen but that nonsurvivors had a lack of increase in oxygen extraction due to blood by-passing the microcirculation of actively respiring tissues.

They then devised an interventional study to examine the effect of prostacyclin infusion on oxygen delivery and uptake in patients with ALF and normal healthy volunteers. Prostacyclin is a microvascular vasodilator and has properties which may improve blood flow through the microcirculation such as inhibition of platelet aggregation and reduction of leucocyte adhesion to vascular endothelium[10]. In ALF patients infusion of prostacyclin for 20 minutes caused a significant decrease in systemic vascular resistance, a compensatory increase in cardiac output, an increased oxygen delivery and an increase in oxygen consumption. Healthy volunteers also had increased oxygen delivery but had no increase in oxygen consumption. This novel finding led the authors to conclude that a state of 'covert tissue hypoxia' exists in ALF and that this results in a state of pathological supply dependency for oxygen and is responsible for the initiation and maintenance of multiple organ failure.

In practice the use of prostacyclin is associated with a fall in mean arterial pressure in some individuals and also arterial hypoxaemia by increasing shunting in the lung by virtue of the vasodilatory effect on the lung vasculature in nonventilated segments. Today it is only used in those patients who demonstrate obvious derangement of microvascular flow such as cold mottled extremities in the presence of a normal or supranormal cardiac output.

N-Acetyl Cysteine in ALF: From Clinical Observation to Randomised Controlled Trials
Harrison et al., Lancet (1990)
Lee et al., Gastroenterology (2009)

In the late 1980s the commonest cause of ALF in the United Kingdom was poisoning with paracetamol, and the routine use of intravenous N-acetyl cysteine (NAC) had become commonplace in the early treatment of poisoned patients[11,12].

In paracetamol poisoning, hepatocytes are damaged by the toxic metabolite N-acetyl-*p*-benzoquinone imine (NAPQI) which is normally removed from the body by conjugation with glutathione. In paracetamol poisoning glutathione stores become rapidly depleted, accumulating large amounts of hepatotoxic NAPQI. The administration of NAC replenishes glutathione stores and prevents hepatotoxicity. NAC can prevent or reduce liver damage even after large overdoses when given early but was not thought to be effective when given later in the course of poisoning, especially after 24 hours[11]. This was challenged by the Kings College group in 1990 when they published their experience of patients with ALF who had been treated with NAC at later time points.

Although this was not a controlled study, the findings suggested that the late administration of NAC reduced mortality from 58% to 37% and appeared to lessen organ failure despite liver disease of similar severity to non-NAC treated patients[13]. At this time there was emerging evidence that NAC could have important effects on the circulation by promoting the relaxation of vascular smooth muscle and reversing tolerance to nitrate[14].

Further studies suggested that NAC could improve oxygen delivery and consumption secondary to a restoration of microcirculatory flow[15]. Even in patients with non-paracetamol-induced liver failure there were improvements noted in systemic haemo-dynamics and oxygen transport, suggesting for the first time that NAC may be beneficial in all types of ALF.

Many units began to treat all ALF patients with NAC, but as the studies were small and uncontrolled, its role remained in a state of clinical equipoise until 1998 when it became the focus of research for the newly formed United States Acute Liver Failure Study Group (USALFSG) led by Professor William Lee.

The USALFSG commenced a clinical trial of NAC in non-paracetamol-induced ALF in late 1998. It enrolled patients from 24 sites and completed in 2006. The findings, published in 2009, have already led to a change in clinical practice. This randomised placebo controlled trial hypothesised that the use of NAC would result in increased survival of ALF patients at 3 weeks compared to placebo. Secondary end points stated *a priori* were that NAC would result in an increase in transplant free survival and a reduction in the need for liver transplantation.

The patients were randomised to NAC or placebo for 72 hours. The majority had quite severe liver injury caused by either drugs or a sero-negative aetiology. There was no difference in overall survival (70% NAC, 66% placebo). However in patients with lower grades of encephalopathy receiving NAC the transplant free survival was 52% compared to only 30% in patients receiving placebo (Figure 19.1). Treatment with NAC was also associated with a longer time to transplantation and transplant free survival but only in patients with lower grades of encephalopathy. Overall the incidence of organ failures and other complications was similar.

The conclusion was that treatment with NAC was associated with an increase in transplant free survival and time to transplantation but only in patients with lower grades of encephalopathy, perhaps representing those patients earlier in their disease course.

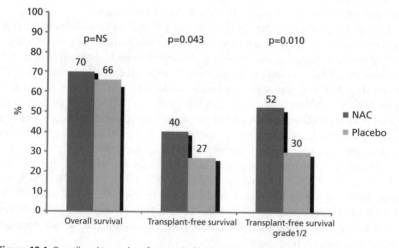

Figure 19.1 Overall and transplant-free survival in ALF patients treated with NAC or placebo. Source: Adapted from data in Lee *et al.*, *Gastroenterology* (2009).

Ammonia: The Key Player in Hepatic Encephalopathy and Cerebral Oedema

Clemmesen et al., Hepatology (1999)

In the early experience of ALF treatment in ICUs the commonest cause of death was CH secondary to ICH. Currently this mode of death is relatively rare and multiple organ failure and sepsis have supervened as the cause of death in the majority of patients[6]. The largest impact has come from rational therapies based on a better understanding of the pathogenesis of ICH in ALF, firstly through animal studies and then through clinical studies.

Animal studies led the way in linking ammonia to cerebral oedema. Ammonia is detoxified in the brain by the enzyme glutamine synthetase. Glutamine is osmotically active and contributes to astrocyte swelling as well as inducing cellular dysfunction. Inhibition of glutamine synthetase ameliorates cerebral oedema and prolongs survival in animal models of ALF[16–19]. These findings led to the formation of the 'ammonia hypothesis' of the pathogenesis of cerebral oedema (Figure 19.2).

In 1999 Clemmeson and colleagues published a paper in Hepatology that confirmed the ammonia hypothesis in humans. In order to confirm these animal data, it was necessary to demonstrate that patients with ALF had hyperammonaemia derived from the hepato-splanchnic circulation due to reduced ammonia extraction by the liver. Secondly, it was necessary to show that ammonia was taken up by the brain and that ammonia levels correlated with the development of CH.

This elegant paper describes a series of experiments performed in patients with ALF, chronic liver disease and healthy controls. All patients had measurements of arterial ammonia and in a subset, hepatic ammonia extraction and blood flow was measured via

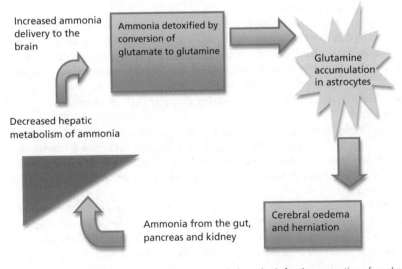

Figure 19.2 Schematic representation of the ammonia hypothesis for the generation of cerebral oedema in ALF. Ammonia which is normally removed from the circulation by the liver accumulates and in conditions of hyperammonaemia is detoxified by the brain. This detoxification process generates glutamine which is osmotically active and causes astrocyte and subsequent brain swelling resulting in cerebral oedema and eventual death through cerebral herniation.

radiographically placed catheters within the hepatic vein. Ammonia concentrations were also measured from the femoral and internal jugular vein to give information about regional ammonia metabolism and then correlated with the development of CH.

The results showed very clearly that ammonia had a pivotal role in the development of ICH and subsequent outcome. There were 14 deaths from CH out of the 44 ALF patients studied. In CH patients the mean arterial ammonia concentration was 230 ± 58 micromol/L compared to 118 ± 48 micromol/L in patients not developing CH. In fact, CH was not seen in any patient with an arterial ammonia of less than 146 micromol/L, even in those with liver and other organ failure as severe as those with higher levels of ammonia who subsequently developed CH.

Measurement of both arterial and internal jugular concentrations of ammonia allows the calculation of the arterial-venous difference in ammonia and the degree of ammonia extraction by the brain. In this study there was a linear relationship between the arterial and internal jugular concentrations of ammonia but as the arterial ammonia increased the difference between the arterial and jugular concentrations also increased consistent with the notion that increased ammonia delivery to the brain caused increased ammonia extraction. This is compatible with the observation that ammonia can cause increased cerebral blood flow further contributing to the development of ICH and CH[20].

Hepatic venous concentrations of ammonia were higher than arterial concentrations in ALF patients demonstrating that the hepato-splanchnic circulation was the source of the excess ammonia secondary to decreased detoxification in the liver. Interestingly this was not observed in chronic liver disease patients where the liver was a net remover of ammonia, perhaps explaining why ammonia levels in patients with chronic liver disease are usually somewhat lower than those in ALF patients and cerebral oedema is rarely observed. Finally, the results also suggested that muscle tissue could act to locally reduce circulating ammonia levels.

This study was a major landmark in the critical care management of ALF for a number of reasons. The most important finding was the confirmation of the animal data that high ammonia levels had a direct clinical impact. Ammonia levels are now used to stratify patients in terms of risk of development of ICH and CH. High risk individuals (ammonia levels greater than 150 micromol/L) may be selected for invasive measurements of intracranial pressure or ammonia lowering therapies such as haemofiltration at an earlier stage.

The finding that high levels of ammonia increases cerebral blood flow which contributes to ICH has resulted in patients with high ammonia levels routinely undergoing interventions to reduce cerebral blood flow, for example tight control of CO_2 levels, avoidance of fever and in those at risk of CH active cooling to moderate hypothermia[21].

Finally the demonstration that muscle can be a secondary site for the removal of ammonia from the circulation has stimulated research in this area and novel compounds such as L-ornithine-phenylacetate, which stimulates the detoxification and subsequent removal of ammonia by muscle, are already entering clinical trials[22,23].

Conclusion

The recognition of the variable aetiologies and outcomes of patients with acute liver failure has led to a concerted international effort to further characterise the factors that influence prognosis. Easily obtained clinical and biochemical data now allow identification of patients who are likely to improve or who are likely to require early consideration of transplantation. Patients at risk of developing complications such as raised intracranial pressure are now identified early and managed in ICUs where appropriate according to strategies based on a better, although incomplete, understanding of the underlying pathophysiology. N-acetyl cysteine had long been used in the early treatment of paracetamol overdose but is now emerging as an important therapy in later presentations and even in other aetiologies. Further international, multicentre studies are needed to develop further effective therapies.

Key Outstanding Questions

1. Are there any simple clinical or biochemical parameters that can be used to better predict an individual's prognosis at the initial presentation of ALF?
2. Can we improve the sensitivity of selection criteria used to identify patients for liver transplantation?
3. Are there any clinically meaningful ways to assess covert tissue hypoxia in patients with ALF?
4. To what extent does covert tissue hypoxia drive and maintain multiple organ failure and are there any interventions that can reverse the process?

Key Research Centres

It should be clear from our selection of papers that, historically, the Kings College Hospital in London has contributed significantly to our understanding and management of ALF. However, there are too many centres internationally to pick out just a few. The following links should provide an appropriate to explore the centres with major ongoing research projects.

1. American Association for the Study of Liver Disease, http://www.aasld.org
2. British Association for the Study of the Liver, http://www.basl.org.uk
3. British Society of Gastroenterology, http://www.bsg.org.uk
4. European Association for the Study of the Liver, http://www.easl.ch

References

Bihari, D., et al. (1985) Lactic acidosis in fulminant hepatic failure: some aspects of pathogenesis and prognosis. Journal of Hepatology, 1, 405–416. http://www.sciencedirect.com/science/article/pii/S0168827885807789

Clemmesen, J.O., et al. (1999) Cerebral herniation in patients with acute liver failure is correlated with arterial ammonia concentration. Hepatology, 29, 648–653. http://onlinelibrary.wiley.com/doi/10.1002/hep.510290309/Abstract

Harrison, P.M., et al. (1990) Improved outcome of paracetamol-induced fulminant hepatic failure by late administration of acetylcysteine. Lancet, 335, 1572–1573. http://www.ncbi.nlm.nih.gov/pubmed/1972496

Lee, W.M., et al. (2009) Intravenous N-acetylcysteine improves transplant-free survival in early stage nonacetaminophen acute liver failure. Gastroenterology, 137, 856–864. http://www.ncbi.nlm.nih.gov/pubmed/19524577

Lucké, B., and Mallory, T. (1946) The fulminant form of epidemic hepatitis. *American Journal of Pathology*, **22**(5), 867–945. http://www.ncbi.nlm.nih.gov/pmc/articles/PMC1934231/?tool= pubmed

O'Grady, J.G., *et al.* (1988) Controlled trials of charcoal hemoperfusion and prognostic factors in fulminant hepatic failure. *Gastroenterology*, **94**, 1186–1192. http://www.gastrojournal.org/article/0016-5085(88)90011-X/Abstract

O'Grady, J.G., *et al.* (1989) Early indicators of prognosis in fulminant hepatic failure. *Gastroenterology*, **97**, 439–445. http://www.gastrojournal.org/article/0016-5085(89)90081-4/Abstract

O'Grady, J.G., *et al.* (1993) Acute liver failure: redefining the syndromes. *Lancet*, **342**, 273–275. http://www.sciencedirect.com/science/article/pii/0140673693918187

Additional References

1. Obstetric acute yellow atrophy (1956) *Lancet*, **267**, 847–848.
2. Kalk, H. (1959) Biopsy findings during and after hepatic coma and after acute necrosis of the liver. *Gastroenterology*, **36**, 214–218.
3. Temple, R.L., *et al.* (1962) Massive hepatic necrosis following general anesthesia. *Anesthesia and Analgesia*, **41**, 586–592.
4. Trey, C., and Davidson, C.S. (1970) The management of fulminant hepatic failure. *Progress in Liver Disease*, **3**, 282–298.
5. Gimson, A.E., *et al.* (1986) Late onset hepatic failure: clinical, serological and histological features. *Hepatology*, **6**, 288–294.
6. Bernal, W., *et al.* (2010) Acute liver failure. *Lancet*, **376**, 190–201.
7. Gimson, A.E., *et al.* (1983) Clinical and prognostic differences in fulminant hepatitis type A, B and non-A non-B. *Gut*, **24**, 1194–1198.
8. McPhail, M.J., *et al.* (2010) Meta–analysis of performance of Kingss College Hospital Criteria in prediction of outcome in non-paracetamol-induced acute liver failure. *Journal of Hepatology*, **53**, 492–499.
9. Bihari, D.J., *et al.* (1986) Cardiovascular, pulmonary and renal complications of fulminant hepatic failure. *Seminars in Liver Disease*, **6**, 119–128.
10. Bihari, D.J., and Tinker, J. (1988) The therapeutic value of vasodilator prostaglandins in multiple organ failure associated with sepsis. *Journal of Intensive Care Medicine*, **15**, 2–7.
11. Prescott, L.F. (1981) Treatment of severe acetaminophen poisoning with intravenous acetylcysteine. *Archives of Internal Medicine*, **141**, 386–389.
12. Prescott, L.F., *et al.* (1977) Treatment of paracetamol (acetaminophen) poisoning with N-acetylcysteine. *Lancet*, **2**, 432–434.
13. Keays, R., *et al.* (1991) Intravenous acetylcysteine in paracetamol induced fulminant hepatic failure: a prospective controlled trial. *British Medical Journal*, **303**, 1026–1029.
14. Laursen, J.B., *et al.* (1996) Nitrate tolerance impairs nitric oxide-mediated vasodilation in vivo. *Cardiovascular Research*, **31**, 814–819.
15. Harrison, P.M., *et al.* (1991) Improvement by acetylcysteine of hemodynamics and oxygen transport in fulminant hepatic failure. *New England Journal of Medicine*, **324**, 1852–1857.
16. Blei, A.T., *et al.* (1994) Ammonia-induced brain edema and intracranial hypertension in rats after portacaval anastomosis. *Hepatology*, **19**, 1437–1444.
17. Ganz, R., *et al.* (1989) Ammonia-induced swelling of rat cerebral cortical slices: implications for the pathogenesis of brain edema in acute hepatic failure. *Metabolic Brain Disease*, **4**, 213–223.

18. Swain, M., *et al.* (1992) Ammonia and related amino acids in the pathogenesis of brain edema in acute ischemic liver failure in rats. *Hepatology*, **15**, 449–453.

19. Cordoba, J., *et al.* (1996) Glutamine, myo-inositol, and organic brain osmolytes after portocaval anastomosis in the rat: implications for ammonia-induced brain edema. *Hepatology*, **24**, 919–923.

20. Chodobski, A., *et al.* (1986) Effect of ammonia intoxication on cerebral blood flow, its autoregulation and responsiveness to carbon dioxide and papaverine. *Journal of Neurology, Neurosurgery & Psychiatry*, **49**, 302–309.

21. Vaquero, J., *et al.* (2005) Keeping cool in acute liver failure: rationale for the use of mild hypothermia. *Journal of Hepatology*, **43**, 1067–1077.

22. Jalan, R., *et al.* (2007) L-Ornithine phenylacetate (OP), a novel treatment for hyperammonemia and hepatic encephalopathy. *Medical Hypotheses*, **69**, 1064–1069.

23. Ytrebo, L.M., *et al.* (2009) L-ornithine phenylacetate attenuates increased arterial and extracellular brain ammonia and prevents intracranial hypertension in pigs with acute liver failure. *Hepatology*, **50**, 165–174.

20   Haemostasis and Thrombosis

Charles Percy and Raza Alikhan

Haemophilia and Thrombosis Centre, University Hospital of Wales, Cardiff, UK

Introduction

The first reference to coagulation was made by Hippocrates (460–377 B.C.), who observed that blood collected from a sacrificed animal congealed on cooling. Aristotle (384–322 B.C.) also noted that blood cooled on leaving the body and surmised that this initiated its decay and subsequent congealing. The cooling hypothesis continued until Hewson (1770) excised a blood-filled vein and, keeping it at body temperature, demonstrated blood clot formation. However, he came up with a new 'air theory' to explain why warm blood in the circulation remained fluid and on exposure to air congealed. Other theories included the 'rest theory' supported by William Harvey (1578–1657) which stated that motion inhibited clotting, seemingly confirmed by Thomas Sydenham (1624–1689) who found that if freshly drawn blood was stirred vigorously it failed to clot. These theories were all rejected by John Hunter (1728–1793), surgeon and anatomist, who demonstrated that blood from cold water fish clotted more rapidly on warming, blood within a vacuum clotted faster than that exposed to air and that stirred blood clotted as quickly as blood left to sit in a cup.

While there was wide debate, for almost two millennia, as to why blood clotted on leaving the body, most denied or ignored the presence of intravascular coagulation. Ambroise Pare (1576) first documented that blood could clot in a vein 'they [the varicose veins] often swell with congealed and dryed bloud and cause pain'. Richard Wiseman (1676), surgeon to Charles II, also described blood clots in relation to varicose veins. He also wrote prolifically on the development of venous thrombosis following childbirth. It is Rudolf Virchow (1821–1902) who has been credited with the description of a triad of factors that are still considered central to the pathogenesis of venous thrombosis (i.e. vessel damage, reduction in venous blood flow and a state of hypercoagulability).

Venous thromboembolism (VTE) – deep vein thrombosis and pulmonary embolism – is a major health problem, the prevalence and seriousness of which are often not fully appreciated. Venous thromboembolic disorders are a common occurrence affecting approximately 1 in 1000 of the population per year. Irrespective of one's clinical speciality, VTE will be encountered both in hospital and in the community setting.

Understanding Medical Research: The Studies that Shaped Medicine, First Edition. Edited by John A. Goodfellow. © 2012 John Wiley & Sons, Ltd. Published 2012 by John Wiley & Sons, Ltd.

The Discovery of Heparin

By 1918 work in various institutions had led to the recognition that there were a number of substances involved in the control of haemostasis: fibrinogen, prothrombin as a precursor of thrombin, calcium, antithrombin and what were termed 'thromboplastic substances'.

Howell and Holt, American Journal of Physiology (1918)

The discovery of heparin is somewhat mired in controversy as to whom the credit should be attributed. A medical student, Jay McLean, working under the physiologist William Howell is often credited with its discovery. Howell and Holt were the first to publish work identifying the water soluble compound they called heparin, 'hepar' or liver, named after the tissue it was first isolated from. They proceeded to demonstrate that when heparin was administered to dogs by intravenous injection the time taken for blood to clot was subsequently prolonged. Furthermore, they demonstrated that this was dose dependent and that the clotting time returned to normal 3–4 hours after the injection.

There then followed a protracted period where fears regarding side effects of the early preparations, including nausea, headaches and fevers, paralysed its clinical use. Consistency of efficacy of the early preparations was also an issue and it was not until the 1930s that animal experiments showed heparin's ability to prevent thrombus formation in the setting of trauma. By the 1940s, case reports were appearing of patients with gangrene and frostbite where heparin had been used successfully. During this period, another anticoagulant was also being investigated.

The Discovery of Warfarin

Aside from the economy, all was not well in the countryside of Wisconsin in the 1920s. During the winter months, cattle had started to die from a mysterious haemorrhagic disease. Efforts to identify the cause led to the finding of a compound produced by sweet clover fermenting in the hay they were eating.

Stahmann et al., Journal of Biological Chemistry (1941)

After a decade of effort, in 1940 Karl Link and his team successfully concentrated the compound in the sweet clover responsible for the haemorrhagic manifestations. They perfected a technique to effectively obtain the coumarin compound they called dicoumarol. This work had been undertaken under the auspices of the Wisconsin Agricultural Research Foundation (WARF). Adding '-arin' to the end of this produced the name of the drug as we now know it, warfarin.

Clinicians now had two anticoagulant agents with clinical applications. Case reports continued to accrue, and President Eisenhower was one of the first patients to receive warfarin following cardiac surgery in the early 1950s. Warfarin is now the most widely used anticoagulant in the world, with at least 1% of the UK population taking it. However, it was more than 40 years after heparin was first described and more than two decades after warfarin was first available that a randomised control trial assessing the efficacy of these drugs was first published.

The Treatment of Pulmonary Embolism
Barritt and Jordan, Lancet (1960)

This team, based at the Bristol Royal Infirmary in England, recruited a total of 73 patients identified by clinical colleagues as potentially suffering from acute pulmonary embolism (PE). Included patients were randomised to both standard care (bed rest with inotropes, antiarrhythmics and oxygen as needed) and anticoagulation with heparin and nicoumalone (acenocoumarol) or to standard care alone. Ten thousand units of heparin were given six hourly for six doses and nicoumalone was started concurrently and continued for 14 days or until the patient was able to mobilise, whichever was the later. No laboratory monitoring was undertaken for heparin; however, the prothrombin time was used to adjust the nicoumalone dose to maintain the patient's result 2–3 times longer than the control. After the first 35 cases, the data were reviewed. Of the 19 patients in the standard treatment arm, five had died and five had suffered a further PE. In the intervention arm, there had been one death due to pneumonia and haemorrhage from a duodenal ulcer and no cases of recurrent PE. In view of these findings, Barritt and Jordan felt it unethical to continue to randomise to the standard treatment arm. The remaining 38 patients therefore all received anticoagulation.

This seminal paper showed beyond doubt that anticoagulation could successfully reduce the mortality and recurrence of PE. The next clinical question was inevitably whether or not venous thromboembolism could be prevented and subsequently whether those at particular risk could be predicted.

Prevention of Venous Thrombosis
Kakkar et al., Lancet (1975)

VV Kakkar published a number of small randomised controlled trials in the late 1960s and early 1970s showing the efficacy of heparin in preventing venous thromboembolism after surgery. In 1975 he published the results of a landmark international multicentre randomised controlled trial which recruited 4121 patients undergoing surgery requiring general anaesthesia and a subsequent hospital stay of at least 7 days. In the intervention arm 5000 units of heparin were administered subcutaneously 2 hours preoperatively and then 8 hourly for 7 days or until ambulant, whichever was longer. Overall there were 100 deaths in the control arm and 80 deaths in the intervention arm. Post-mortem examination was carried out in 72% of the patients in the control arm and in 66% of the intervention arm. Deaths from PE accounted for 22% of those in the control arm compared to only 4% in those receiving heparin. In addition, 220 cases of DVT were recorded in control patients compared to 65 DVTs in those receiving heparin. DVT was confirmed either by venography, isotopic fibrinogen measurement or post mortem. Clearly there was a significant reduction in both fatal PE and DVT in those patients receiving heparin. Finally they looked at the perennial question of whether or not there was excess bleeding in those receiving heparin. Of 2045 patients receiving heparin, treatment was discontinued due to blood loss in 53 (2.6%). Aware that such clinical assessment can be prone to subjectivity, they looked at the fall in haemoglobin and total blood transfusion in 1475 patients (744 controls and 731 receiving heparin). There was no significant difference. Furthermore there was no significant difference in the number of deaths attributable to haemorrhage (7% versus 8%).

Warfarin and Heparin in the Initial Treatment of Thromboembolic Disease

Brandjes et al., New England Journal of Medicine (1992)

There continued to be international heterogeneity in clinical practice with some using coumarin anticoagulants alone to treat venous thromboembolism rather than the combination with heparin such as used by Barritt and Jordan. This was based on the argument that high doses of coumarins were equivalent to heparin. A lack of robust trial evidence to support one approach over the other led Brandjes and colleagues to devise their study. They undertook a randomised, double-blind study comparing continuous intravenous heparin plus acenocoumarol with acenocoumarol alone in the initial treatment of outpatients with proximal DVT. The primary endpoint was a confirmed symptomatic extension or recurrence of VTE during 6 months of follow-up. They also assessed asymptomatic thrombus extension or PE by repeating venography and lung ventilation/perfusion scanning after the first week of treatment. Due to an excess of symptomatic events in the group that received acenocoumarol alone [in 12 of 60 patients (20%)], as compared with [4 of 60 patients (6.7%)] in the combined-therapy group, the study was terminated early. Recurrent thrombotic episodes were observed in 39.6% of the patients in the acenocoumarol group and in 8.2% of patients treated with heparin plus acenocoumarol. There was no significant difference in haemorrhagic events between the two groups. As a result of these findings and further confirmatory studies it is now standard practice to initiate treatment for venous thromboembolic events with heparin for a minimum of 5 days and continue with an oral anticoagulant, such as warfarin, for the duration of a patient's treatment.

Activated Protein C Resistance and the Discovery of the Factor V Leiden Mutation

In 1965 Egberg described a hereditary thrombophilia due to antithrombin III deficiency. Over the next 20 years, patients with hereditary deficiencies of Protein C and S were described. Yet there continued to be families where there was clearly an underlying predisposition to thrombosis but testing revealed normal levels of antithrombin III, Protein C and S.

Dahlback et al., Proceedings of the National Academy of Sciences (1993)

Dahlback and colleagues reported a series of experiments on the plasma from a family whose members had suffered numerous thrombotic episodes. No hitherto identifiable cause could be found. The team hypothesised that a poor anticoagulant response to activated protein C (aPC) could predispose to thrombosis. To investigate this further they devised the tests that now form the basis for the aPC resistance (aPCR) ratio often reported when a thrombophilia screen is requested. The activated partial thrombo-plastin time (APTT) was measured for the patient and normal control, in the presence and absence of aPC. These tests were repeated with increasing doses of aPC. The results showed that irrespective of the dose of aPC, the APTT prolongation was significantly less in the patient than the control. They went on to test a total of 19 family members, 14 of whom yielded similar results. The experiments were also performed using activated factor IX and factor X assays, again showing similar findings, although with a less marked difference in the factor X assay. The factor VIII gene was sequenced to look for known mutations in the aPC cleavage site and none were found. These findings led the team to conclude that it was unlikely that the underlying defect lay in factor V as the results of the factor X assay showed less pronounced prolongation. As a result they did not sequence the factor V gene. A group in the Netherlands, led by Bertina, drew a different conclusion.

Bertina et al., Nature (1994)

The mounting evidence for inherited activated protein C resistance spurred Bertina and colleagues to sequence the factor V gene. Looking for mutations in the postulated site of cleavage by activated protein C revealed a substitution of glutamine for arginine at position 506. The team then looked at other patients recorded in their database as having aPC resistance and found that overall 80% with aPCR ratio <0.84 and 100% of those with aPCR ratio <0.73 had this mutation present. They went on to estimate the overall prevalence of this mutation in the Dutch population to be 2%. This research was undertaken in Leiden hence the name given to this mutation, Factor V Leiden mutation, the most common of the hereditary thrombophilias.

The Introduction of Low Molecular Weight Heparin
Koopman et al., New England Journal of Medicine (1996)

Clinical treatment continued to progress on pragmatic grounds while the underlying mechanisms of VTE were being investigated. Intravenous heparin administration inevitably required hospital administration. The advent of low molecular weight heparins which could be given subcutaneously with predictable efficacy raised the possibility of being able to manage VTE in the community. Avoiding intravenous administration also had potential safety benefits such as avoiding over- and under-anticoagulation due to difficulties with monitoring the effect of heparin.

To answer the question of whether low molecular weight heparin was as effective as intravenous heparin, Koopman and colleagues devised a multicentre randomised control trial. A total of 400 patients were randomised between standard treatment (198 patients) or low molecular weight heparin (202 patients). Follow-up was for a total of 2 years. The primary endpoint of recurrent VTE was similar between the two groups 17 (8.6%) in the intravenous heparin arm versus 14 (6.9%) in the low molecular weight heparin arm. Bleeding occurred in a small number of patients – four in the intravenous heparin arm and one in the LMWH arm. Furthermore, 44 (22%) patients in the LMWH arm were discharged within 48 hours of treatment initiation, providing further support to the argument for ambulatory treatment.

Mechanical Methods of Preventing Pulmonary Emboli

Despite the success of treating VTE with heparin and coumarins not all patients can receive an anticoagulant. The most common contraindications to anticoagulation are an increased risk of bleeding or active bleeding. There have been more than a hundred case reports and case series on the use of vena caval filters to prevent PE in patients with VTE but it was not until the late 1990s that a randomised controlled trial was undertaken.

Decousus et al., New England Journal of Medicine (1998)

Decousus and colleagues set out to resolve the question as to whether insertion of an inferior vena caval (IVC) filter conferred any benefit over anticoagulation alone in patients suffering from an isolated proximal DVT with or without PE. A total of 400 patients with proximal DVT were recruited, 145 (36%) with symptomatic PE and 52 (13%) with asymptomatic PE. They were randomised equally to receive a permanent IVC filter or not. In addition the study randomised patients to receive either LMWH and a coumarin or intravenous unfractionated heparin and a coumarin. There was a reduction in the incidence of PE in those who received a filter; an effect most pronounced in the first 3 months. However, by 24 months of follow-up there had been a significant increase in the incidence of DVT in the filter arm (20.8% versus 11.6% in the anticoagulation only arm). Overall mortality at 24 months was no different between the two groups. Analysis of LMWH and unfractionated heparin randomisation revealed no significant differences.

An 8-year follow-up of the above study was performed to assess the long-term effect of permanent IVC filter insertion (PREPIC 2005). The studies overall findings were that vena cava filters reduce the risk of PE but increase the risk of DVT and have no long-term effect on post-thrombotic syndrome or survival.

The conclusion drawn is that permanent IVC filters confer no overall long term benefit in patients in whom there is no contraindication to anticoagulation. As a result, the use of IVC filters is now generally restricted to those in whom there is a contraindication to anticoagulation. For such patients temporary filters are preferable due to the increased long term incidence of DVT seen with permanent filters.

Predicting Venous Thrombosis

Wells et al., New England Journal of Medicine (2003)

With the introduction of LMWH allowing outpatient management of VTE the pressure for rapid diagnosis increased. Clinical assessment is fallible and diagnostic imaging resources finite. Development of a D-dimer assay of sufficient reproducibility allowed its application in the clinical setting. Mounting evidence from the mid-1990s had shown that the D-dimer test had a high negative predictive value. To assess whether the D-dimer result could be used as part of a predictive algorithm in the diagnosis of DVT, Wells and colleagues devised a randomised trial. Patients with suspected DVT were recruited from five centres, yielding a total of 1096 patients. In one arm patients were first assessed clinically as to the likelihood of DVT and then underwent ultrasound scanning. In the second group, a D-dimer test was performed. If clinically assessed as likely to have had a DVT, they underwent an ultrasound scan irrespective of the D-dimer result. In those assessed on clinical grounds as being unlikely to have had a DVT, ultrasound scanning was only performed if the D-dimer was positive. Patients were then followed up for 3 months. In patients where DVT was initially excluded, 0.4% of those where the D-dimer test had been used went on to have an episode of VTE by the end of 3 months compared to 1.4% where ultrasound had been used. The importance of clinical assessment in utilising the D-dimer result was highlighted by the finding that the negative predictive value where there was a low clinical likelihood of DVT was 99.1%, falling to 89% where there was a high clinical probability.

These findings have allowed patients with suspected VTE to be assessed and unnecessary imaging and treatment pending imaging to be avoided.

Conclusion

Over the past 100 years, our ability to treat and prevent thrombosis has improved significantly. It is likely that the use of heparin and warfarin will diminish with time as the newer generation of injectable and oral anticoagulants (fondaparinux, rivaroxaban, dabigatran) now enter clinical practice. However, our understanding of the mechanisms of thrombosis remains incomplete. Certainly we have identified various acquired and hereditary risk factors, but this fails to explain the numerous cases of venous thrombosis where these known factors are absent. In hereditary thrombophilias it remains unclear why there is heterogeneity in the severity of thrombotic events between families with the same defect. There is clearly still much to learn.

Key Outstanding Questions

1. What factors are responsible for apparently idiopathic venous thromboembolism?
2. After a first venous thrombotic event, in which patients can anticoagulation be safely stopped and in which patients should anticoagulation be continued long term?
3. Why is there a variation in the severity of the phenotype of hereditary thrombophilia between families with the same condition?

Key Research Centres

1. Addenbrooke's Hospital Haemostasis Unit, Cambridge, United Kingdom
2. Department of Haematology, Ottawa Hospital, Ottawa, Canada
3. Department of Vascular Medicine, Academic Medical Centre, Amsterdam, Netherlands
4. Division of Angiology and Haemostasis, Geneva University Hospital, Geneva, Switzerland
5. Haemostasis and Thrombosis Research Centre, Leiden University Medical Centre, Leiden, Netherlands
6. Haemophilia and Thrombosis Centre, IRCCS Maggiore Hospital, University of Milan, Milan, Italy
7. Haemostasis Research Unit, University College London, London, United Kingdom
8. Haemophilia and Thrombosis Centre, Royal Hallamshire Hospital, Sheffield, United Kingdom
9. Thrombosis Research Group, University Hospital of Saint-Etienne, Saint-Etienne, France
10. McMaster Medical Centre, Hamilton, Canada
11. Thromboembolism Unit, University of Padua, Padua, Italy

References

Barritt, D.W., and Jordan, S.C. (1960) Anticoagulant drugs in the treatment of pulmonary embolism: a controlled trial. *Lancet*, **1**, 1309–1312. http://www.sciencedirect.com/science/article/pii/S0140673660922996

Bertina, R.M., *et al.* (1994) Mutation in blood coagulation factor V associated with resistance to activated protein C. *Nature,* **369**, 64–67. http://www.ncbi.nlm.nih.gov/pubmed/8164741

Brandjes, D.P., *et al.* (1992) Acenocoumarol and heparin compared with acenocoumarol alone in the initial treatment of proximal-vein thrombosis. *New England Journal of Medicine,* **327**, 1485–1489. http://www.ncbi.nlm.nih.gov/pubmed/1406880

Dahlback, B., *et al.* (1993) Familial thrombophilia due to a previously unrecognised mechanism characterised by poor anticoagulant response to activated protein C: prediction of a cofactor to activated protein C. *Proceedings of the National Academy of Sciences of the USA,* **90**, 1004–1008. http://www.ncbi.nlm.nih.gov/pubmed/8430067

Decousus, H., *et al.* (1998) A clinical trial of vena caval filters in the prevention of pulmonary embolism in patients with proximal deep-vein thrombosis. Prévention du Risque d'Embolie Pulmonaire par Interruption Cave Study Group. *New England Journal of Medicine,* **338**, 409–415. http://www.ncbi.nlm.nih.gov/pubmed/9459643

Howell, W.H., and Holt, E. (1918) Two new factors in blood coagulation – heparin and proantithrombin. *American Journal of Physiology,* **47**, 328–341. http://ajplegacy.physiology. org/content/47/3/328.full.pdf.html

Kakkar, V.V., *et al.* (1975) Prevention of fatal postoperative pulmonary embolism by low doses of heparin. An International Multicentre Trial. *Lancet,* **306**, 45–51. http://www.thelancet. com/journals/lancet/article/PIIS0140-6736(75)90494-8/Abstract

Koopman, M.M., *et al.* (1996) Treatment of venous thrombosis with intravenous unfractionated heparin administered in the hospital as compared with subcutaneous low-molecular-weight heparin administered at home. The Tasman Study Group. *New England Journal of Medicine,* **334**, 682–687. http://www.ncbi.nlm.nih.gov/pubmed/8594426

Stahmann, M.A., *et al.* (1941) Studies on the haemorrhagic sweet clover disease. *Journal of Biological Chemistry,* **138**, 513–527. http://www.jbc.org/content/138/2/513.full.pdf.html

Wells, P.S., *et al.* (2003) Evaluation of D-dimer in the diagnosis of suspected deep-vein thrombosis. *New England Journal of Medicine,* **349**, 1227–1235. http://www.ncbi.nlm.nih. gov/pubmed/14507948

Additional References

1. Comp, P.C., and Esmom, C.T. (1984) Recurrent venous thromboembolism in patients with a partial deficiency of protein S. *New England Journal of Medicine,* **311**, 1525–1528.
2. Egeberg, O. (1965) Inherited antithrombin deficiency causing thrombophilia. *Thrombosis et Diathesis Haemorrhagica,* **13**, 516–530.
3. Griffin, J.H., *et al.* (1981) Deficiency of protein C in congenital thrombotic disease. *Journal of Clinical Investigation,* **68**, 1370–1373.
4. Lyttleton, J.W. (1954) The antithrombin activity of human plasma. *Biochemical Journal,* **58**, 8–15.
5. PREPIC (2005) Eight–year follow-up of patients with permanent vena cava filters in the prevention of pulmonary embolism. *Circulation,* **112**, 416–422.
6. Virchow, R.L.K. (1856) Thrombose und Embolie. Gefässentzündung und septische Infektion. In: *Gesammelte Abhandlungen zur wissenschaftlichen Medicin,* 219–732. Von Meidinger & Sohn, Frankfurt am Main. Translation in Matzdorff, A.C., and Bell, W.R. (1998). *Thrombosis and embolie (1846–1856).* Science History Publications, Canton, MA.

21 The Inherited Disorders of Haemoglobin

Sir David Weatherall

Weatherall Institute of Molecular Medicine, University of Oxford, Oxford, and Keele University, Keele, UK

Introduction

The inherited disorders of haemoglobin are the commonest monogenic diseases. It is estimated that over 300,000 babies are born each year with a severe form of these diseases. There are two main groups. Firstly, there are the structural haemoglobin variants, by far the commonest of which is sickle cell disease. Secondly, there are the inherited defects in haemoglobin synthesis which form a heterogeneous group of disorders called the thalassaemias.

Sickle cell anaemia was first identified in 1910 by James Herrick of Chicago. His patient was a student from the Caribbean who had a severe haemolytic anaemia associated with curious elongated, sickle-shaped red cells. Further cases in patients of African background were described and it became clear that the condition, as well as being associated with a haemolytic anaemia, is also characterised by intermittent attacks of severe bone pain due to blockage of small vessels, a marked propensity to infection, and a wide variety of other complications. Many years after its first description, it was found to be inherited as a Mendelian recessive disorder.

The severe form of thalassaemia was first described by Thomas Cooley of Detroit in 1925. He described several young children with profound anaemia, splenomegaly, a curious 'Mongoloid appearance' of the skull, and remarkable radiological changes of the skull and long bones. The disease was later called 'thalassaemia', from the Greek word for sea, because all the early cases that were described in the United States appeared to be of Mediterranean origin. In the same year that Cooley described the first severe cases of thalassaemia milder forms of what appeared to be the same condition were described quite independently by workers in Italy. Like sickle cell anaemia, the thalassaemias turned out to be inherited in a Mendelian recessive fashion and it slowly became apparent that they are a heterogeneous group of diseases ranging in severity from profound anaemia and death in the first few years of life to disorders of varying severity, at least some of which are compatible with survival into adult life.

In the early years following their discovery, it was thought that sickle cell anaemia was confined to those of African origin and thalassaemia to Mediterranean races, but later it became apparent that sickle cell disease also occurs in the Mediterranean region, Middle East and the Indian subcontinent, and that the thalassaemias are spread widely across Africa, the Middle East, the Indian subcontinent and Southeast Asia. Although the haemoglobin disorders occur at their highest frequencies in tropical countries, due to

Understanding Medical Research: The Studies that Shaped Medicine, First Edition. Edited by John A. Goodfellow. © 2012 John Wiley & Sons, Ltd. Published 2012 by John Wiley & Sons, Ltd.

widespread emigration from these regions they are now seen in almost every country of the world.

These diseases pose a major global health problem, particularly for the developing countries. As the first genetic diseases to be explored at the molecular level, they have played an important role in the development of molecular medicine and because of their high frequency they are also of interest to evolutionary biologists. Hence the field has gathered a large and diverse literature. The ten papers that follow were not selected necessarily as the 'best' or most original in the field, but simply to illustrate different phases and aspects of its development.

Molecular and Cellular Pathology
Pauling et al., Science (1949)

The discovery that sickle cell disease results from the production of an abnormal haemoglobin followed a chance conversation between the haematologist William Castle and the protein chemist Linus Pauling in 1945. Castle told Pauling that when he had been examining the blood of patients with sickle cell disease he had noticed that when their red cells were deprived of oxygen and formed a sickle shape they showed unusual properties when examined under polarized light. As a chemist, Pauling realised that this might reflect some form of molecular reorganisation and that it might therefore indicate that the haemoglobin of patients with sickle cell disease could be in some way abnormal. At about this time the Swedish chemist Tiselius had developed a technique called electrophoresis which made it possible to separate proteins of different structure and charge in an electric field. Pauling, together with a post-doctoral student Harvey Itano, set about building a Tiselius apparatus and examined the haemoglobin of patients with sickle cell anaemia. Remarkably they found that it moved in an electric field at a different rate to the haemoglobin of normal persons and, equally importantly, that the red cells of unaffected carriers of the sickle cell gene contained both normal and abnormal haemoglobin. Their paper in *Science*, published in 1949 and entitled 'Sickle cell anaemia, a molecular disease', is often regarded as the beginning of the era of molecular medicine.

Within a few years a much simpler method for searching for haemoglobin variants was developed using filter paper and a small power-pack to supply the current. Soon laboratories all over the world were using this technique and new abnormal haemoglobins were reported at regular intervals. Initially they were designated by letters of the alphabet; normal haemoglobin was called haemoglobin A (HbA), sickle haemoglobin haemoglobin S (HbS) and numerous others followed until the alphabet was used up and haemoglobins had to be named after their place of origin.

Although hundreds of abnormal haemoglobins were discovered in subsequent years only three, Hbs S, C and E, reached extremely high frequencies in certain populations.

Ingram and Stretton, Nature (1959)

In the ten years after the discovery of sickle cell haemoglobin, remarkable progress was made towards an understanding of the structure and genetic control of human haemoglobin. It was found that it is composed of two unlike pairs of globin chains each of which is wound round a porphyrin ring, or haem, which is the oxygen binding site. Hence adult haemoglobin was designated $\alpha_2\beta_2$. This intimated that there must be at least two sets of genes involved in the control of adult haemoglobin synthesis, α genes and β genes. Ingram then discovered that the difference between normal haemoglobin and sickle-cell haemoglobin is a single amino acid substitution; glutamic acid in normal haemoglobin is replaced by valine in the β chain of sickle haemoglobin. Clearly, sickle cell anaemia must result from a mutation of the β globin gene. It had also been known for some time that haemoglobin in fetal life is different from that of adult haemoglobin and it was designated haemoglobin F (HbF). HbF was shown to consist of α chains combined with different chains from adult haemoglobin which were called γ chains; it therefore has the structure $\alpha_2 \gamma_2$. It was also found that normal adults have a minor haemoglobin called haemoglobin A_2 and that this has the structure $\alpha_2 \delta_2$. Hence there must be at least four sets of genes that regulate human haemoglobin, α, β, γ and δ.

At the same time as these seminal studies were being carried out, the haemoglobin constitution of patients with thalassaemia was investigated. No abnormal haemoglobins could be detected but at least some children with severe thalassaemia had persistently elevated levels of fetal haemoglobin, the synthesis of which normally declines rapidly after birth and which is only present in trace amounts in normal adults. It was also found that the level of Hb A_2 is elevated in a high proportion of the parents, or carriers, of thalassaemic children. Furthermore some patients with thalassaemia have curious homotetramer haemoglobins in their blood, that is haemoglobins that consist of either four β or four γ chains; when the former was discovered H was the next letter available in the alphabet to name a haemoglobin so it was called Hb H, but by the time the γ_4 molecule was discovered there were no letters left and it was named Hb Bart's after its discovery at St Bartholomew's hospital in London.

But the most remarkable finding in the thalassaemias was that many patients who had inherited a thalassaemia gene from one parent and the sickle cell gene from the other had approximately 70 – 80% HbS in their red cells and only about 20% HbA; carriers for the sickle cell gene usually have just the opposite (i.e. about 70% HbA and 30% HbF). Since it was now known that the sickle cell mutation involves the β globin gene this suggested that the action of the thalassaemia gene was to depress the synthesis of normal β chains. It was also found that in babies who have Hb Bart's or older patients with Hb H the blood picture is typical of that of thalassaemia.

In their seminal paper of 1959 Ingram and Stretton analysed all these findings, which were the work of many scientists, and produced a theoretical model for the genetic basis of the thalassaemias. In short, they suggested that there were two types, α and β thalassaemia. The β thalassaemias are those that are associated with high levels of HbF in severe cases and raised levels of HbA$_2$ in the symptomless carriers, both reflecting a defect in β chain production. They used the model of the reversed HbA to S ratios in patients with HbS β thalassaemia as further evidence for the existence of defective β chain production and interpreted forms of thalassaemia in which no interaction of this type occurs, or in which Hbs Bart's or H are found, as reflecting defective α chain synthesis.

This paper set the scene for research in the thalassaemia field from the 1960s onwards.

Weatherall et al., Nature (1965)
Although the studies of the haemoglobin patterns of patients with thalassaemia had suggested that there might be two varieties, α and β thalassaemia, it was necessary to prove that these conditions result from defective α or β globin chain synthesis. It had

been known for several years that it is possible to incorporate radioactive amino acids into haemoglobin in red cells incubated *in vitro*, provided there are sufficient numbers of reticulocytes with the capacity to make haemoglobin in the blood samples. The main problem, however, was how to separate the α and β chains to assess their individual rates of synthesis in experiments of this type. To achieve this end a method was developed in which the globin chains could be fractionated quantitatively by chromatography on a specific cellulose in a strong buffered solution of urea. The key to the successful separation of the chains was the addition of 2-mercaptoethanol to the buffer, which prevents aggregation of the α and β chains by inhibiting bonding between them.

In the first description of the application of this method to the study of thalassaemia it was possible to obtain a reasonably complete picture of the pattern of normal globin synthesis and of its abnormal synthesis in both α and β thalassaemia. It was found that in normal reticulocytes α and β chain production is almost synchronous. On the other hand, in β thalassaemia there is a marked imbalance of globin chain production and, overall, a variable excess of α chains are produced In the moderately severe form of α thalassaemia, HbH disease, there is a marked deficit of α chain synthesis. Further work using this system showed that the excess of α chains produced in β thalassaemia undergo two fates; some are degraded by the proteolytic enzymes of the red cell, while others become associated with the red cell membrane. It was also found that in some forms of β thalassaemia there is a complete absence of β chain production, while in others there is only a partial defect, and that babies who are stillborn with very severe α thalassaemia produce no α chains whatever.

It was now clear that the thalassaemias are not so much disorders of haemoglobin production but rather of imbalanced globin chain production. In subsequent years it was possible to relate the profound anaemia and ineffective erythropoiesis of this disease to the deleterious effects of the particular globin chains that are produced in excess. In β thalassaemia the ineffective erythropoiesis is due to damage to the red cell precursors in the bone marrow; the shortened survival of such red cells that do reach the peripheral blood results from both the damaging effect of precipitated α chains during their passage through the spleen and also direct oxidant damage by the degradation products of these α chains on the structure and function of the red cell membrane. The severe bone changes in this disease and associated splenomegaly and other features can be ascribed to a remarkable erythropoietin response to the profound anaemia, with massive expansion of red cell precursors, many of which die within the bone marrow.

One of the pleasing outcomes of this study was that within only a few years it was possible to apply *in vitro* globin synthesis for the prenatal diagnosis of both α and β thalassaemia using fetal blood samples, with a remarkable reduction in the births of cases of babies with thalassaemia in many countries.

Ottolenghi et al., Nature (1974)
Taylor et al., Nature (1974)

These papers, which appeared back to back in the same edition of *Nature* in 1974, described completely independent studies by two groups which were the first to demonstrate directly a defect in a human gene at the DNA level.

When it was found that babies who were stillborn with a very severe form of α thalassaemia produced no α chains it was suggested that their α globin genes might be either completely or partially deleted, that is they had no functional α genes. In the early 1970s methods for searching for genes with radioactively labelled probes became available. In 1970 Baltimore and Temin independently discovered an enzyme in certain tumour viruses which they called reversed transcriptase, a finding that made it possible to synthesise complementary DNA (cDNA) from mRNA templates. Hence by obtaining RNA from normal reticulocytes, that is young red cells that can retain the capacity for synthesising haemoglobin and which therefore must contain α and β globin mRNA, and by adding radioactive nucleotides to the reaction, it became possible to synthesise radioactively-labelled α or β globin cDNA. Because of the strict rules of pairing between nucleotide bases, these could only bind, or hybridise, to α or β globin mRNA or DNA of the same sequence. It was postulated therefore that it should be possible to use these probes to determine whether babies with severe α thalassaemia had α globin genes in their DNA.

These experiments entailed obtaining DNA from the tissues of a stillborn baby in whom a complete absence of α chain synthesis had been demonstrated and then to compare the pattern of cDNA hybridisation using an α globin gene probe with that of a stillborn infant with no evidence of thalassaemia. The experiments showed that DNA obtained from the liver of a thalassaemic baby contained β globin DNA sequences but a more or less complete absence of α globin DNA, while in DNA prepared from the tissues of stillborn infants with no evidence of thalassaemia the expected α and β DNA sequences were present. These findings showed beyond any reasonable doubt that the severe form of α thalassaemia which the thalassaemic infant had inherited from both parents was due to a major deletion of the α globin genes.

These findings were confirmed only a few years later when further methods were developed for both mapping the globin genes and for sequencing them directly. It turned out that the β thalassaemias are the result of literally hundreds of different mutations in the β globin genes, and that the α thalassaemias result from many different sized deletions of one or both of the α globin genes or point mutations similar to those in the β globin genes.

Improvements in the Prevention and Treatment of the Thalassaemias and Sickle Cell Disease
Wolman, Annals of the New York Academy of Science (1964)

From its first discovery in 1925 until after the Second World War the management of thalassaemia was completely unsatisfactory and most affected children died early in life. Although attempts had been made to maintain these children by blood transfusion there was no consistency in the way this was organised. At a meeting of the Cooley's Anaemia Blood and Research Foundation for Children Inc in New York in 1963 the results of an enquiry sent to more than 12 centres, caring for over 150 patients with severe thalassaemia, was presented. It appeared that there were no consistent criteria for determining when a child should be transfused. Rather, transfusions were administered either when a particular haemoglobin level was reached or when a child became symptomatic; when symptomatic treatment was administered the haemoglobin level before transfusion was often as low as 3.0 g/dl and even if a particular haemoglobin level was chosen it tended to be no higher than 7.0 g/dl.

At the same meeting, Irving Wolman of the Children's Hospital in Philadelphia presented findings of a preliminary study in which he had set out to determine whether children with severe thalassaemia who had been maintained by blood transfusion at a near-normal haemoglobin level were better off than those who had only received transfusion when they were symptomatic. The findings suggested that children maintained at a relatively high haemoglobin level were taller, had smaller livers and spleens, showed less skeletal deformities, fewer fractures and much better dental development, and had less cardiomegaly. In short, it was clear that a more aggressive transfusion regimen was able to reverse many of the more distressing features of severe thalassaemia.

Wolman's results were confirmed at a meeting held in 1969, by which time there was no doubt that patients maintained at a relatively high haemoglobin level had grown and developed well during their early years, although it was noted that they did not show the usual adolescent growth spurt. They had continued to have less skeletal deformity and bone disease, and their spleens and livers had remained small. However, a serious problem had arisen; of a total of 17 children who had received the high transfusion regimen for long enough for adequate evaluation, six had died, all from disorders that could be related to the damaging effects of excess iron in the body. This was not surprising of course. We have no way of excreting iron and every unit of blood adds at least 200 mg of iron to the body iron stores. Hence by the time these children were becoming teenagers they had already accumulated in excess of 20–30 grams of iron, and this had an extremely damaging effect on their livers, their endocrine glands and in particular their hearts. So although this transfusion regimen provided a much better childhood, unless the problem of excessive iron loading could be overcome they were all likely to die of the effects of iron loading before they reached the age of 20 years.

Sephton-Smith, Annals of the New York Academy of Science (1964)

A major problem which faced those who were trying to develop drugs that might remove excess iron from the body, iron-chelating agents, was specificity. Many agents can bind iron, but they also bind other metals and hence cannot be used for treating iron-loaded patients. In the early 1960s the pharmaceutical company CIBA explored the possibility of developing chelating agents from sideramines, naturally occurring iron-binding agents that are required by bacteria to incorporate iron which is important for their growth. This led to the development of a strong iron-chelating agent, desferrioxamine. At the same meeting in New York in 1963, Sephton-Smith described his experiences with this agent and another chelating agent with a high affinity for iron, diethylenetriamine-pentaacetate (DTPA). He reported studies in which he had administered these agents either orally, intramuscularly or intravenously. They had no effect after oral administration but were able to remove varying amounts of iron, depending on the iron status of the particular patients, by either intramuscular or intravenous administration. Sephton-Smith concluded that perhaps the best way forward would be to use daily intramuscular injections of DTPA or desferrioxamine combined with an intravenous infusion of desferrioxamine at the time of transfusion. However, DTPA injections proved to be extremely painful and the field slowly evolved using desferrioxamine as its major chelating agent.

For several years it was believed that it was not going to be possible to control iron accumulation with desferrioxamine because of difficulties with compliance and other factors but the results of a controlled trial at Great Ormond Street Hospital suggested that it might be effective. Later, by using prolonged subcutaneous infusions driven by clockwork pumps, it became possible to maintain many children in iron balance with remarkable improvements in the prognosis for the disease. However, difficulties with compliance remained, leading to the development of several oral chelating agents. It still took many years to prove the efficacy of desferrioxamine and there remain uncertainties about the true role of these newer drugs in the long-term management of iron loading, a problem that became even more important when, in order to prevent strokes, many patients with sickle cell anaemia began to be maintained on blood transfusion.

Charache et al., New England Journal of Medicine (1995)

Over the years, many different forms of treatment were attempted to control the painful crises and other complications of sickle-cell disease but none of them stood up to critical evaluation. In the event, it was an experiment of nature which pointed the way towards the better control of this condition. It was observed that patients with sickle cell anaemia who had unusually high levels of fetal haemoglobin in their red cells appeared to run a milder course than those with lower levels. This was most vividly demonstrated in patients with sickle cell anaemia in Saudi Arabia and India; the sickle cell mutation appeared to have arisen independently in these populations and for reasons that are still not absolutely clear the disease is associated with a much higher level of Hb F production than in African patients and a significantly milder clinical phenotype.

It had been known for some time that patients recovering from bone marrow depression tend to go through a phase of increased Hb F production. Early studies with the drug decitabine produced moderate increases in Hb F, probably reflecting hypomethylation of DNA as the mechanism for Hb F elevation. Because of a variety of concerns about this agent it was suggested that it might be worth attempting to increase Hb F by the administration of hydroxyurea, a drug which might increase Hb F production by accelerating the differentiation rate of red cell precursors. This concept was confirmed experimentally by showing a marked elevation in Hb F production in phlebotomised monkeys who had been treated with hydroxyurea. This agent was given to small numbers of patients with sickle cell disease and a modest increase in fetal haemoglobin was observed.

The paper by Charache et al, published in 1995 describes the results of a relatively large randomised, placebo-controlled trial of hydroxyurea with well-defined clinical end points. Remarkably, this study had to be terminated prematurely when an interim analysis revealed a significant reduction in the frequency of painful crises and other life threatening complications of patients with sickle cell disease in the treated as compared with the control group.

Following this promising result hydroxyurea was licensed in many countries for the treatment of sickle cell disease. It appears to be effective in the control of many of the unpleasant side effects of the condition, but not all, and so far there is no evidence of any increase in haematological malignancies which of course were always a possibility with the long-term administration of an agent like hydroxyurea. The administration of this agent for improving β thalassaemia by elevating Hb F levels has been much less effective.

One of the intriguing questions is why this drug actually works. It undoubtedly does increase the level of fetal haemoglobin production but not to a very high level and several studies have suggested that its effect, at least in part, may be mediated by a reduction in white blood cells and hence modification of the complex interactions between sickled erythrocytes and the microcirculation. Regardless of how it works, it was the first relatively effective agent for the treatment of this disease and so far no better approaches have been developed with the exception of long-term transfusion, which has been found to be effective in reducing the rate of strokes which are an increasingly common complication in older patients.

Alter, Annals of the New York Academy of Science (1990)

During the late 1960s and early 1970s it was found that, although the main type of haemoglobin that is produced during fetal life is Hb F, small amounts of adult haemoglobin are present quite early during fetal development. *In vitro* studies of haemoglobin synthesis showed that adult β chain synthesis is activated at about the tenth week of gestation and reaches a steady state of about 10% of haemoglobin synthesised up to about 30 weeks gestation, after which it begins to rise rapidly as the level of fetal haemoglobin begins to fall. These observations suggested that if it were possible to obtain fetal blood samples during midgestation, it might be possible to identify fetuses with homozygous β thalassaemia or sickle cell disease. Following improvements in fetal blood sampling, by the end of 1978 workers in the United States, England and the Mediterranean region were able to publish results of early attempts at the prenatal diagnosis of β thalassaemia. At this stage, based on an experience of over 100 attempts, the technique appeared to be feasible for identifying β thalassaemia and sickle cell anaemia; there had been remarkably few diagnostic errors and the only worrying feature was the relatively high fetal loss attributable to the procedure.

During the next 10 years, Alter maintained an international register and in 1990 was able to present data on 13,921 prenatal diagnoses for thalassaemia and sickle cell anaemia that had been carried out in 20 centres in different countries using fetal blood sampling between 1974 and 1989. Although these results varied between different countries, particularly in those like Cyprus and Sardinia where prenatal diagnosis programmes had been accompanied by extremely effective public education programmes, the resulting fall in the births of babies with severe β thalassaemia was quite dramatic.

The smaller overall numbers of diagnoses for sickle cell anaemia reflect continued uncertainty about how to predict its degree of severity in individual families.

The problem with this approach was that using fetal blood sampling and *in vitro* haemoglobin synthesis analysis the diagnosis had to be carried out relatively late in pregnancy which meant that, if the parents decided to terminate a pregnancy carrying an affected fetus, it was a particularly unpleasant experience for the mother. However, in the early 1980s it became possible to obtain fetal DNA by chorion villus sampling, which could be carried out at about 12 weeks of pregnancy, and this new technology gradually replaced *in vitro* globin synthesis as an approach to prenatal diagnosis. In this paper Alter was also able to summarise data on the first 750 diagnoses of this type. Currently, prenatal diagnosis is carried out in countries all over the world, mainly for thalassaemia. Because of the continued uncertainties about how to predict the prognosis for patients with sickle cell disease it is still used much less widely for its prenatal detection.

Thomas et al., Lancet (1982)

This paper described the first successful cure of a patient with thalassaemia by bone marrow transplantation by E. Donnall Thomas and his team in Seattle.

Thomas was the main pioneer of bone marrow transplantation, an approach which followed many years of experimental work in mice and outbred dogs. After innumerable setbacks his team had their first successes in treating patients with aplastic anaemia and, later, leukaemia, remarkable achievements which depended on the development of better ways of suppressing the recipient's bone marrow, the application of improved tissue typing and, not in the least, the meticulous after care of patients whose bone marrows had been suppressed during the procedure and who were therefore at high risk for infection.

The first successful bone marrow transplant for thalassaemia was carried out on a 14-month-old child who had never received a blood transfusion; the results were remarkably successful. Shortly afterwards, a 14-year-old child with thalassaemia who had already received 150 red cell transfusions received a bone marrow transplantation in Italy but this was followed by recurrence of the patient's thalassaemia after the donor marrow had been rejected.

In subsequent years Lucarelli's centre in Pesaro carried out over 1000 marrow transplants for thalassaemia, and other centres around the world started to gain experience of the procedure. There was a steady improvement in the results which followed more effective pre-transplantation regimens, the introduction of more potent immunosuppressant drugs, and improved treatment of infection. It also became clear that the best results were obtained if the procedure was carried out early in life and before the children had begun to develop the complications of thalassaemia, particularly iron overload.

Of course, because only one in four siblings will be HLA compatible, this approach has its limitations but it was undoubtedly a major advance in the management of thalassaemia in particular. Many successful transplants for sickle cell disease have also been carried out.

Why Are the Inherited Haemoglobin Disorders So Common?
Haldane, Proc. VIII Int. Cong. Genetics Hereditas (1949)

In the early population studies that were carried out in the 1940s, workers on both sides of the Atlantic were puzzled as to why the thalassaemias seemed to occur at an extraordinarily high frequency in persons from the southern Mediterranean countries yet not in northern Europeans. These findings were particularly difficult to understand since most serious genetic diseases occur at low frequencies throughout different populations. In order to explain them, the American workers Neel and Valentine proposed that there is a particularly high mutation rate for thalassaemia and even suggested that mutation rates might vary between different ethnic groups.

These issues were discussed at the Eighth International Congress of Genetics in Stockholm in 1948, which was attended by one of the great founders of statistical genetics, J.B.S. Haldane. Haldane did not like the idea of these high mutation rates and his alternative explanation for the high frequency of thalassaemia, which is summarised in the Proceedings of the meeting, formed the basis for future work in this important aspect of human evolutionary biology. In short, Haldane suggested that the small red cells of carriers for thalassaemia might be a less attractive environment for malarial parasites. Up to the Second World War there had been a high mortality from malaria in the southern Mediterranean and Haldane suggested that carriers for thalassaemia, because of relative malaria resistance, might have survived longer than normal people in a malarial environment and hence the frequency of the β thalassaemia gene would have increased until it was balanced by loss through the death of homozygous children.

Curiously, it was work on sickle cell anaemia by Allison in the early 1940s, which showed that the sickle cell trait offered considerable protection against malaria, that was the first evidence that Haldane was correct. It was only many years later that it was established that the extraordinarily high frequencies of α thalassaemia, β thalassaemia, and Hbs C and E also reflect heterozygote protection against malaria. Although it turned out that Haldane's concept that the small red cells in thalassaemia are an unattractive home for malarial parasites is an over-simplification, in terms of population distribution and numbers Haldane's malaria hypothesis has stood the test of time.

Summary

The haemoglobinopathies have turned out to be by far the commonest human monogenic diseases. There is now no doubt that they will present an increasingly severe health burden for the developing countries, particularly those that are going through an epidemiological transition with improvements in public health and living conditions such that babies who would have died early in life with these conditions are now surviving to present for treatment.

These diseases were the first to be examined at the molecular level. It is now clear that the thalassaemias result from literally hundreds of different mutations of the α or β globin genes and that the sickle cell mutation has arisen at least twice in different populations. Some progress has been made in determining why the phenotypes of these conditions vary so much, reflecting layer upon layer of modifier genes together with variation in the pattern of adaptation to the disease and the effects of the environment. Screening and prenatal diagnosis programmes in many countries have reduced the birth rate of babies affected with these conditions and there have been genuine improvements in their symptomatic management. For those with suitable donors, marrow transplantation is now a successful therapeutic option. Unfortunately, in many of the poorer countries of the world where these conditions are particularly common, facilities for their symptomatic management and population control are still extremely limited.

The population genetics and dynamics of the haemoglobin disorders have also provided a remarkable model of the complex evolutionary basis for the varying frequency and distribution of different human diseases.

Key Outstanding Questions

1. What are the precise mechanisms and therapeutic potential for the developmental switch from fetal to adult Hb production?
2. What are the precise mechanisms by which the carrier states for different haemoglobin disorders afford protection against severe malaria?
3. Will somatic-cell gene therapy approaches ultimately offer a cure for the haemoglobin disorders?

4. To what extent is the remarkable phenotypic variation of the haemoglobin disorders in different parts of the world the result of genetic modifiers compared with the environment?

5. When will the major international health agencies and funding bodies, and the governments of many of the developing countries, finally realise that the inherited disorders of haemoglobin are an increasingly serious global health problem?

Acknowledgements

My thanks to Jeanne Packer and Liz Rose for their help in preparing this chapter.

References

Alter, B.P. (1990) Antenatal diagnosis: summary of results. *Annals of the New York Academy of Science*, **612**, 237. http://onlinelibrary.wiley.com/doi/10.1111/j.1749-6632.1990.tb24311.x/Abstract

Charache, S., *et al.* (1995) Effect of hydroxyurea on the frequency of painful crises in sickle cell anemia. *New England Journal of Medicine*, **332**, 1317–1322. http://www.ncbi.nlm.nih.gov/pubmed/7715639

Haldane, J.B.S. (1949) The rate of mutation of human genes. *Proc. VIII Int. Cong. Genetics Hereditas*, **35**, 267–273. http://www.springerlink.com/content/v572t14418w42167/

Ingram, V.M., and Stretton, A.O.W. (1959) Genetic basis of the thalassemia diseases. *Nature*, **184**, 1903–1909. http://www.nature.com/nature/journal/v184/n4703/pdf/1841903a0.pdf

Ottolenghi, S., *et al.* (1974) The severe form of a thalassaemia is caused by a haemoglobin gene deletion. *Nature*, **251**, 389–392. http://www.nature.com/nature/journal/v251/n5474/abs/251389a0.html

Pauling, L., *et al.* (1949) Sickle-cell anemia, a molecular disease. *Science*, **110**, 543–548. http://www.sciencemag.org/content/110/2865/543.extract

Sephton-Smith, R. (1964) Chelating agents in the diagnosis and treatment of iron overload. *Annals of the New York Academy of Science*, **119**, 776. http://onlinelibrary.wiley.com/doi/10.1111/j.1749-6632.1965.tb54079.x/Abstract

Taylor, J.M., *et al.* (1974) Genetic lesion in homozygous a-thalassaemia (hydrops foetalis). *Nature*, **251**, 392–393. http://www.nature.com/nature/journal/v251/n5474/abs/251392a0.html

Thomas, E.D., *et al.* (1982) Marrow transplantation for thalassaemia. *Lancet*, **ii**, 227–229. http://www.thelancet.com/journals/lancet/article/PIIS0140-6736(82)90319-1/Abstract

Weatherall, D.J., *et al.* (1965) Globin synthesis in thalassemia: an in vitro study. *Nature*, **208**, 1061–1065. http://www.nature.com/nature/journal/v208/n5015/pdf/2081061a0.pdf

Wolman, I.J. (1964) Transfusion therapy in Cooley's anemia: growth and health as related to long-range hemoglobin levels, a progress report. *Annals of the New York Academy of Science*, **119**, 736–747. http:// onlinelibrary.wiley.com/doi/10.1111/j.1749-6632.1965.tb54075.x/Abstract

Additional References

1. Serjeant, G.R. (2001) *Sickle cell disease*. 3rd ed. Oxford University Press, New York.
2. Steinberg, M.H., Forget, B.G., Higgs, D.R., and Weatherall, D.J., eds. (2008) *Disorders of hemoglobin*. 2nd ed. Cambridge University Press, New York.
3. Weatherall, D.J., and Clegg, J.B. (2001) *The thalassaemia syndromes*. 4th ed. Blackwell Science, Oxford.

22 Diabetes Therapy and the Prevention of Vascular Damage

Philip Home

Institute of Cellular Medicine, Newcastle University, Newcastle upon Tyne, UK

Introduction

Diabetes mellitus is a series of medical conditions grouped together by the single diagnostic finding of raised plasma glucose concentrations. These conditions have a diverse aetiology, with type 2 diabetes becoming a major scourge affecting over 280 million people. Western lifestyle habits are being taken up by industrialising low- and middle-income countries and increasing its prevalence.[1] Type 2 diabetes occurs when the liver can no longer cope with the caloric load presented to it, inducing a state of insensitivity which then overtaxes compensatory pancreatic insulin production in some people. By contrast, type 1 diabetes is a pure hormonal deficiency disease of autoimmune origin.

In all forms of diabetes, specific complications of a similar kind occur, notably retinopathy, nephropathy and neuropathy. Atherosclerosis indistinguishable from that affecting people without diabetes has an approximately doubled incidence compared to the background population. It might be thought that if a specific biochemical abnormality (here hyperglycaemia) is associated in a number of conditions of different aetiology with later development of specific complications, then it will be obvious that the metabolic abnormality must be causative of those complications, and that normalisation of biochemistry will reduce the risk of later complications. Medical scepticism, clinical inertia, and the tenets of evidence-based medicine prevent such easy conclusions, and the tools for treatment of diabetes remained too primitive for years to set and test the hypothesis easily. This review tells the story of the last 30 years, a story which presently ends in some controversy.

Urinary Glucose Control and Microvascular Complications in Clinical Practice
Pirart, Diabetes & Metabolism (1977)

The state of the art in 1978 was summarised in a scholarly review by Tchobroutsky in which he noted that 'The ideal study [of glucose control and diabetes complications] is impossible to do in man for practical and ethical reasons', having noted that 'Definite criteria are lacking for the quantification of both complications and the degree of [glucose] control'.[2] While this set the challenge for the following decades, the power of careful and complete data collection and analysis was demonstrated in a three-paper effort by Pirart, a physician in Brussels. Some 4398 people with a mixture of types of

Understanding Medical Research: The Studies that Shaped Medicine, First Edition. Edited by John A. Goodfellow. © 2012 John Wiley & Sons, Ltd. Published 2012 by John Wiley & Sons, Ltd.

diabetes were followed for up to 25 years with glucose control being assessed largely by urinary glucose excretion. By dividing people according to the degree of glycosuria, Pirart and his colleagues were able to show that worse long-term glucose control was associated with higher risk of microvascular complications, and indeed that the more severe forms of retinopathy were likewise associated.

The leap of faith from such associations to using therapy to improve glucose control with the intent of preventing vascular damage is large. Further it was made worse by the very poor therapeutic ratio of insulin administration, which causes significant hypo-glycaemia at around half the dose needed to obtain good blood glucose control.

Subcutaneous Pumped Insulin: Better Glucose Control in Type 1 Diabetes
Pickup et al., BMJ (1978)

Tchobroutsky's comment as to the poor state of diabetes therapy and measurement technology was already changing as he wrote. In April 1976, a woman with type 1 diabetes in a ward at Guy's Hospital in London was begun on an experimental form of subcutaneous insulin delivery using an insulin pump. The idea was coined by three senior professors in the back of a London taxi, the concept being to use mini-pumps designed for endocrinological animal experiments to deliver insulin to people and replace insulin injections. The attraction would be as a tool for studies on insulin absorption, but it soon became obvious that the potential for better blood glucose control could be realised too. Insulin pumps used only dissolved unmodified animal insulin (later human insulin and then insulin analogues), thus avoiding the problems of delivery and absorption of the intermediate-acting insulins. In a series of studies, Pickup and colleagues were able to show sustainability of good blood glucose control for long periods of therapy in the ambulant patient and more comprehensive improvements in other aspects of metabolic control.

But pumps themselves were not the only innovation in insulin delivery about that time. In Glasgow, Ireland came up with the idea of replacing the insulin syringe and vial with a combined insulin pen-injector,[3] technical developments of which are now used by tens of millions of people with diabetes worldwide for administration of most forms of insulin. Pump and pen regimens stimulated interest in which could give better blood glucose control. This could now be better assessed for two developments in the late 1970s enabled its more accurate measurement. Across the river from Guy's, Boucher promoted the use of glycated haemoglobin (GHb, a non-enzymatic product of glucose and haemoglobin) as a clinical test of recent blood glucose control, while the crude Eyetone meter used to monitor the first pumps at Guy's evolved into an ever-expanding range of finger-prick blood glucose strips and meters. With these four technological advances (pumps, pens, GHb and self-test strips and meters), the scene was set to perform Tchobroutsky's impractical study.

A Feasibility Study of Glucose Control and Complications
Kroc Collaborative Study Group, NEJM (1984)

Ethically it was still impossible to randomise people to poor blood glucose control, and then wait to see if they went blind, lost a limb, or developed progressive kidney disease.

At that time the availability to intervene in the microvascular complications once they had become evident was unproven and in some instances unknown. Accordingly the trial would have to be of ordinary day-to-day blood glucose control against near-normoglycaemia, and there was no evidence that this could be achieved on the wide scale needed for such a clinical trial, and therefore no prospect of getting funding. Major clinical trials at that time were tiny: human insulin was introduced to the market in the early 1980s, with its largest randomised study of around 100 people with type 1 diabetes. Together these issues resulted in a short-term collaborative feasibility study in a limited number of centres on both sides of the Atlantic, funded in part by the owner of the McDonald's restaurant chain. Though secretly hoping for astounding results, the investigators were faced with early worsening of retinopathy with improved blood glucose control, and in the pre-DHL days the attempt to measure GHb in a central laboratory with samples crossing the ocean was a fiasco of evaporated dry ice and leaked blood samples. Importantly, the measurement of retinopathy had also become possible in the previous decade thanks to some careful grading work notably by the Wisconsin group, though obtaining multiple 35 mm photographs of each eye and having them expertly graded were tedious and subject to error.

The Ultimate Type 1 Diabetes Study
Diabetes Control and Complications Trial (DCCT) Research Group, NEJM (1993)

The DCCT was the first of the major diabetes clinical trials, although the 1441 people studied now seem a modest number. Nevertheless 6.5 years duration is still longer than for many metabolic outcome studies, and from first recruitment this means some data may be available for as long as 7–8 years in a few participants. The DCCT was conducted on one continent, with centres in the United States and Canada, and planning that now seems merely normal but at that time seemed meticulous. Thus participating centres were all closely monitored, special attention was paid to the central assay of GHb and retinopathy and the participants with type 1 diabetes in the intensive group were given pumps, pen-injectors, self-monitoring equipment, dietary education, weekly phone calls, incentivising communications and the like. By this time HbA_{1c}, the more specific glycated fragment of haemoglobin, was being standardised across laboratories, and indeed the standardisation developed for the DCCT became the global *de facto* standard in use up to 2009. Change in retinopathy grade with time was the primary outcome measure, again centrally assessed by graders working in pairs in Wisconsin. The study probably remains the most significant performed in diabetes ever.

The results, in terms of microvascular disease, were unequivocal. Firstly the intensive therapy successfully separated glucose control by around 2.0 % HbA_{1c} (a reduction of around 22% in blood glucose levels), and this was sustained throughout the study. Secondly, while it appeared that people who had had poor glucose control for some time did have some worsening of retinopathy when first moved to good blood glucose control, the endpoint finding was unequivocally that retinopathy was reduced by a large margin (around 75%) from 2 years onwards (Figure 22.1). Other microvascular disease findings were supportive. But the news was not all good; in some centres the institution of tighter blood glucose control increased hypoglycaemia and severe hypoglycaemia rates, overall by some two to three times. While there was no evidence of safety issues

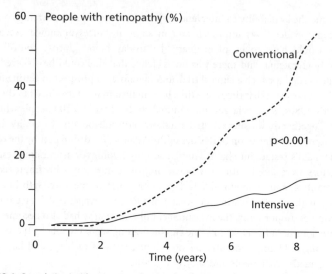

Figure 22.1 Cumulative incidence curves for the development of significant retinopathy in those with no prior retinopathy on entry into the Diabetes Control and Complications study (1993), comparing intensive to conventional glucose control. Hazard ratio 0·24 (95% CI 0.15, 0.38). Reproduced with permission from *NEJM*, 1993, **329**, 977–986.

from that, the observation that after the study around a third of the improvement in good glucose control in the intensive group was quickly lost implied poor tolerability.

In diabetes studies, the kinds of questions that can be asked address whether there is any glucose threshold below which complications do not develop, questions subject to unknown bias when applied to cross-sectional populations. In the DCCT, the initial analysis as published was unsatisfactory and was very recently repeated.[4] In the intensive group in whom glucose control would have been relatively steady over 6+ years, the complication incidence showed no rise up to an updated average HbA_{1c} level of 8.0 %. In the standard therapy group, with presumably less stable control, microvascular complications increased with time at levels below 8.0 %, implying that although if you always remain below this level you will be safe, any fluctuations around this as an average level may be detrimental.

Persistent Effects of Glucose Control on Arteriosclerotic Outcomes
Diabetes Control and Complications Trial/Epidemiology of Diabetes Interventions and Complications (DCCT/EDIC) Study Research Group, NEJM (2005)

The DCCT did not show any effect of good blood glucose control on macrovascular disease. Interpretation of that needs to be very cautious, however, as no such effect would have been expected given the small number of such events in what was a relatively young adult population.

As noted above, after the study glucose levels in the intensive group deteriorated such that within 2 years the HbA_{1c} means were the same. The authors were interested in how

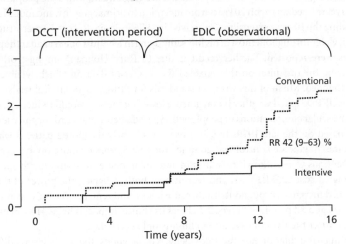

Cumulative incidence of major CVD (%)

Figure 22.2 Cumulative incidence curves for the occurrence of a first major cardiovascular event in the EDIC follow-up study of the Diabetes Control and Complications Trial (2005). Note that blood glucose control was only different between the randomised cohorts for the original period of the DCCT, 6.5 years. Reproduced with permission from *NEJM*, 2005, **353**, 2643–2653.

quickly the effects of good blood glucose control would be lost, and indeed whether a period of good glucose control of 5 years duration would delay the development of other complications. The 'whole' population was therefore followed for a further 12 years. The results were astounding.

From around 3 years after the end of the intervention study, cardiovascular disease (CVD) rates diverged steadily, despite the similar blood glucose control (Figure 22.2). The difference was large: relative risk in the previously intensive group was 42% of that in the prior standard control group. This 'legacy effect' is unexplained but is important in demonstrating that amelioration of glucose control can reduce cardiovascular events, and that this is achievable when the therapy used is insulin. Type 1 diabetes is a much purer form of glucose disorder than type 2 diabetes, and there is evidence that glucose is the primary early toxin which damages endothelium and makes it susceptible to other metabolic risk factors. The 8-year delay may reflect this observation, perhaps coupled to a delay from when vascular damage was beginning linked to the rising background incidence of CVD with age.

Type 2 Diabetes: A Study That Took 20 Years
United Kingdom Prospective Diabetes Study (UKPDS) Group, *Lancet (1998)*

'Study' is perhaps the wrong word for the UKPDS. It is more of a research institution in its own right. In a provocatively titled book, *UKPDS – the first 30 years*, Holman and Watkins list some 78 numbered UKPDS papers, many in major journals, and a list of other papers. Like the DCCT, the UKPDS has spawned a useful follow-up paper and a number of epidemiological analyses. The study statistics are gargantuan, with 5102 people followed for 10 years (median), with 20 years from inception to primary report, and indeed 30 years including the 10-year extension. Conceived in 1976 in India, Robert Turner struggled to keep it viable throughout most of his life, sadly dying in 1999 just one year after the primary results were reported. Further credit is due to Rury Holman, amongst others, for delivering the organisation that enabled the quality of data on which reliable results were founded. Much of this work set standards for future major clinical trials.

The UKPDS asked whether blood glucose lowering therapy would reduce arterial and microvascular complications in people with type 2 diabetes. Standards of glucose control were based on the late 1970s but, because it was newly diagnosed patients who were randomised, glucose control was good for the first 5 years or more on average. Study interventions were sulfonylureas, insulin and (in an obese substudy) metformin. With funding (it cost £23M/$37M) and recruitment both struggles, the power of the study remained marginal throughout, but because it was, and remains, the only such study in newly diagnosed people with type 2 diabetes its clinical impact is huge. How many other studies affect the lives of over 200 million people every day?

On microvascular disease the study delivered the goods: the 0.9 % HbA_{1c} difference (an 11% reduction), giving a 25% (95% CI 7–40%) risk reduction in microvascular endpoints, notably including the need for laser photocoagulation to the retina. This was achieved with sulfonylurea–insulin therapy but not with metformin in the obese substudy, probably due to underpowering.

The study also confirmed that the major impact of diabetes in people with type 2 diabetes was not microvascular damage but arterial disease. The major endpoint for this was myocardial infarction, and predetermined mortality endpoints again had confidence intervals that indicated underpowering. The central estimate for myocardial infarction reduction was 16%, right on the limit of study power, so the 95% confidence intervals were 0–29%. For many physicians, even academics, brought up in a era before confidence estimation, the key figure was the p value, 0.052, leading to the statement, blind to Bayesian probability, of 'not statistically significant'. A statistician later observed that only physicians, and not statisticians, could tell the differences between p = 0.05 and p = 0.052.

Some rescue of the situation came from the metformin study, where central estimates for diabetes death reduction and myocardial infarction were around an unlikely 40%, albeit with wide confidence intervals which overlap the central estimates for sulfonylureas and insulin. As a result, many physicians came to believe that metformin alone reduced macrovascular disease in type 2 diabetes, and this observation cemented its role as first-line therapy in most clinical guidelines. Some subsequent studies have not found metformin any better than sulfonylureas or the thiazolidinedione rosiglitazone.[5]

Other data from UKPDS has had a major impact on core diabetes thinking and clinical guidelines. The epidemiological analyses are the basis of data used to populate mathematical models of diabetes used for health economic modelling. Baseline epidemiological analysis showed almost equal importance of LDL cholesterol, HDL cholesterol, blood glucose control, smoking, and blood pressure in predicting coronary disease outcomes, with little effect of obesity. The blood pressure study showed that therapy had a profound effect on microvascular disease progression, including retinopathy, as well as arterial disease. But a marked and important outcome was the observation that type 2 diabetes was a progressive condition in terms of glucose control, worsening on average by around 0.15 % HbA_{1c} per year. This has profound implications for clinical care in terms of continued monitoring and up-titration of intensity of therapy. Furthermore, this was shown to be due to progressive loss of insulin secretion, independent of the therapies used, spawning an industry dedicated to preventing such decline in islet B-cell function. Only the thiazolidinediones have as yet shown any impact in this area.

The Glucose Legacy Effect Wins Again
Holman et al., NEJM (2008)

This had to come, and as with the EDIC study after the DCCT, participants in the UKPDS study showed rapid convergence of HbA_{1c} after the main study was completed, the better controlled group worsening and the conventional group improving. An extension study accumulates more events, so statistical power goes up such that if central estimates of risk advantage remain unchanged, the confidence limits narrow, and the chances of statistically significant findings improve. This was the case with UKPDS, such that the diabetes-related death and myocardial infarction measures changed little but became highly statistically significant. Not surprisingly, the metformin findings remained largely unchanged but with the central estimates of risk reduction becoming less extreme, best interpreted as regression to the mean. To many of us, these findings closed the glucose control and complications debate: improving glucose control reduces both microvascular and macrovascular complications. However, other issues remained, such as how tight glucose control should be.

Also of interest is that the legacy effect demonstrated in the EDIC extension of the DCCT is seen again; this perhaps emphasises the early role glucose has in initiating endothelial and therefore vascular damage, enabling other risk factors to cause structural damage over later years. The corollary of this is also important clinically: diagnosis and good glucose control must start early and be maintained long. In the era of statins, effective blood glucose control, better lifestyle advice and better salvage therapy, people with diabetes are living longer, and can so benefit.

The Power of Multifactorial Intervention in Type 2 Diabetes
Gæde et al., NEJM (2008)

Steno 1 was an attempt to do a DCCT-type study in the 1980s in a much smaller population, and it is now largely forgotten. This study was Steno 2 and is, however, important, though again rather small. Indeed, it should not really have delivered a useful result, as the population studied was very small (n = 160) and the control group was managed to a reasonable standard of care by Danish general practitioners. However, the participants were chosen as high risk, giving a high event rate to improve study power, and the intensive management group was subject to multifactorial intervention targeted at blood glucose, blood pressure, LDL cholesterol, triglycerides and hypercoagulability. As a result, by the time the extension study was completed (13.3 years, being 7.8 years for the main study, then 5.5 years of observation), the hazard ratio for cardiovascular events was HR 0.41 (95% CI 0.25–0.67), thus a hefty 59% reduction.

Hazard ratios and relative risks can mean little if the absolute event rates are low, but that is not the case here such that the absolute risk reduction is 29%, meaning the number needed to treat (NNT) is just 3.4 people. Furthermore, in the study nearly every other outcome was massively reduced, from death to progression of renal failure, all with NNTs of less than eight (death was five). Taken together, the NNT for preventing one such outcome must be around two people.

The authors subjected the primary part of the study to health economic analysis.[6] The health gains were judged to be cost saving, largely because of the expensive complications prevented: a health care bargain.

Intensive Glucose Control or Over-Intensive Glucose Control?
Action to Control Cardiovascular Risk in Diabetes (ACCORD) Study Group, NEJM (2008)

The ACCORD study has generated considerable controversy but cannot be ignored. The issues are complicated, medically and statistically, and not easy to summarise.

The issue addressed comes from UKPDS, and is simply stated as whether it would be possible to maintain blood glucose control at very tight levels in the intervention group and whether that would improve vascular outcomes further. The study was carefully designed and supervised, and recruited >11,000 participants, who, unlike UKPDS, had a long duration of diabetes and were often high risk. A study duration of over 5 years was planned, but the study was stopped early due to excess mortality in the intensively managed cohort.

It can be debated whether the increased death rate was statistically significant (the safety monitoring group was testing a series of outcomes and testing recurrently, so that the usual standard for judging p values does not apply). Chance may have been the explanation: the death event curves varied from year to year as to which group was higher risk. Nevertheless, it is difficult in this environment to continue a study. As a result, an explanation has been sought through data snooping within the results. Some of the resulting findings have been counter-intuitive, but probably real.

An immediate question was whether any one therapy used was the culprit (if there was a culprit). ACCORD used very heavy glucose lowering therapy. Many people reportedly got onto high doses of multiple insulin injection therapy in combination with multiple-tablet therapy, a strategy that indeed proved capable of achieving a mean HbA_{1c} of 6.5 %, with no deterioration with time in contrast to UKPDS. But only insulin therapy showed any sign of being associated with increased mortality risk. Because insulin is often a last-resort therapy, it is almost usual to find it associated with adverse outcomes of any kind, so the observation is probably not useful.

Could hypoglycaemia be the culprit? Hypoglycaemia can trigger an adrenergic or sympathetic response, and at least theoretically this could cause dysrhythmia in people with low glucose supply to cardiac conducting tissue. Certainly in this study and others published the same year [the Veterans Affairs Diabetes Trial (VADT) from the US Veterans Administration[7] and the Action in Diabetes and VAscular disease: preterax and diamicroN modified release Controlled Evaluation (ADVANCE)[8] trial], a history of hypoglycaemia was a risk factor for death, but hypoglycaemia is associated with the presence of other illness such as renal impairment. Detailed within-study epidemiological analysis failed to pin down an increased association of hypoglycaemia with death in the intensively managed cohort. It did, however, appear to be a lesser risk factor in this group. Furthermore, it turned out that hypoglycaemia was higher within both groups in the participants with higher HbA$_{1c}$ levels, and in those whose glucose control did not improve quickly in response to intensification of therapy. This meant the simplistic hypothesis 'Tight control = more hypoglycaemia = more death' is untenable; indeed, better glucose control was a marker for lower risk. The message seems to be 'If glucose control can be improved with the tools available, then that is a good thing, but if HbA$_{1c}$ becomes stuck at higher levels (e.g. 8.0 % or above) despite appropriate therapy including moderate insulin doses, do not try too hard to reduce it further'.

Unfortunately, stopping ACCORD early means that it accumulated too few events overall to have sufficient power to address the question of whether tight blood glucose control reduced cardiovascular outcomes, even though the central hazard ratio was appropriately reduced. VADT delivered a similar result, being always too small to be adequately powered. ADVANCE, a global study reporting at the same time, had the power but recruited a rather unusual diabetic population and returned only nonstatistically significant results. Students of statistics will note a common theme here, in that a series of studies had central hazard or risk estimates below 1.00, but were not statistically significant by themselves. This then sets the scene for meta-analysis.

Meta-Analysis to the Rescue
Ray et al., Lancet (2009)

In fact, there were four such studies published in 2009. Two are worth discussion (one of the others is concordant, and one not). Ray and colleagues took the five large studies in people with type 2 diabetes [UKPDS, Prospective Pioglitazone Clinical Trial in Macrovascular Events Study (PROactive), ACCORD, VADT, and ADVANCE] comprising some 33,000 participants, achieving an average difference of 0.9% HbA$_{1c}$ between groups and having a total of around 1500 myocardial infarction results. Myocardial infarction presents the easiest outcome to meta-analyse between studies, with all recording it and with seeming reasonable concordance of definition and ascertainment. The estimated reduction was 17% [odds ratio 0·83 (95% CI 0·75–0·93)] (Table 22.1). For ischaemic heart disease, with less concordance of definition and ascertainment, the odds were 0·85 (0·77–0·93). In conventional terms, these findings are highly statistically significant.

Table 22.1 Meta-analysis results from the major glucose-lowering cardiovascular outcome studies

Meta-analysis	Outcome	Odds ratio (95% CI)
1	IHD	0·85 (0·77–0·93)
2	Major CV events	0·91 (0·84–0·99)
3	Major CV events	0·91 (0·84–0·99)
1	MI	0·83 (0·75–0·93)
2	MI	0·85 (0·78–0·93)
3	MI	0·85 (0·78–0·93)

Meta-analyses: [1]Ray, *et al., Lancet* (2009); [2]Turnbull, *et al., Diabetologia* (2009); [3]Mannucci, *et al, Nutrition, Metabolism & Cardiovascular Diseases* (2009).

Turnbull and colleagues performed a superficially similar analysis,[9] but being the investigators on four of the studies (not including PROactive) they had access to patient-level data. Their results for major cardiovascular events were 0.91 (0.84–0.99), but for myocardial infarction they were 0.85 (0.76–0.94), essentially the same as those found by Ray and colleagues.

Concluding Comment

It might be thought that this 30-year-long story has come to an end. But science generates more questions than it ever answers. Left undone are issues related to which people benefit most from tighter blood glucose control, particularly in those with more limited life expectancy and those at risk from therapy-related side effects such as hypoglycaemia. The issue of particular therapies remains an enigma, particularly as new therapies with effects on reducing body weight come onto the market. Some reassurance from a study in people with proven coronary artery disease (BARI-2D) is useful – a cohort mostly using metformin and rosiglitazone did similarly over 5 years to a cohort using mainly insulin and sulfonylureas.[10] A series of cardiovascular outcome trials on the weight-neutral DPP-4 inhibitors are already underway.

Meanwhile evidence-based guidelines are adopting something like the following summary: 'Monitor and improve blood glucose control to a target of 6.5 % or to 7.0 % where this can be achieved, if necessary with insulin therapy, without pushing glucose-lowering therapies too hard, especially in those with other illness'.

References

Action to Control Cardiovascular Risk in Diabetes (ACCORD) Study Group (2008) Effects of intensive glucose lowering in type 2 diabetes. *New England Journal of Medicine*, **358**, 2545–2559. http://www.ncbi.nlm.nih.gov/pubmed/18539917

Diabetes Control and Complications Trial/Epidemiology of Diabetes Interventions and Complications (DCCT/EDIC) Study Research Group (2005) Intensive diabetes treatment and cardiovascular disease in patients with type 1 diabetes. *New England Journal of Medicine*, **353**, 2643–2653. http://www.ncbi.nlm.nih.gov/pubmed/16371630

Diabetes Control and Complications Trial (DCCT) Research Group (1993) The effect of intensive treatment of diabetes on the development and progression of long-term complications in insulin-dependent diabetes mellitus. *New England Journal of Medicine*, **329**, 977–986. http://www.ncbi.nlm.nih.gov/pubmed/8366922

Gìde, P., *et al.* (2008) Effect of a multifactorial intervention on mortality in type 2 diabetes. *New England Journal of Medicine*, **358**, 580–591. http://www.ncbi.nlm.nih.gov/pubmed/12556541

Holman, R.R., *et al.* (2008) 10-year follow-up of intensive glucose control in type 2 diabetes. *New England Journal of Medicine*, **359**, 1565–1576. http://www.ncbi.nlm.nih.gov/pubmed/18784090

Kroc Collaborative Study Group (1984) Blood glucose control and the evolution of diabetic retinopathy and albuminuria: a preliminary multicenter trial. *New England Journal of Medicine*, **311**, 365–372. http://www.ncbi.nlm.nih.gov/pubmed/6377076

Mannucci, E., *et al.* (2009) Prevention of cardiovascular disease through glycemic control in type 2 diabetes: a meta-analysis of randomized clinical trials. *Nutrition, Metabolism & Cardiovascular Diseases*, **19**(9), 604–612.

Pirart, J. (1977) Diabetes mellitus and its degenerative complications: a prospective study of 4.400 patients observed between 1947 and 1973 (in three parts). *Diabetes & Metabolism*, **3**, 97–107, 173–182, 245–256. http://www.ncbi.nlm.nih.gov/pubmed/892130, http://www.ncbi.nlm.nih.gov/pubmed/913749 and http://www.ncbi.nlm.nih.gov/pubmed/598565

Pickup, J.C., *et al.* (1978) Continuous subcutaneous insulin infusion: an approach to achieving normoglycaemia. *British Medical Journal*, **i**, 204–207. http://www.ncbi.nlm.nih.gov/pmc/articles/PMC1602534/?tool¥pubmed

Ray, K.K., *et al.* (2009) Effect of intensive control of glucose on cardiovascular outcomes and death in patients with diabetes mellitus: a meta-analysis of randomised controlled trials. *Lancet*, **373**, 1765–1772. http://www.thelancet.com/journals/lancet/article/PIIS0140-6736(09)60697-8/fulltext

United Kingdom Prospective Diabetes Study (UKPDS) Group (1998) Intensive blood glucose control with sulphonylureas or insulin compared with conventional treatment and risk of complications in patients with type 2 diabetes. *Lancet*, **352**, 837–853. http://www.thelancet.com/journals/lancet/article/PIIS0140-6736(98)07019-6/Abstract

Additional References

1. International Diabetes Federation (2009) *IDF atlas*. 4th ed. International Diabetes Federation, Brussels.
2. Tchobroutsky, G. (1978) Relation of diabetic control to development of microvascular complications. *Diabetologia*, **15**, 143–152.
3. Paton, J.S., *et al.* (1981) Convenient pocket insulin syringe. *Lancet*, **1**(8123), 189–190.
4. Lachin, J.M., *et al.*, for the DCCT/EDIC Research Group (2008) Effect of glycemic exposure on the risk of microvascular complications in the Diabetes Control and Complications Trial – revisited. *Diabetes*, **57**, 995–1001.
5. Home, P.D., *et al.* (2009) Rosiglitazone evaluated for cardiovascular outcomes in oral agent combination therapy for type 2 diabetes (RECORD), a multicentre, randomised, open-label trial. *Lancet*, **373**, 2125–2135.
6. Gæde, P., *et al.* (2008) Cost-effectiveness of intensified versus conventional multifactorial intervention in type 2 diabetes: results and projections from the Steno-2 study. *Diabetes Care*, **31**, 1510–1515.
7. Duckworth, W., *et al.*, for the VADT Investigators (2008) Glucose control and vascular complications in veterans with type 2 diabetes. *New England Journal of Medicine*, **360**, 129–139.
8. The ADVANCE Collaborative Group (2008) Intensive blood glucose control and vascular outcomes in patients with type 2 diabetes. *New England Journal of Medicine*, **358**, 2560–2572.
9. Turnbull, FM., *et al.* (2009) Intensive glucose control and macrovascular outcomes in type 2 diabetes. *Diabetologia*, **52**, 2288–2298.
10. The BARI 2D Study Group (2009) A randomized trial of therapies for type 2 diabetes and coronary artery disease. *New England Journal of Medicine*, **11**(360), 2503–2515.

23 Rheumatoid Arthritis

Jonathan C.W. Edwards and Maria J. Leandro

Centre for Rheumatology, Division of Medicine, University College London,
London, UK

Introduction

Rheumatoid arthritis is the commonest non-organ-specific autoimmune disease and has been a major source of disability in younger adults. Research into pathogenesis and treatment has been particularly rewarding over recent years. What was once a largely untreatable progressive disorder is now in most cases well controlled by targeted therapies. Moreover, there are reasons to be optimistic that research over the next decade may allow the development of strategies for more or less indefinite remission.

Throughout the history of research into rheumatoid arthritis, we have been faced with the puzzle of an association between a systemic disturbance of lymphocyte behaviour and the predominant clinical features of synovitis and suppressed erythropoiesis. Clues to possible answers can be found in histological studies going back into the 19th century. But it was not until the 1980s, when monoclonal antibody and gene-cloning technologies allowed the identification of the molecular pathways of the immune response, that detailed solutions to the puzzle could be formulated. Controversy still dominates the field but the same technologies have both tested hypotheses and provided direct benefit in the clinic. Arguably we are about halfway to a full understanding of the disease with the exciting prospect that the final pieces of the puzzle can be brought into place in the near future.

What Is the Tissue Pathology?
Hoffa and Wallenburg, Stuttgart, 1908

Hypotheses about pathogenesis do not arise in a vacuum. The recognition of rheumatoid arthritis as a systemic inflammatory disease arose partly from clinical observation, but also from painstaking histopathological description. It is salutary to note that observations on rheumatoid synovium heralded as new discoveries in the 1990s can be found in the German histopathological literature of 100 years earlier. Hoffa and Wallenberg were familiar in 1908 with the formation within synovium of lymphoid follicles and what came to be known as germinal centres, together with extensive infiltrates with plasma cells. They were not to know that both features represented stages in development of antibody-producing B lymphocytes but these early observations formed the foundations for our understanding of rheumatoid

Understanding Medical Research: The Studies that Shaped Medicine, First Edition. Edited by John A. Goodfellow. © 2012 John Wiley & Sons, Ltd. Published 2012 by John Wiley & Sons, Ltd.

arthritis as an aberration of the immune response. Classical histological studies of rheumatoid arthritis by pathologists such as Fassbender and Gardner[1] continued to explore the extent of the disease up until the 1980s when immunohistochemical techniques took over. Involvement of serosae, lung interstitium, spleen, liver and bone marrow and the structure of the unique nodular lesions of the disease were documented. The challenge was to explain all these features.

What Mediates the Systemic Process?
Waaler, Acta Pathologica Microbiologica Scandinavica (1940)
In 1940 Waaler reported the ability of sera from rheumatoid arthritis patients to agglutinate sheep red cells coated with rabbit gamma globulin. It may now seem strange that the experiment was even done. Nevertheless, whether or not by serendipity, the observation was made that rheumatoid serum contained a factor that interacted in an abnormal way with gamma globulin. The 'rheumatoid factor' turned out itself to be in the gamma globulin fraction and ultimately proved to be a population of antibodies of all classes reactive with the constant fragment of antibodies of IgG class. It took several years for the potential significance of this observation to be recognised but a clue had been established to the systemic immunological abnormality underlying the clinical disease.

How Might Rheumatoid Factors Be Pathogenic?
Kunkel et al., Journal of Clinical Investigation (1959)
Rather than select a particular paper, it might be appropriate to consider as a whole the work of Henry Kunkel and his many eminent students. With legendary thoroughness, Kunkel applied the techniques of analytical physical chemistry to a wide range of phenomena documented in sera over previous decades. Kunkel's group took Waaler's rheumatoid factors (RF) and showed that they formed complexes with IgG in the circulation. Conditions of association and dissociation and interaction with complement were precisely documented.

Small complexes based on IgG RF were found almost exclusively in rheumatoid sera, and it seemed likely that these might be the mediators of tissue inflammation. An answer seemed to be in sight; however, by the mid-1970s an apparent paradox arose. Immune complexes were thought to generate inflammation through the fixation of complement and release of the vasoactive and chemotactic fragments C3a and C5a, yet small IgG RF-based complexes fixed complement poorly if at all[2]. By the mid-1970s, interest in immunology had been caught by the newly discovered roles of T cells and faith in the pathogenic role of small immune complexes began to falter. In 1983 Nardella, working with Mannik who continued to champion the role of small complexes, demonstrated that RF-based complexes had the ability to stimulate monocytes to produce a newly discovered type of inflammatory mediator[3]. What was then called mononuclear cell factor proved to be a mixture of potent pro-inflammatory cytokines that included tumour necrosis factor (TNF) and interleukin-1. But the fashion for T cells had taken over and Nardella's study remained largely ignored for a dozen years.

What Is the Basis of Genetic Susceptibility to RA?
Stastny, New England Journal of Medicine (1978)

Work on histocompatibility antigens in the early 1970s led to the chance finding of an association between ankylosing spondylitis and HLA-B27[4]. Further exploration of disease associations led to the discovery by Stastny of an association between RA and what was then described as 'B lymphocyte antigen Dw4'. This turned out to be an allele of HLA-DR, which is expressed at high level on macrophages and dendritic cells, in addition to B cells. It became clear that HLA-DR is involved in presentation of antigen to CD4 T cells. This fuelled the shift of interest from B cells to T cells, despite the fact that HLA-DR was first identified on B cells! Twenty years later, antigen presentation by B cells was to be hailed as a new discovery by those perhaps unfamiliar with the title of Stastny's paper.

What Stastny's study did indicate was that the disordered immune response in RA was likely to be dependent on interaction with T cells. A role for interactions with T cells has recently been confirmed by the therapeutic benefit of blockade of T cell co-stimulation with a fusion protein of CTLA-4 and IgG Fc (CTLA-4Ig; abatacept[5]). This is consistent with a role for autoantibody since antigen presentation by B cells to T cells is a crucial step in the generation of antibody responses. It was also possible that the inflammatory effector mechanism was mediated directly by T cells. Obtaining evidence for such a T cell effector mechanism then became a major aim of research and T cells became the target of therapeutic strategies.

Although in empirical terms Stastny's major contribution was to demonstrate a genetic factor in the cause of RA he also brought to people's attention the possibility that much of the remaining causality might be stochastic rather than environmental, a concept of considerable relevance to subsequent therapeutic strategies.

What Is the Crucial Inflammatory Mediator in RA?
Elliott et al., Lancet (1994)

Studies of T cell behaviour in rheumatoid synovium dominated research in the 1980s. Interest also focused on the roles of newly identified inflammatory cytokines derived from macrophages. Originally identified as stimulators of tissue catabolism through collagenase[6], interleukin-1, TNF and interleukin-6 were found to have a wide range of pro-inflammatory properties.

In 1989 Brennan[7] reported that in cultures of cells from rheumatoid synovium, TNF appeared to be the critical pro-inflammatory signal. This led to the proposal that blockade of TNF might be of therapeutic value. In what is perhaps the single most informative clinical interventional experiment in RA, Maini and colleagues administered the chimaeric monoclonal anti-TNF antibody infliximab to a group of RA patients in this study. A significant proportion showed a dramatic response, and a randomised controlled trial confirmed the potency of this approach. For patients without contra-indications of malignancy or infection, TNF inhibition became the gold standard of management of severe disease.

An interesting caveat to the original concept of TNF as pivotal mediator in RA is the finding that inhibition of interleukin-6 (and less convincingly interleukin-1) are also effective. The anti-interleukin-6 receptor antibody (which blocks IL-6) is of comparable efficacy to TNF inhibitors[8]. It seems that there is no single crucial mediator involved.

Does Smoking Contribute to the Causation of RA?
Silman et al., Arthritis and Rheumatism (1996)

The search for environmental factors in the causation of RA was for many years focused on infective agents. However, the stochastic epidemiological pattern of RA noted by Stastny mitigated against a concept of an infective 'trigger' at the time of disease onset. What came as something of a surprise was that a quite different environmental factor, cigarette smoking, was associated with a significantly increased risk of development of RA. The finding was first suggested by a study by Voigt[9] in 1994, and formally confirmed by a study of twins by Silman in 1996.

The role of smoking in RA remains unknown, but it has been suggested that it may be linked into the association with antibodies to citrullinated proteins. Nevertheless, the appreciation that smoking is a major risk factor has had a significant impact on our approach to the disease. It has provided a strong motivation to discourage smoking in RA sufferers, because smoking is associated both with incidence and subsequent severity. Moreover, it focused attention on the increased cardiovascular risk associated with RA. Increased mortality in RA is largely due to an increase in atherosclerosis, suggesting that the inflammatory process contributes to changes in arterial wall. Detailed assessment of cardiovascular risk is now routine in RA.

Why Do RA Patients Have Antibodies to Keratin?
Schellekens et al., Journal of Clinical Investigation (1998)

Despite a general loss of interest in autoantibodies in RA after 1980 a few laboratories continued to work on autoantibody biology. The ability of antibodies in RA sera to bind to keratin (and also perinuclear material) had been known for some time. Of interest, the anti-keratin reactivity appeared to be more specific to RA than rheumatoid factor itself. In this study in 1998 van Venrooij and colleagues showed that the antibodies responsible were binding to citrullinated arginine residues. These residues occur naturally on mature keratin but can occur as a post-translational modification on a wide range of proteins. Thus it seemed likely that the binding to keratin was not in itself of significance. If these antibodies had a pathogenic role it might be through binding to any citrullinated protein. Subsequently interest has focused on citrullinated fibrin in inflamed joints, although it is still unclear what role the antibodies do play.

What New Insights Can Immunohistochemistry Provide?
Kraan et al., Arthritis and Rheumatism (1998)

Immunohistochemical techniques were first applied to rheumatoid synovial tissue in the late 1970s, but it was not until the early 1990s that techniques were developed for dissecting synovial cell populations in detail[10]. It became clear that synovial fibroblasts were significantly specialised in their gene expression repertoire, with intimal fibroblasts characterised by high levels of expression of the adhesion molecule VCAM-1 and the complement regulatory protein CD55. Both of these molecules are found in micro-environments conducive to B lymphocyte survival. Bhatia also showed in 1996[11] that synovial intimal macrophages had a high level of expression of the immune complex binding receptor FcγRIIIa, as did macrophages at extra-articular sites targeted by RA. These findings sparked a renewed interest in the role of B cells and antibody in generating synovitis.

The full potential of immunohistochemical analysis of inflamed synovium was explored by Tak and colleagues in a series of systematic studies aimed at reviewing the cellular dynamics of the disease. Of particular interest are studies by Kraan and Smeets looking at different stages of disease development[12]. It had been observed since the 1960s that the earliest identifiable structural changes in RA synovium were an increase in number and size of intimal macrophages and signs of activation of endothelial cells, in the absence of significant T lymphocyte infiltrate. This observation was confirmed using immunohistochemical markers. Evidence of intimal macrophage activation was confirmed by the presence of macrophage-derived cytokines. It was also found that the pathological changes in early disease were essentially the same as those in late disease in character and moreover that such changes could often be found in asymptomatic joints.

These findings set the stage for a reappraisal of the historic model of RA as a systemic immune disturbance in which synovium and other tissues suffer as downstream targets as a result of circulating soluble factors, the most likely of which remained the small immune complexes described by Kunkel and colleagues. The failure of these complexes to engage complement now posed less of a problem because it had become clear that complexes generate inflammation largely through the activation of macrophages via FcRIIIa, leading to the secretion of cytokines such as TNF and IL-1 (the mechanism identified by Nardella in 1983).

When Does the Immunopathology Begin?
Rantapää-Dahlqvist et al., Arthritis and Rheumatism (2003)
Pathodynamic studies in synovial tissue were soon to be complemented by long-term studies of autoantibody populations. Jonsson and Valdemarston had, in 1992, already provided evidence that rheumatoid factors were present in the serum of patients several years before clinical disease became apparent[13]. This was established by studying rheumatoid factor levels in blood from healthy individuals (at the time) donating blood and then following up these individuals for the presence of RA. In 2003 Rantapää-Dahlqvist reported similar and more detailed findings relating to both rheumatoid factors and antibodies to citrullinated peptides. Confirmation came from other centres. Increasingly the evidence appeared to suggest that RA arose from a systemic immunological disturbance characterised by autoantibody production that only subsequently led to disseminated pathology when the extent of autoantibody production had risen above some form of threshold.

Sequential studies suggest that antibodies to citrullinated peptides precede rheumatoid factors, raising the possibility that their genesis is interrelated. However, a proportion of patients with rheumatoid factors do not have antibodies to citrullinated peptides. The reasons why some autoimmune disorders are associated with more than one autoantibody response and the apparently partial interdependence of these poses a major continuing puzzle.

Is RA Due to Self-Perpetuating Autoreactive B Cells?
Edwards et al., New England Journal of Medicine (2004)
The return to an interest in B lymphocytes in the pathogenesis of RA came about for a variety of reasons. Scepticism about a dominant role for T cells had always had adherents, fuelled by the difficulty in finding evidence for T cell effector mechanisms in synovium[14].

Early speculation on a specific role for TH1 cells in RA shifted to an interest in TH17 cells, partly fuelled by animal systems of uncertain relevance to RA. Evidence of T cell autoreactivity remained lacking in RA. The T cell activation that could be documented appeared not to be through T cell receptor signalling[15]. In contrast, several new observations pointed towards B cell and antibody-mediated mechanisms.

The potential role of VCAM-1 expression by synovial fibroblasts in supporting B cell survival in synovium was the first motivation for considering B cell-targeted therapy. By 1998 the potential relevance of Kunkel's small RF-based complexes in local TNF production via FcγRIIIa was appreciated and a well-defined rationale for depletion of B lymphocytes was formulated. This included the idea that the survival of autoreactive B cells in RA might be in a sense self perpetuating, via antibody products (RFs) that subvert survival control mechanisms both by acquiring help from T cells recognising foreign antigen (see also chapter on autoimmunity) and by self-associating to form complexes capable of acquiring complement C3d and cross-linking B cell receptor and CD21[16]. This view avoids the need to invoke steps for which evidence has not been found: triggering infective agents or loss of T cell tolerance.

The self-perpetuating autoreactive B cell hypothesis generated the prediction that short term B cell depletion with an anti-CD20 antibody might induce persistent remission, as aimed for in the treatment of lymphoma. Both B cell lymphoma and RA involve uncontrolled proliferation of B cell clones (one in lymphoma and several in autoimmune disease) associated with disadvantageous gene translocations. The translocations in autoimmunity are stochastic physiological immunoglobulin gene re-arrangements rather than the unprogrammed translocations of lymphomata. Nevertheless, the dynamic objective is comparable.

By chance, precisely at the time of formulation of this hypothesis (1996) the anti-CD20 monoclonal antibody rituximab had been shown in early clinical trials to be an effective B cell depleting agent. Moreover, it showed much less in the way of immunosuppressive problems than expected. Protective immunoglobulin levels were well maintained. An open pilot study of B cell depletion in five patients with RA was set up by 1998, and following positive results this led on to a formal randomised controlled trial in 2001. B cell depletion with rituximab proved to be approximately as effective in controlling inflammatory disease as TNF inhibition and by 2006 had become a licensed therapy.

Two aspects of the results of B cell depletion in RA turned out not quite as expected. In view of the minimal early fall in total immunoglobulins seen in lymphoma patients, it might have been expected that any improvement in RA due to fall in autoantibody levels might be very slow or marginal. In practice rheumatoid factor levels fell much more rapidly than total immunoglobulins and clinical improvement paralleled this fall over a period of approximately 3 months. While slower in onset than with TNF inhibition this meant that good levels of disease control could be achieved relatively quickly. On the negative side, it rapidly became clear that improvement was rarely if ever permanent, with disease relapse occurring at any time from 6 months to 5 years after treatment. In retrospect this is not so surprising since it was known that B cell depletion with rituximab is not complete. Moreover, there are reasons to think that residual plasma cells secreting rheumatoid factors may provide feedback signals that would tend to encourage the re-emergence of new autoreactive clones (as part of the proposed vicious cycle).

Conclusions and Key Outstanding Questions

Within the working lifetime of present-day rheumatologists, RA has gone from being a more or less mysterious untreatable condition to something that is reasonably well understood and in most cases very controllable. The elements of the pathogenic process seem reasonably clear. What remains uncertain is which components are critical to the long term propagation of the disease. If that was known we are entitled to think that strategies for induction of long-term remission should be formulable and translatable into real therapy. The current task facing researchers in this area is perhaps best illustrated by the state of a patient who one year after treatment with rituximab is free of clinical evidence of disease and may even no longer have autoantibody levels outside the normal range but for whom return of both clinical disease and autoantibodies at some time in the next few months or years is apparently inevitable. It may be that the problem is a residue of autoreactive B cells not cleared by rituximab. It may be that surviving plasma cells are providing signals that can re-engage new B cells in affinity maturation to autoreactivity. It may also be that at some stage of the process, either as an initial step or along the line, the T cell repertoire has been skewed in a such a way that 'disease memory' resides in the T cell compartment. It is unclear what such T cell reactivities might be, but they might have to do with proteins that undergo citrullination. There are also more subtle possibilities relating to changes in lymph node architecture and sequestration of antigens (perhaps citrullinated proteins) in follicle centres.

To date, no clear answer to the 'disease memory' question has emerged, despite several years of trawling of immunodynamic data. Nevertheless the availability of an increasingly wide range of targeted biologic agents suggests that we should be optimistic that clinical experiments can be designed that will both reveal these mechanisms and provide a means to overcome them.

References

Edwards, J.C.W., *et al.* (2004) Efficacy of the novel B cell targeted therapy, rituximab, in patients with active rheumatoid arthritis. *New England Journal of Medicine*, **350**, 2572–2581. http://www.ncbi.nlm.nih.gov/pubmed/15201414

Elliott, M.J., *et al.* (1994) Randomised double-blind comparison of chimeric monoclonal antibody to tumour necrosis factor alpha (cA2) versus placebo in rheumatoid arthritis. *Lancet*, **344**(8930), 1105–1110. http://www.thelancet.com/journals/lancet/article/PIIS0140-6736(94)90628-9/Abstract

Hoffa, A., and Wallenberg, G.A. (1908) *Arthritis deformans und sogennanter, chronische Gelenkrheumatismus.* Enke, Stuttgart.

Kraan, M.C., *et al.* (1998) Asymptomatic synovitis precedes clinically manifest arthritis. *Arthritis and Rheumatism*, **41**(8), 1481–1488. http://onlinelibrary.wiley.com/doi/10.1002/1529-0131(199808)41:8%3c1481::AID-ART19%3e3.0.CO;2-O/Abstract

Kunkel, H.G., *et al.* (1959) Studies on the isolation and characterization of the 'rheumatoid factor'. *Journal of Clinical Investigation*, **38**(2), 424–434. http://www.ncbi.nlm.nih.gov/pmc/articles/PMC293171/?tool$^{1}/_{4}$pubmed

Rantapää-Dahlqvist, S., *et al.* (2003) Antibodies against cyclic citrullinated peptide and IgA rheumatoid factor predict the development of rheumatoid arthritis. *Arthritis and Rheumatism*, **48**(10), 2741–2749. http://www.ncbi.nlm.nih.gov/pubmed/14558078

Schellekens, G.A., *et al.* (1998) Citrulline is an essential constituent of antigenic determinants recognized by rheumatoid arthritis-specific autoantibodies. *Journal of Clinical Investigation*, **101**(1), 273–281. http://www.ncbi.nlm.nih.gov/pmc/articles/PMC508564/?tool$^{1}/_{4}$pubmed

Silman, A.J., *et al.* (1996) Cigarette smoking increases the risk of rheumatoid arthritis. Results from a nationwide study of disease-discordant twins. *Arthritis and Rheumatism*, **39**(5), 732–735. http://onlinelibrary.wiley.com/doi/10.1002/art.1780390504/Abstract

Stastny, P. (1978) Association of the B-cell alloantigen DRw4 with rheumatoid arthritis. *New England Journal of Medicine*, **298**(16), 869–871. http://www.ncbi.nlm.nih.gov/pubmed/147420

Waaler, E. (1940) On occurrence of factor in human serum activating specific agglutination of sheep blood corpuscles. *Acta Pathologica Microbiologica Scandinavica*, **17**, 172–175. http://onlinelibrary.wiley.com/doi/10.1111/j.1600-0463.2007.apm_682a.x/Abstract

Additional References

1. Gardner, D.L. (1992) *Pathological basis of connective tissue diseases*. Edward Arnold, London.

2. Winchester, R.J., *et al.* (1969) The joint-fluid gammaG-globulin complexes and their relationship to intraarticular complement diminution. *Annals of the New York Academy of Science*, **168**(1), 195–203.

3. Nardella, F.A., *et al.* (1983) Self-associating IgG rheumatoid factors stimulate monocytes to release prostaglandins and mononuclear cell factor that stimulates collagenase and prostaglandin production by synovial cells. *Rheumatology International*, **3**(4), 183–186.

4. Brewerton, D.A., *et al.* (1973) Ankylosing spondylitis and HLA-27. *Lancet*, **1**(7809), 904–907.

5. Kremer, J.M., *et al.* (2003) Treatment of rheumatoid arthritis by selective inhibition of T-cell activation with fusion protein CTLA4Ig. *New England Journal of Medicine*, **349**(20), 1907–1915.

6. Dayer, J.-M., *et al.* (1976) Production of collagenase and prostaglandins by isolated adherent rheumatoid synovial cells. *Proceedings of the National Academy of Sciences of the USA*, **73**(3), 945–949.

7. Brennan, F.M., *et al.* (1989) Inhibitory effect of TNF alpha antibodies on synovial cell interleukin-1 production in rheumatoid arthritis. *Lancet*, **29**(8657), 244–247.

8. Maini, R.N., *et al.* (2006) Double-blind randomized controlled clinical trial of the interleukin-6 receptor antagonist, tocilizumab, in European patients with rheumatoid arthritis who had an incomplete response to methotrexate. *Arthritis and Rheumatism*, **54**(9), 2817–2829.

9. Voigt, L.F., *et al.* (1994) Smoking, obesity, alcohol consumption and the risk of rheumatoid arthritis. *Epidemiology*, **5**(5), 522–532.

10. Edwards, J.C.W. (2003) The synovium. In: *Rheumatology*, ed. Hochburg, M.C., Silman, A.J., Smolen, J.S., Weinblatt, M.E., and Weisman, M.H. 3rd ed. Mosby Year Book, London.

11. Bhatia, A., *et al.* (1998) Differential distribution of FcRIIIa in normal human tissues. *Immunology*, **94**, 56–63.

12. Smeets, T.J., *et al.* (1998) Poor expression of T cell-derived cytokines and activation and proliferation markers in early rheumatoid synovial tissue. *Clinical Immunology and Immunopathology*, **88**(1), 84–90.

13. Jonsson, T., *et al.* (1992) Population study of the importance of rheumatoid factor isotypes in adults. *Annals of the Rheumatic Diseases*, **51**(7), 863–868.

14. Firestein, G.S., and Zvaifler, N.J. (1990) How important are T cells in chronic rheumatoid synovitis? *Arthritis and Rheumatism*, **33**, 768–773.

15. Brennan, F.M., *et al.* (2002) Evidence that rheumatoid arthritis synovial T cells are similar to cytokine-activated T cells: involvement of phosphatidylinositol 3-kinase and nuclear factor kappaB pathways in tumor necrosis factor alpha production in rheumatoid arthritis. *Arthritis and Rheumatism*, **46**(1), 31–41.

16. Edwards, J.C.W., *et al.* (1999) Do self-perpetuating B lymphocytes drive human autoimmune disease? *Immunology*, **97**, 1868–1876.

24 Osteoarthritis

Kirsten White, Alexander S. Nicholls, Anushka Soni and Nigel Arden

Botnar Research Centre, Institute of Musculoskeletal Sciences, University of Oxford, Oxford, UK

Introduction

Osteoarthritis (OA) is a complex disease involving both bone and soft-tissue of a joint. It most commonly affects the synovial joints of hands, hips, knees and spine and is primarily related to age, weight and previous trauma. OA is a steadily increasing global health burden due to the rise of obesity and the aging population of many countries. The economic cost for both healthcare and missed work due to disability are also on the rise, with $11.6 billion spent solely on hip and knee replacements in a single year in the United States[1]. This figure does not include primary health care costs such as doctor's visits, pain medication, physiotherapy or lost work.

In this chapter, we highlight some key papers that have addressed the recurrent issues in OA research, namely, identifying risk factors, understanding pain, correlating radiological features and symptoms and traditional and emerging surgical therapies.

Risk Factors for Osteoarthritis
Cooper et al., Arthritis and Rheumatism (2000)

The nature of OA, with varying types of pain, pathology, joint location and disability, makes it an extremely difficult disease to define for both research and clinical purposes. Radiographic features of OA are often used to define incidence and progression for the purposes of drug trials, as well as a way to understand the disease epidemiologically.

Various risk factors have been identified for osteoarthritis however they vary considerably depending on several factors of the study design. The temporal association (cross-sectional and longitudinal), the definition of OA utilised (radiographic, painful and combination) as well as the type of disease occurrence (prevalence, incidence and progression) used in the study will result in different risk factors being identified. For clinical purposes, the most useful of these would likely be a longitudinal study which identifies predictive risk factors for radiographic and/or clinical OA.

In this 2000 study, the authors used a longitudinal study design and distinguished risk factors for incident radiographic knee OA from risk factors for progressive OA. Part of the rationale for this separation was an attempt to explain the known difference between knee OA prevalence in a population and the percentage of people requiring knee replacements. 354 subjects were included with and without knee pain at baseline and

Understanding Medical Research: The Studies that Shaped Medicine, First Edition. Edited by John A. Goodfellow. © 2012 John Wiley & Sons, Ltd. Published 2012 by John Wiley & Sons, Ltd.

were radiographed, clinically examined and administered a comprehensive question-naire at both baseline and an average of 5 years later. Definitions for incidence and progression were primarily based on the Kellgren and Lawrence (K&L) radiographic scoring system. Both the traditional cut-off for disease presence (grade 2) and the more recently recognised clinically significant grade 1 were analysed separately as indicators of incidence. Progression was defined as an increase of one grade or more from either cut-off score. The results showed that subjects in the top third BMI category had a 9-fold risk of developing incident OA (K&L grade 1) and an 18-fold risk of developing K&L grade 2 or above as compared to the lowest third BMI category. Oddly, the risk factors for incident K&L 1 included knee pain at baseline, Heberden's nodes, and previous injury, while K&L 2 incident only included the latter (in addition to BMI). Obesity was also found to be a risk factor for progression, although it was not as significant as its association with incidence. Knee pain at baseline and Heberden's nodes appeared to double the risk of progression, but did not reach significance due to the small number in this group.

While this study thoroughly addresses the risk factors for radiographic OA, more often in clinical settings it is the risk factors for pain and disability that are of a greater importance. This discrepancy occurs because the radiographic features of OA have not been definitively associated with symptomatic OA. In 2009 a Japanese group found that varus-valgus knee alignment was found to be the only significant risk factor for pain out of age, BMI, gender, radiographic grade and quadriceps muscles torque[2], while Rogers and Wilder found a positive association of BMI with pain in a cross-sectional study of subjects with radiographic OA[3].

Focus on Pain
Hawker et al., Osteoarthritis and Cartilage (2008)

The tendency when studying both diagnosis and progression of OA has been to focus on factors contributing to the development of certain structural features usually measured on radiographs. There is a recognised discordance between structural joint abnormalities and pain reported by patients, especially in early stages of OA, highlighting an incomplete understanding of the underlying pain mechanisms. Pain is the number one reason people with OA choose to have replacement surgery, and yet relatively little is known about quality and characteristics of the knee pain. In this context Gilliam Hawker and colleagues conducted a qualitative study with the ultimate aim of developing a new knee osteoarthritis pain measure which would better capture the patient pain experience.

English-speaking patients with knee or hip OA, recruited from North America, Europe and Australasia participated in focus group discussions and one-to-one inter-views. This qualitative research revealed important new information about the nature of pain experienced by patients with lower limb OA; in particular the discovery of two distinct types of pain as the symptoms progressed. Patients clearly described a dull, aching, throbbing pain at the outset which gradually became more constant in nature. Over time this initial pain was punctuated by episodes of more intense, unpredictable and emotionally draining pain predominantly associated with social and recreational activity avoidance. This improved qualitative understanding of patient symptoms subsequently led to improved quantitative assessment as the group went on to design and validate the Measure of Intermittent and Constant Osteoarthritis Pain (ICOAP) and its use is being encouraged at an international level[4,5].

This study is an excellent example of the advantage of using qualitative and quantitative approaches in conjunction in order to more fully understand a disease process. A key aim in research into knee OA is to explain the aetiology of pain, which may well differ between patients. Emerging evidence suggests that a process known as central sensitisation may well be relevant in lower limb OA. In this process CNS plasticity results in increased sensitivity to stimuli such as pressure, heat and light touch with corresponding change in the symptom quality with numbness, tingling and electric shock type pain being more common. Qualitative studies may be able to distinguish patients in whom central sensitisation is key and ultimately improving our ability to target therapeutic strategies[6].

Linking Radiological OA and Clinical Symptoms
Arden et al., Arthritis and Rheumatism (2009)

The association between radiographic features of OA and pain, the main problem for patients, is notoriously disparate. Too often, studies focus on defining progression/incidence in *either* radiographic OA *or* symptomatic (painful) OA which further widens the gulf between the two most common ways of defining OA. Furthermore the majority of epidemiology studies on OA focus on structural features, with pain and disability sometimes included in a composite definition of disease, but are not often used as the main outcome of disease. Many studies have attempted to close the gap between radiological features and pain, with varying degrees of success.

In 2009 Arden and colleagues analysed various definitions of radiographic hip OA using combinations of structural features in order to determine which definitions best correlated with cross-sectional symptoms as well as identified progression to a total hip replacement (THR). They considered a wide variety of individual structural features such as osteophytes, joint space narrowing, subchondral cysts, subchondral sclerosis in addition to composite scores of the above features. They also included common radiographic scoring systems such as K&L[7] and a modified Croft[8] system. Because of the absence of a 'gold standard' for defining clinical hip OA, construct validity for cross-sectional association between radiographic features and clinical OA was based upon the presence and location of pain in five locations; groin/inside leg, outside leg, front of leg, buttocks and lower back. Predictive validation criteria included a combination of new pain, pain on internal rotation, physician diagnosed hip OA, and THR surgery not present at the previous examination. Radiographic features and composite scores were then compared with the incidence established by clinical examination. Results showed little overlap with the validation criteria (i.e. pain) when using individual radiographic features alone; only 27% of patients would have been identified by osteophytes and only 26% of those would have been identified by joint space narrowing. Composite definitions fared better, identifying 51–84% of hips with clinically established incident OA. The strongest predictive validity for a THR was a Croft grade greater than three and any of the composite definitions that used both osteophytes and joint space narrowing as part of the definition. The definitions for predicting pain on walking were slightly different with those using osteophyte presence alone, or a composite definition which included osteophytes, having the strongest association.

Neogi et al., British Medical Journal (2009)

Another key 2009 study addressed the discordance between pain and radiographic features of knee OA by conducting a cross-sectional analysis in two large cohorts. A novel feature of this study was using subjects with discordant knee pain as a within-person case-control study. Subjects from the MOST (Multicenter OA study) and the Framingham OA study had bilateral weight bearing fixed flexion AP radiographs which were scored for both global K&L grades (0–4), as well as individual scores for osteophytes and joint space narrowing. Three pain measures were also used to assess the subjects, which included the presence of frequent knee pain aching or stiffness during the previous month. The consistency and severity of pain were also assessed using the WOMAC questionnaire in the MOST cohort. Subjects who had frequent pain in one knee, but not in the contralateral knee were included in the final analysis. Results showed that knees with pain were more likely to have higher K&L scores than knees without. In the MOST cohort, knees with K&L 1 were 1.5 times more likely to have pain than a knee with K&L 0, while K&L 2 was 3.9 times more likely. Both K&L 3 and 4 showed high risk ratios when compared with K&L 0 for pain, 3 being 9 times more likely and 4 being 151 times more likely to be painful. Subjects from the Framingham cohort showed a similar trend. Other findings included a positive correlation between the severity of radiographic OA and the severity of pain. Importantly however, 45.7% of patients in the MOST study and 57.7% in the Framingham study were non-informative, having the same K&L grade in both knees. Furthermore, in 10.5% and 8.3% of patients had worse K&L grades in their non-painful knee, and were therefore mis-informative. Similar associations were seen with individual radiographic features, although the effect was greater in joint space narrowing than osteophytes.

Other studies addressing radiographic and painful OA discordance have suggested that either the type of imaging used or the views selected for imaging may be at fault. Raynauld and colleagues in 2006 found that using quantitative MRI identified progression of cartilage loss in less than two years and found that it was modestly associated with the WOMAC pain measure[9]. Duncan and colleagues, also in 2006, decided to look at several radiographic views in addition to the traditional AP view and found that 68% of their subjects with painful knees were identified when also using skyline and lateral radiographic views[10]. Only 38% of the painful knees were identified as radiographic OA by the AP view alone.

Surgical Treatment of Osteoarthritis
Charnley, Journal of Bone and Joint Surgery (1972)

Following army service in the Middle East during the Second World War, John Charnley returned to Manchester and continued his practice of orthopaedic surgery. It was during the early 1960s at the Writington Centre for Hip Surgery that he developed, tested and revised his idea of the low friction hip arthroplasty for severe OA. In his tireless pursuit of this goal, he produced this milestone paper outlining the prospective study of 773 low-friction arthroplasty cases. This study gives comprehensive descriptions of the individuals' preoperative clinical severity, complication rates associated with the procedure and postoperative results, quantified by pain, mobility and range of movement of the hip joint. Not only does Charnley's 1972 paper report on the arrival and implementation of newly invented implants and bearing surfaces, but also its comprehensive longitudinal follow-up of all cases gives us full appreciation of the benefits and risks of arthroplasty in clinically severe cases of hip OA.

Each individual recruited for THA during 1962 and 1965 was assessed preoperatively for clinical severity using a scoring system. Pain, range of motion and walking ability were constituent measurements in the grading of each patient's OA severity. This is reflected in contemporary clinical outcome measures used to monitor outcomes in arthroplasty today. Low-friction arthroplasty using high-density polyethylene bearing surfaces were conducted in 582 hips. Of this group, 379 were followed-up for greater than 4 years. Complications encountered during this follow-up period were addressed systematically by the author, including pulmonary embolism (3.2%), deep vein thrombosis (5.5%), death (1.4%) and infection (3.8%). In total, success rate was 92.7% and in this group of patients 90% returned to excellent function whilst 10% return to good function. This very high success rate, and the corresponding quality of results within that group, abrogated the need for the classification of an 'intermediate' grade to be assigned between those cases that were a success and those that were failures. The surgical technique described was still being routinely used by surgeons in the United Kingdom when this article was published in 1972.

The invention, implementation and development of the low-friction THA is widely regarded as one of the greatest surgical achievements in the treatment of severe OA. The excellent functional results achieved today with THA were made possible by the meticulous foundations laid by this study.

Dawson et al., Journal of Bone and Joint Surgery (1998)

Prior to this paper, the success of lower limb arthroplasty had traditionally been measured by relying on the technical surgical result, encompassing clinical and radiological components. Typically the need for revision surgery was quoted as a major outcome measure, overlooking the degree of symptomatic relief achieved: 'While a surgeon may judge a hip replacement successful because the procedure has been performed perfectly on the day, the patient will rightly disagree if they are still in pain and continue to have a poor quality of life six months down the line' (Prof. Lord Darzi, Paul Hamlyn Chair of Surgery, Imperial College London).

As the approach to measuring treatment success evolved, a greater emphasis was placed on factors that are important to and can be reported by patients themselves. Accordingly in 1998, Professor Andrew Carr and colleagues in Oxford reported on a new questionnaire developed to measure outcome following total knee replacement (TKR). This subsequently named Oxford Knee Score (OKS) has been adopted by numerous observational and interventional studies to date and in April 2008 was selected by the UK Department of Health to be the Patient Reported Outcome Measure for nationally assessment of primary unilateral TKR.

In contrast to the traditional approach, the content for this questionnaire was primarily identified by interviewing patients about the problems they experienced with the aim of devising a short, patient oriented, self-administered disease and site-specific measurement. The original draft contained 20 items, which was trialled on a group of new patients and following further refinement, the final tool comprising only 12 simple questions, was found to be reliable, valid, reproducible and sensitive to clinically important change over time.

Although this type of score is very convenient to use, it still does not provide a complete representation of the pain experienced by the patient peri-operatively[4,6,11,12]. Specific limitations, identified by patients themselves, include the intermittent and variable nature of pain making it difficult to select one response, the fact that pain elsewhere in the body influences the experience of joint pain, the difficulty in separating pain and function, and the fact that adaptation and avoidance strategies modify the experience of pain[12]. Furthermore it has been shown that the overall score is influenced by both psychological and constitutional status[13]. These factors may contribute to the apparent discrepancy between quantitative scores and qualitative assessment of patients symptoms[14]. The information gained from qualitative assessment can be used to improve quantitative assessment. For example, constant and intermittent pain have been identified as two distinct types of pain in lower limb OA, with the latter having a greater impact in quality of life. Subsequently, the Measure of Intermittent and Constant Osteoarthritis Pain (ICOAP) has been developed and its use is being encouraged at an international level[4,5].

D'Antonio et al., Journal of Bone and Joint Surgery (2009)

Since the development and vast implementation of the THA for severe OA, there has been an enormous amount of money and scientific energy channelled into the further development of these surgical implants. More specifically, new generation bearing surfaces have been the focus of much contemporary literature in this field as they have gained increasing popularity over traditional polyethylene. This juncture of medicine, surgery and biomedical engineering is developing rapidly, however long term follow-up studies of these new biomaterials are still in gestation. The selected paper, moderated by James D'Antonio, consists of four separate vignettes, each of which aims to give a current overview of new generation bearing surfaces used in THA.

Three new-generation bearing surfaces (ceramic-on-ceramic, metal-on-metal and high cross-linked polyethylene) each demonstrated significant reduction in wear following mechanical testing compared to traditional polyethylene. Furthermore, ceramic-on-ceramic (CoC) and metal-on-metal (MoM) surfaces show even significantly less wear than high cross-linked polyethylene (HCLP). However, HCLP remains very useful in practice due to its limited risk profile. Fracture of ceramic bearing surfaces and systemic sequelae due to elevated serum metal ions are serious risks that must be considered in the context of the individual patient being treated. Large amounts of volumetric wear debris from ceramic bearing surfaces can also cause local osteolysis, subsequent implant loosening and failure. Additionally, elevations in serum and local metal ions have been demonstrated to have associations with complications such as pseudotumor, metal allergy and osteolysis.

In a large THA follow-up study where subsequent revision for any reason was measured as the endpoint, CoC bearings were found to have a significantly greater 10-year survival rate (96.6%) when compared to metal-on-conventional polyethylene (91.3%). Specific problems, other than loosening and failure, that were identified with CoC bearing surfaces included squeaking (~1%) and chip fractures and cracks at the acetabular rim (0.5%).

As a guide, all three new generation bearing surfaces (HCLP, MoM and CoC) have reduced wear rates relative to traditional polyethylene. Attention must be paid to the individual patient's activity levels and also their ability to tolerate possible side effects such as squeaking and metal ion sequelae. There is particularly a place for CoC bearing surfaces in active women of child-bearing ages and MoM bearing surfaces in some very active men. However, with all of these new-generation bearing surfaces it will take time for large studies with long follow-up periods to clarify their risk profiles against traditional polyethylene.

Individual surgeons' practices vary. There are those who select one bearing surface they believe to be superior and apply it to all patients, and there are others who labour extensively over selecting the most evidence-based bearing surface for each individual.

Autologous Chondrocyte Implantation: The Future of OA Therapuetics?
Gikas et al., Journal of Bone and Joint Surgery (2009)

Advances in operative treatments for full-thickness chondral injuries to articular surfaces in the knee have led to the development of a new surgical technique known as autologous chondrocyte implantation (ACI). In this two-stage technique, arthroscopic harvest of healthy non-weight-bearing chondrocytes (often from the trochlear groove) is performed and these cells are then cultured for between 4 and 6 weeks. During this culture phase, an optional tissue scaffold may be incorporated into the chondrocytes, allowing for a variation of ACI known as matrix-induced autologous chondrocyte implantation (MACI). The second stage of the technique requires another operation involving arthrotomy of the knee joint, at which point the edges of the chondral defect are debrided and then the cultured chondrocytes are implanted. Depending on surgeon preference, the area is then secured with either a periosteal flap taken from the proximal tibia or, as is the case in MACI, the cells are covered by a collagen membrane. Rehabilitation protocols vary between study centers, however all are tailored to involve a period for a (1) proliferative phase, when the implanted cells adhere to subchondral bone, (2) transition phase, when there is an expansion of the collagenous matrix released by the chondrocytes, and (3) matrix remodeling phase, when the new cartilage tissue progressively acquires similar histological appearance to the surrounding articular surface. The selected paper provides a recent review of ACI and MACI techniques and outcomes, whilst also reporting on the experiences within a large UK orthopaedic centre over the past 9 years.

The optimum method for post-operative outcome evaluation of ACI is arthroscopic assessment, usually around one year post-implantation. This allows the repair site to be visualised directly, probed for stiffness and finally biopsied for histological evaluation. Magnetic resonance imaging (MRI) has also proved to be useful in assessing articular cartilage quality, with advances in delayed gadolinium-enhanced scans improving this avenue of outcome evaluation. Clinical outcome measures in most previous studies are categorised using subjective scoring methods that assess pain, function and locking.

In a review of 14 previous studies into ACI efficacy, each with less than 100 patients, there was a good to excellent outcome in 82–94% of cases. This was with an average follow-up period of 4.4 years. There was no evidence for the treatment of small (<1 cm^2) asymptomatic defects. The most common indications for ACI were trauma, osteochondritis dissecans and chondromalacia, each of which is associated with discrete chondral defects. In addition to treating the chondral lesion, preoperative assessment must involve assessment and, if needed, correction of any alignment or stability problems in the knee. Failure to detect such issues results in poorer outcomes.

ACI has become a popular technique for repairing isolated chondral defects with the view to reducing symptoms and in the longer term, preventing OA. Several recent studies have reported good to excellent clinical and histological results. Further development of surgical techniques and additional growth stimulating factors such as bone morphogenic protein and transforming growth factor-beta, may offer further improvement from present results. Larger studies with longer follow-up periods are needed to assess the impact on OA prevention, however early results from over 10,000 patients treated with ACI are promising.

Key Outstanding Questions

1. Which criteria are best for defining OA – radiological, clinical or a combination?
2. Can we consistently identify significant risk factors for the development of OA?
3. How central is neuropathic pain in the pain cycle in OA?
4. Do any of the new generation of surgical bearing surfaces offer an advantage?
5. Will autologous chondrocyte implantation be useful in treating and preventing OA?

Key Research Centres

1. Botnar Research Centre, Institute of Musculoskeletal Sciences, University of Oxford, United Kingdom
2. MRC Epidiemology Resource Centre, Southampton General Hospital, Southampton, United Kingdom
3. Kennedy Institute of Rheumatology, Imperial College London, London, United Kingdom

References

Arden, N.K., *et al.* (2009) Defining incident radiographic hip osteoarthritis for epidemiologic studies in women. *Arthritis and Rheumatism*, **60**, 1052–1059. http://onlinelibrary.wiley.com/doi/10.1002/art.24382/abstract

Charnley, J. (1972) The long-term results of low-friction arthroplasty of the hip performed as a primary prevention. *Journal of Bone and Joint Surgery (British Volume)*, **54-B**, 61–76. http://web.jbjs.org.uk/cgi/content/abstract/54–B/1/61

Cooper, C., *et al.* (2000) Risk factors for the incidence and progression of radiographic knee osteoarthritis. *Arthritis and Rheumatism*, **43**, 995–1000. http://onlinelibrary.wiley.com/doi/10.1002/1529-0131(200005)43:5%3c995::AID-ANR6%3e3.0.CO;2-1/abstract

D'Antonio, J.A., *et al.* (2009) Controversies regarding bearing surfaces in total hip replacement. *Journal of Bone and Joint Surgery (American Volume)*, **91**(Suppl. 5), 5–9. http://www.ncbi.nlm.nih.gov/pubmed/19648612

Dawson, J., *et al.* (1998) Questionnaire on the perceptions of patients about total knee replacement. *Journal of Bone and Joint Surgery (British Volume)*, **80-B**, 63–69. http://web.jbjs.org.uk/cgi/content/abstract/80-B/1/63

Gikas, P.D., *et al.* (2009) An overview of autologous chondrocyte implantation. *Journal of Bone and Joint Surgery (British Volume)*, **91-B**, 997–1006. http://web.jbjs.org.uk/cgi/content/abstract/91-B/8/997

Hawker, G.A., *et al.* (2008) Understanding the pain experience in hip and knee osteoarthritis-an OARSI/OMERACT initiative. *Osteoarthritis and Cartilage*, **16**, 415–422. http://www.oarsijournal.com/article/S1063-4584(07)00403-7/abstract

Neogi, T., *et al.* (2009) Association between radiographic features of knee osteoarthritis and pain: results from two cohort studies. *British Medical Journal*, **339**, b2844. http://www.ncbi.nlm.nih.gov/pmc/articles/PMC2730438/?tool$^{1}/_{4}$pubmed

Additional References

1. Merrill, C.T., and Elixhauser, A. (2007) Hospital stays involving musculoskeletal procedures. Healthcare Cost and Utilization Project (HCUP), Agency for Healthcare Research and Quality Statistical Brief #34. http://hcup-us.ahrq.gov/reports/statbrief/sb34.pdf

2. Miura, H., *et al.* (2009) Varus-valgus laxity correlates with pain in osteoarthritis of the knee. *The Knee*, **16**, 30–32.

3. Rogers, M.W., and Wilder, F.V. (2008) The association of BMI and knee pain among persons with radiographic knee osteoarthritis: a cross-sectional study. *BMC Musculoskeletal Disorders*, **9**, 163.

4. Hawker, G.A., *et al.*, (2008) Development and preliminary psychometric testing of a new OA pain measure – an OARSI/OMERACT initiative. *Osteoarthritis Cartilage*, **16**(4), 409–414.

5. Maillefert, J.F., *et al.* (2009) Multi-language translation and cross-cultural adaptation of the OARSI/OMERACT measure of intermittent and constant osteoarthritis pain (ICOAP). *Osteoarthritis Cartilage*, **17**(10), 1293–1296.

6. Hawker, G.A. (2009) Experiencing painful osteoarthritis: what have we learned from listening? *Current Opinion in Rheumatology*, **21**(5), 507–512.

7. Kellgren, J.H., and Lawrence, J.S. (1957) Radiologic assessment of osteoarthrosis. *Annals of the Rheumatic Diseases*, **16**, 494–502.

8. Croft, P., *et al.* (1990) Defining osteoarthritis of the hip for epidemiological studies. *American Journal of Epidemiology*, **132**, 514–522.

9. Raynauld, J.P., *et al.* (2006) Long term evaluation of disease progression through the quantitative magnetic resonance imaging of symptomatic knee osteoarthritis patients: correlation with clinical symptoms and radiographic changes. *Arthritis Research and Therapy*, **8**(1), R21.

10. Duncan, R.C., *et al.* (2006) Prevalence of radiographic osteoarthritis – it all depends on your point of view. *Rheumatology*, **45**, 757–760.

11. Hawker, G.A., *et al.* (2008) Understanding the pain experience in hip and knee osteoarthritis – an OARSI/OMERACT initiative. *Osteoarthritis and Cartilage*, **16**(4), 415–422.

12. Gooberman-Hill, R., *et al.* (2007) Assessing chronic joint pain: lessons from a focus group study. *Arthritis and Rheumatism*, **57**(4), 666–671.

13. Wolfe, F. (1999) Determinants of WOMAC function, pain and stiffness scores: evidence for the role of low back pain, symptom counts, fatigue and depression in osteoarthritis, rheumatoid arthritis and fibromyalgia. *Rheumatology (Oxford)*, **38**(4), 355–361.

14. Woolhead, G.M., *et al.* (2005) Outcomes of total knee replacement: a qualitative study. *Rheumatology (Oxford)*, **44**(8), 1032–1037.

25 Systemic Vasculitis

Joanna Robson, Ravi Suppiah and Raashid Luqmani

Nuffield Department of Orthopaedics, Rheumatology and Musculoskeletal Sciences, University of Oxford, Oxford, UK

Introduction

The systemic vasculitides are a group of conditions characterised by inflammation of blood vessels which can lead to occlusion and subsequent tissue damage. The current nomenclature and classification criteria use vessel size and pathological features as the defining characteristics. Systemic upset, weight loss, myalgia and arthralgia are common among the whole group, but expression of the more specific features are dependent on the size and distribution of blood vessels involved. Clinical, laboratory, radiographic and histologic features play an important role in diagnosis. For most forms of primary vasculitis, the aetiology is unknown with the exceptions of hepatitis B-related polyarteritis nodosa and hepatitis C-associated mixed cryoglobulinemia which should now be considered infectious diseases.

Giant cell arteritis is the most common form of systemic vasculitis. It usually affects patients older than 50, and involves large and medium sizes vessels with a predilection for the cranial arteries. The incidence of giant cell arteritis in populations of northern European ancestry is approximately 150–500 per million for people over the age of 50. The preferred method of diagnosis remains the temporal artery biopsy, but this is imperfect and can miss the diagnosis if a portion of artery that is not involved is sampled. New developments in diagnostic radiology such as Doppler ultrasound may supersede biopsy in the future. The other relatively common form of vasculitis is a group associated with Anti Neutrophil Cytoplasm Antibodies (ANCA), including Wegener's granulomatosis, microscopic polyangiitis and Churg Strauss syndrome; all of which involve small vessels including the capillaries of the lung and kidneys. The overall incidence of the ANCA associated vasculitides is approximately 10–20 per million, and can affect individuals of any age. The remainder of the systemic vasculitides are much rarer. The severity of vasculitis can range from mild and not require active therapy, to severe, which if untreated would result in death or severe organ dysfunction. Therefore, there is a need to rationalise and identify safer and more effective therapeutic strategies.

We review the first description of primary systemic vasculitis and the development of a classification system, and highlight progress that has been made in understanding the aetiology and how this has led to improvement in treatment for some of these disorders.

Understanding Medical Research: The Studies that Shaped Medicine, First Edition. Edited by John A. Goodfellow. © 2012 John Wiley & Sons, Ltd. Published 2012 by John Wiley & Sons, Ltd.

Describing the Disease
Kussmaul and Maier, Deutsches Archiv für klinische Medizin (1866)

The first comprehensive clinical and pathological description of primary systemic vasculitis was given in 1866 by Professor Adolf Kussmaul, a distinguished German physician, and his pathologist colleague Rudolf Maier. Other descriptions of vasculitis may have existed at the time but the detailed 35-page article written by Kussmaul and Maier is considered the classic description. They described a 27-year-old tailor who presented with fever, productive cough, myalgia, anorexia, muscle wasting, weakness, paresthesia, abdominal pain, cutaneous nodules, haematuria and oliguria. The patient died within 1 month of presentation. The autopsy revealed multiple nodular thickenings of arteries in many different tissues, especially at branching points of vessels the calibre of the hepatic and coronary arteries; histologically shown to be areas of inflammation and necrosis. In addition the authors observed glomerular lesions and inflammation in the smallest branches of the coronary arteries. Kussmaul and Maier concluded that they were dealing with a new disease attacking small and medium sized arteries and named it *periarteritis nodosa*.

Periarteritis nodosa became the default term used to describe a wide spectrum of systemic vasculitic disorders including conditions that manifested as arterial aneurysms and those that caused diffuse necrotizing glomerulonephritis. The term was subsequently changed to polyarteritis nodosa (PAN) in the mid-1900s to better reflect the transmural rather than perivascular inflammation of vessels caused by this disorder. The original description made by Kussmaul and Maier has been the cornerstone for understanding the pathophysiology of other forms of idiopathic vasculitis and forms the basis by which we currently characterise other vasculitidies.

Classification of Vasculitis
Zeek, American Journal of Clinical Pathology (1952)

Soon cases with a large variety of vascular inflammatory lesions which were loosely or wrongly labelled as *periarteritis nodosa* began to appear in the medical literature. By the 1940s it was clear that there were patients with different types of vasculitis, including patients who had additional features such as upper airways granulomatous inflammation or asthma and peripheral blood eosinophilia and that a classification system was desperately needed. The first person to recognise this need was Pearl Zeek, an American pathologist, who published the first widely accepted classification system in 1952. Her system was based on the predominant vessel size involved and this principle has been applied ever since. She was able to describe in detail the characteristic vessel wall changes at the microscopic level, and used the term 'necrotizing angiitis' to describe vascular lesions, both arterial and venous, which included fibrinoid necrosis and inflammation involving the full thickness of the vessel wall. In addition she separated small vessel vasculitis from periarteritis nodosa and other conditions affecting larger vessels. The classification imposed order in a field where chaos and confusion previously prevailed. The types of necrotizing angiitis proposed were: (1) hypersensitivity angiitis, (2) allergic granulomatous angiitis, (3) rheumatic arteritis, (4) periarteritis nodosa and (5) temporal arteritis. It is not clear whether Zeek was unaware of Wegener's granulomatosis or had grouped it together with allergic granulomatous angiitis in this classification. The method of using the predominant vessel size as the main discriminator is not perfect because there are a number of conditions where there is no predominant vessel size, but the principle has allowed progress in the understanding of vasculitis pathogenesis and outcome.

The modern classification systems including the 1990 American College of Rheumatology (ACR) criteria and the 1994 Chapel Hill Consensus Conference (CHCC) definitions have retained the concept of dominant vessel size as the main discriminating feature. Unfortunately one of the key disadvantages of the current ACR criteria was not to distinguish polyarteritis from microscopic polyangiitis, despite the recognition that these were separate entities in 1948.

Davson et al., QMJ (1948)

In 1948 Davson and colleagues described 14 cases that fitted the clinical description of periarteritis nodosa which came to autopsy. They divided the cases into two groups based on the histological findings in the kidneys. The clinical presentations of both groups were similar with rheumatic pains, chest symptoms and fever. The first group developed uraemia and haematuria or albuminuria but not hypertension. In these nine patients the kidneys showed a pathologically distinctive pattern of necrotizing glomerulonephritis with no arterial aneurysms. In contrast the second group (five patients) showed no extensive glomerular lesions in the kidney. They did, however, have proteinuria, uraemia and, in some patients, severe hypertension. The main pathological findings were widespread aneurysmal development (see Figure 25.1) and renal infarctions. This is the first time that a clear distinction was made between the microscopic

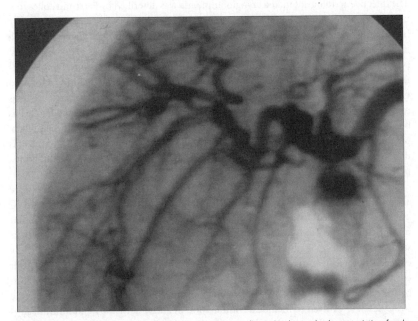

Figure 25.1 Renal angiogram showing aneurysms in medium-sized vessels characteristic of polyarteritis nodosa.
Source: Private collection of Raashid Luqmani.

form of polyarteritis nodosa (now called microscopic polyangiitis) and classical polyarteritis nodosa.

This distinction between microscopic polyangiitis and polyarteritis nodosa is recognised in the CHCC definitions. Polyarteritis nodosa is restricted to a medium vessel disease, and microscopic polyangiitis is considered a small vessel disease. However, this has resulted in inconsistency between our current disease definitions and classification criteria. There is a high level of dissatisfaction about the ACR classification criteria and the CHCC definitions among experts for most of the diseases. Updated definitions and new criteria consistent with modern diagnostic testing and our understanding of these diseases are needed. In response to the perceived current need The European League against Rheumatism (EULAR) systemic vasculitis classification and diagnostic criteria working group have recently (2010) proposed several points to consider when developing new classification and diagnostic criteria[1]. The points to consider are listed alongside the ACR (1990) classification criteria[2,3] in Table 25.1.

Aetiology and Pathogenesis

The aetiology of the 'primary' systemic vasculitis is idiopathic with the exceptions of hepatitis C-related mixed cryoglobulinemia and hepatitis B-related polyarteritis nodosa, both of which should probably now be considered infective diseases.

Ferri et al., Infection (1991)

The infective aetiology of mixed cryoglobulinemia was described by Ferri and colleagues in 1991. Cryoglobulins are immune complexes that precipitate when cooled below core body temperature and re-solubilise when warmed. These immune complexes are able to induce a systemic small vessel vasculitis. There are three distinct types of cryoglobulins: type I is due to monoclonal immunoglobulins which occur in relation to lymphoproliferative disorders; type II is polyclonal IgG with a monoclonal rheumatoid factor; and type III is due to polyclonal IgG and rheumatoid factor. Type II and III are referred to as mixed cryoglobulins. The association between cryoglobulins and a clinical syndrome has been known since 1966 when Metzer described a series of patients with arthralgia, purpura and weakness. We now know that the clinical syndrome described by Metzer is due to a cryoglobulinemia induced small vessel vasculitis that involves the skin, joints, peripheral nerves and kidneys.

Soon after the cloning of the hepatitis C virus in 1989 Ferri and colleagues were attributed as being the first group to describe the strong association between hepatitis C infection and mixed cryoglobulinemia, however several other authors showed similar findings about the same time. Ferri demonstrated that 41/45 (91%) patients in their study with mixed cryoglobulinemia were positive for hepatitis C. The results of this study changed our view of mixed cryoglobulinemia being an idiopathic vasculitis, to our current understanding that it is a complication of an infectious disease. As a result of our better understanding of the pathophysiology of mixed cryoglobulinemia, therapeutic strategies have evolved to include a combination of antiviral therapy and immunosuppression, occasionally with the addition of plasma exchange to remove the circulating immune complexes.

Table 25.1 American College of Rheumatology (ACR) 1990 classification criteria for the primary vasculitides and the European League Against Rheumatism (EULAR) 2010 points to consider when developing new classification or diagnostic criteria

ACR (1990) classification criteria for vasculitis	EULAR (2010) points to consider when developing new criteria in systemic vasculitis (Source: Basu et al. Modified with permission)

Hypersensivity vasculitis (3 of 5 criteria required)	**Churg-Strauss Syndrome** (4 of 6 criteria required)	**Wegener's granulomatosis** (2 of 4 criteria required)	**Biopsy**
1. Age at disease onset >16 years 2. Medication at disease onset 3. Palpable purpura 4. Maculopapular rash 5. Biopsy including arteriole and venule	1. Asthma 2. Eosinophilia >10% 3. Neuropathy, mono or poly 4. Pulmonary infiltrates, non fixed 5. Paranasal sinus abnormality 6. Extravascular eosinophils	1. Nasal or oral inflammation 2. Abnormal chest radiograph 3. Urinary sediment 4. Granulomatous inflammation on biopsy	1. Although histology is fundamental to the diagnosis of vasculitis and exclusion of its mimics, biopsy of affected organs is not always possible and yields vary significantly according to conditions and target organs 2. Temporal artery biopsy (TAB) is an important tool in the diagnosis of GCA. 3. Cases of Henoch Schönlein Purpura (HSP) usually have IgA deposits present on biopsy.

Henoch-Schonlein purpura (2 of 4 criteria required)	**Giant cell arteritis** (3 of 5 criteria required)	**Takayasu's arteritis** (3 of 6 criteria required)	**Laboratory Testing**
1. Palpable purpura 2. Age ≤20 at disease onset 3. Bowel angina 4. Wall granulocytes on biopsy	1. Age at disease onset ≥50 years 2. New headache 3. Temporal artery abnormality 4. Elevated erythrocyte sedimentation rate 5. Abnormal artery biopsy	1. Age at disease onset ≤40 years 2. Claudication of extremities 3. Decreased brachial artery pulse BP difference >10 mm Hg 4. Bruit over subclavian arteries or aorta 5. Arteriogram abnormality	1. ANCA testing plays an important diagnostic role in suspected small vessel vasculitis. 2. In suspected polyarteritis nodosa (PAN), the absence of ANCA has diagnostic value. 3. The role of clinical features and additional surrogate biomarkers for vasculitis is likely to have an important role in the development of future diagnostic criteria. **Diagnostic Radiology** 1. Computer-aided tomography (CT) and magnetic resonance angiography (MRA) techniques can replace standard angiography in the diagnosis of Takayasu's disease (TAK). 2. Ultrasound and high resolution MRI may have a role in the diagnosis of GCA. 3. The role of abdominal angiography in the diagnosis of adult PAN is unclear.

(continued)

Table 25.1 (*Continued*)

Polyarteritis nodosa (3 of 10 criteria required)
1. Weight loss ≥4 kg 2. Livedo reticularis 3. Testicular pain or tenderness 4. Myalgias, weakness, or leg tenderness 5. Mononeuropathy or polyneuropathy 6. Diastolic BP > 90 mm Hg 7. Elevated BUN or creatinine 8. Hepatitis B virus 9. Arteriographic abnormality 10. Biopsy of small or medium-sized artery containing PMN
4. CT and MRI may be useful in diagnosing ENT involvement associated with WG/CSS. 5. The role of radiology in the diagnosis of central nervous system (CNS) vasculitis is unclear. *Nosology* 1. The nomenclature in use for distinguishing between 'disease definitions', 'classification' and 'diagnostic' criteria is confusing and should be clarified wherever possible. 2. Nosology of different forms of vasculitis should be a reflection of their aetiopathogenesis wherever this has been determined. In the absence of this, definition must rely on a clear accurate description of the salient features of the condition. 3. The use of eponyms should be reviewed if a more rational approach to nomenclature can be developed, based on aetiopathogenesis, but their retention is necessary at present to avoid confusion. *Definitions* 1. Age is worthy of inclusion in the definitions of some forms of vasculitis, but its role should not be overstated. *Research agenda* 1. Future criteria initiatives should include all forms of vasculitis, providing definitions of less common syndromes not covered by CHCC. 2. The development of a classification tree will provide the foundations to future criteria.

Guillevin et al., Medicine (2005)

The association between HBV infection and PAN was made in 1970. Since this first association, it has been Professor Loic Guillevin and the French Vasculitis Study Group (FVSG) who have provided us with the main source of knowledge about this disease. Their work has included the epidemiology of PAN (including HBV-PAN), describing the clinical features, investigating the pathophysiology in addition to testing innovative therapies and creating prognostic tools (the five-factor score). The 2005 paper highlights some of the work they have done in the preceding 35 years by reviewing the clinical characteristics and outcome of 115 patients with HBV-PAN that were part of their clinical trials over several decades.

The epidemiology of PAN has changed over time with PAN becoming progressively less common and is now an exceptionally rare disorder. One of the main impacts on the incidence and prevalence has been changes to the definition of PAN, where prior to the 1994 Chapel Hill Consensus Conference (CHCC)[4], the term PAN encompassed the entity of microscopic polyangiitis (MPA), whereas after the CHCC, MPA (which is a small-vessel disease) was considered a separate entity, and PAN was restricted to a medium vessel disease. Guillevin showed that in addition to the overall prevalence of PAN decreasing over time, the relative proportion of HBV-PAN has fallen. HBV-PAN accounted for approximately 50% of PAN in the late 1970s and early 1980s but had fallen to 17% by the turn of the century. Public health initiatives such as widespread immunisation programs and improved blood screening for HBV are the likely cause of this reduction. Their paper also described the treatment strategies over the past 4 decades, especially with regard to the benefit of antiviral therapy in combination with immunosuppression and plasma exchange versus immunosuppression alone.

van der Woude et al., Lancet (1985)

Anti-neutrophil cytoplasm antibodies (ANCA) were first described in this classic *Lancet* paper by the nephrologist and scientist Professor Fokko J. van der Woude. He had originally suspected the involvement of an infectious agent in Wegener's granulomatosis. His search for infection was unsuccessful but instead he discovered IgG auto-antibodies against extranuclear components of polymorphonuclear granulocytes. This was present in the sera of patients with active Wegener's granulomatosis and he proposed a pathogenic role for ANCA in this disease.

ANCA positivity, specifically against proteinase 3 (PR3) has since been demonstrated to be very suggestive of a diagnosis of Wegener's granulomatosis with a sensitivity of 70–80%. There is also an association between myeloperoxidase (MPO) ANCA and microscopic polyangiitis with a 60% sensitivity, and Churg Strauss Syndrome (CSS) with a sensitivity of 40%. Collectively, these diseases are now known as the ANCA-associated vasculitides.

The evidence for pathogenicity in the ANCA-associated vasculitides is however still controversial, with generally more evidence for MPO-ANCA than PR3-ANCA. *In vitro*, neutrophils primed with tumour necrosis factor express PR3 and MPO on their cell surface and have been shown to release reactive oxygen series and lytic enzymes with the addition of ANCA. In patients with MPA and also WG, neutrophils constitutively express more PR3 on their membranes than controls. There is also a suggestion that rising ANCA titres predict an increase in disease activity although conflicting results have been published and in clinical practice levels are not used to guide treatment.

Table 25.2 Treatment of ANCA associated vasculitis based on disease severity

Clinical subgroup	Constitutional symptoms	Typical ANCA status	Threatened organ function	Serum creatinine	Treatment induction
Localised/ early systemic	Yes	−/+	No	<150 μmol/L	Methotrexate or cyclophosphamide
Generalised	Yes	+	Yes	<500 μmol/L	Cyclophosphamide
Severe	Yes	+	Yes	>500 μmol/L	Cyclophosphamide/ plasma exchange/ methylprednisolone

Source: Modified from Lapraik et al. (2007) with permission.

Treatment

Depending on the severity and type of vasculitis, therapy ranges from low dose glucocorticoids and the use of disease-modifying anti-rheumatic drugs (DMARDS), through to heavy duty immunosuppression with agents such as cyclophosphamide. An example of how treatment is stratified according to severity is shown in Table 25.2, which is adapted from the BSR guidelines on the management of ANCA associated vasculitis[5].

Leib et al., American Journal of Medicine (1979)

The treatment and outcome of vasculitis have changed dramatically in the last 70 years. Prior to this, 5-year survival was 10%, increasing to almost 50% by the 1960s with the introduction of corticosteroids. This paper published by Leib and colleagues in 1979 was the first to demonstrate that the use of corticosteroids plus immunosuppressive agents prolongs survival when compared with the use of corticosteroids alone.

The authors retrospectively reviewed the medical and pathological records of 139 patients with the diagnosis of polyarteritis from 1955 to 1977 at the UCLA hospital in California. Patients were excluded if an alternative diagnosis such as a primary collagen vascular disease or subacute bacterial endocarditis was present. Of the 64 patients accepted, biopsies were positive in 34 patients, 13 autopsies were positive and 10 angiograms. Patients were then actively sought to determine their outcome. The patients were divided into three groups based on their previous treatment; the first group had received no steroids or immunosuppressives, the second had received steroids alone and the third had received both steroids and immunosuppressives. There was no significant difference in the three groups in terms of sex, age at onset, steroids dose (second and third group only), hypertension, renal or liver disease, neuromuscular involvement, anaemia or erythrocyte sedimentation rate. Fourteen of the 22 patients on immunosuppressives received azathioprine, 4 oral cyclophosphamide, and 1 each of intravenous cyclophosphamide, busulphan, methotrexate and 6-mercaptopurine. Median survival time in the patients on no steroids or immunosuppressants was 3 months, if steroids were used this increased to 63 months, and in the steroids plus immunosuppressants group medium survival was 149 months. The 5-year survival percentages were 12%, 53% and 80% respectively. These results were statistically significant.

This was the first demonstration of a significant survival benefit to using immunosuppressives and corticosteroids in the treatment of vasculitis. It revolutionised the routine management of patients with vasculitis, which had previously been piecemeal and at the physicians' discretion, and is still the basic principle behind ongoing trials seeking the optimum treatment regimen for these patients.

Jayne et al., New England Journal of Medicine (2003)

In 1994 a group of investigators interested in vasculitis obtained a grant from the European Union to develop clinical trial methodology and conduct randomised controlled trials in ANCA associated vasculitis. This was called the ECSYSVASTRIAL project. The aim was to design and standardise data collection, disease scoring, and to rationalise treatment by facilitating therapeutic trials in this area. The investigators, who constitute the European Vasculitis Study Group (EUVAS), launched their first three randomised controlled trials in 1995. The trials were stratified by extent and severity of disease. The first of the trials to be published was CYCAZAREM, which compared azathioprine to cyclophosphamide for maintenance therapy in patients with a new diagnosis of generalised Wegener's granulomatosis or microscopic polyangiitis and a serum creatinine concentration $\leq 500\,\mu mol/L$. Prior to CYCAZAREM, the standard therapy for ANCA associated vasculitis of similar severity was glucocorticoids and cyclophosphamide for at least one year duration, with a high risk of disease relapse after withdrawal of treatment. The risks associated with cyclophosphamide are substantial and include haemorrhagic cystitis, bladder cancer, other malignancy, infection and infertility. Azathioprine is a less toxic medication which was shown in the CYCAZAREM trial to be as effective as cyclophosphamide in preventing disease relapse, once remission had been achieved with cyclophosphamide. Therefore instead of using cyclophosphamide for a year or more, patients are now treated with cyclophosphamide to induce remission (usually for around 3 months) and then switched to azathioprine to maintain remission, resulting in much lower exposure to the toxic and cumulative side effects of cyclophosphamide.

Several of the other EUVAS trials have now been published; they have all had major impacts on optimizing the treatment of ANCA vasculitis[6–8]. In addition to the knowledge gained from each of the individual trials, the patients from all the different EUVAS trials can be combined into one large cohort because of the standardised data collection and trial protocols. Together these patients form the largest ever group of patients with ANCA associated vasculitis to be prospectively followed; long-term follow-up (≥ 5 years) for the first four studies is now available.

Yazici et al., New England Journal of Medicine (1990)

Behçet's disease is a vasculitis of small and large blood vessels with a unique geographical association with the old Silk Route. It commonly presents with the classical triad of recurrent oral and genital ulcers and uveitis and is also a multisystem disease. Behçet's uveitis is potentially sight-threatening, with a 10-year risk of losing useful vision at 30% for males and 17% for females.

In 1990 the first randomised controlled trial to demonstrate the efficacy of a DMARD in Behçet's uveitis was published by Yazici and colleagues. This double-blinded trial compared the effectiveness of azathioprine, to placebo in 73 Turkish men with Behçet's disease. At the start of the trial, 48 patients had eye disease and 25 did not. All patients were allowed corticosteroids and were followed for 2 years. In those without initial eye involvement, azathioprine was significantly better at preventing new eye disease than placebo. In the patients with eye disease, those treated with azathioprine were significantly less likely to progress to bilateral eye involvement or to have an episode of hypopyon uveitis. No serious side effects were noted due to azathioprine during this trial, and the six patients who were withdrawn due to severe eye disease were all receiving the placebo. Later the authors reported their 8-year follow-up data from the patients in this trial[9]. Despite post-trial treatment, patients treated during the trial with placebo had an increased rate of blindness and decreased visual acuity. The effect of the initial randomisation to azathioprine was most pronounced in those patients who had been diagnosed less than 2 years before the start of the trial, indicating a benefit to starting azathioprine early. Although there has since been evidence to support the use of cyclosporine, interferon-alpha and even anti-TNF therapy in resistant cases, azathioprine, in combination with corticosteroids in the acute phase, is still the recommended first line treatment for Behcet's uveitis.

Newburger et al., New England Journal of Medicine (1986)

Kawasaki syndrome is an acute vasculitis of small and medium sized blood vessels, which affects young children and infants. It presents with a syndrome of self-limiting fever, rash, cervical lymphadenopathy, desquamation of extremities, haemorrhagic erythema of the tongue and conjunctivitis. Of greatest concern is the 15–25% of untreated patients who go on to develop coronary artery aneurysms, which can be fatal.

The historical treatment of Kawasaki syndrome was aspirin, which has both anti-inflammatory and antiplatelet effects, but does not reduce the frequency of coronary artery aneurysms. In 1986 Newburger and colleagues published a randomised trial comparing treatment with intravenous gamma globulin (400 mg/kg/day for 4 days) plus aspirin versus aspirin alone in 168 children with the syndrome. Echocardiograms were performed at baseline and repeated at 2 and 7 weeks, with the cardiologists blinded to the treatment received. At 2 weeks, 23% of children who received aspirin alone had coronary-artery abnormalities versus only 8% in the aspirin plus gamma globulin group. At 7 weeks, only 4% of patients who had received aspirin and gamma globulin had coronary-artery changes, compared with 18% of those who received only aspirin. These results were statistically significant, as was the finding that gamma globulin plus aspirin also rapidly reduced systemic inflammation. There were also no serious adverse effects from the intravenous gamma globulin treatment.

A later randomised controlled trial (RCT) from the same group demonstrated that treatment with a single, high dose of gamma globulin (2 g/kg over 10 hours) with aspirin was more effective again at reducing inflammation and preventing coronary-artery abnormalities than the 4-day regime of 400 mg/kg/day, and this is now the standard treatment[10]. Most experts would also recommend a repeat treatment in patients who fail to respond to the first dose of intravenous gamma globulin. A small RCT of repeated intravenous gamma globulin dosing versus Infliximab in intravenous gamma globulin-resistant cases demonstrated that both approaches were safe and reduced markers of inflammation[11]. Cases of treatment-resistant patients responding to pulsed intravenous methyprednisolone have also been published but routine use of steroids for initial management is not encouraged, with a RCT in new patients involving the routine addition of a pulse of intravenous methyprednisolone to intravenous gamma globulin and aspirin finding no additional benefit[12].

Summary

There has been substantial progress made in our understanding of the primary systemic vasculitides since the first description by Kussmaul and Meier. Zeek's classification remains relevant to our current methods of classification and has allowed us to group and study these relatively rare diseases with greater effectiveness. None of the classification systems are perfect and a number of less common types of vasculitis which do not conform to the restriction of vessel size tend to be excluded. As a result therapeutic trials have been difficult in these unclassified types of vasculitis. In the future our classification of vasculitis may focus on aetiology and incorporate genetic or proteomic biomarkers rather than rely on vessel size.

For the few diseases where the underlying aetiology has been recognised, targeted therapy has definitively changed outcome. In the remainder empiric immunosuppressive therapies are used. The medication of choice depends on the severity of disease and the extent of organ involvement including reliance on potentially toxic treatments such as cyclophosphamide for patients with severe disease. The emergence of newer biologic therapies such as Rituximab, which are presumed safer, remain to be fully evaluated and work is ongoing in this area. More rapid and less invasive diagnostic techniques are also needed, such as the use of ultrasound in giant cell arteritis. Another issue is predicting relapse of disease for which the role of serial ANCA measurements using new sensitive methods of detection is being evaluated.

Despite the advances in the past 150 years, there is an enormous amount we do not know about vasculitis. For future investigators interested in this area there is tremendous scope for more study, especially in elucidating the aetiopathogenesis for most forms of vasculitis and developing and testing targeted less toxic therapies.

Key Outstanding Questions

1. What is the aetiology of the vasculitidies?
2. Is there a genetic contribution to the pathogenesis of these disorders?
3. What is the best way to classify these disorders?
4. Can we better target and reduce the toxicity of therapy?
5. How can we reduce the disease morbidity?
6. What role does infection play and can this be addressed to improve outcome?

Key Research Groups

1. European Vasculitis Study Group (EUVAS): http://www.vasculitis.org
2. French Vasculitis Study Group (FVSG): http://www.vascularites.org
3. Vasculitis Clinical Research Consortium (VCRC): http://rarediseasesnetwork.epi. usf.edu/vcrc/index.htm

References

Davson, J., *et al.* (1948) The kidney in periarteritis nodosa. *Quarterly Journal of Medicine*, **17**(67), 175–202. http://qjmed.oxfordjournals.org/content/17/3/175.full.pdf+html

Ferri, C., *et al.* (1991) Antibodies against hepatitis C virus in mixed cryoglobulinemia patients. *Infection*, **19**(6), 417–420. http://www.springerlink.com/content/l54637411483110l/

Guillevin, L., *et al.* (2005) Hepatitis B virus-associated polyarteritis nodosa: clinical characteristics, outcome, and impact of treatment in 115 patients. *Medicine (Baltimore)*, **84**(5), 313–322. http:// journals.lww.com/md-journal/Abstract/2005/09000/Hepatitis_B_Virus_Associated_Polyarteritis_ Nodosa_.6.aspx

Jayne, D., *et al.* (2003) A randomized trial of maintenance therapy for vasculitis associated with antineutrophil cytoplasmic autoantibodies. *New England Journal of Medicine*, **349**(1), 36–44. http://www.ncbi.nlm.nih.gov/pubmed/12840090

Kussmaul, A., and Maier, R. (1866) Ueber eine bisher nicht beschriebene eigenthumliche Arterienerkrankung (Periarteritis nodosa), die mit Morbus Brightti und rapid fortschreitender allgemeiner Muskellahmung einhergeht. *Deutsches Archiv fr klinische Medizin*, **1**, 484–518.

Leib, E.S., *et al.* (1979) Immunosuppressive and corticosteroid therapy of polyarteritis nodosa. *American Journal of Medicine*, **67**(6), 941–947. http://www.amjmed.com/article/0002-9343 (79)90634-X/abstract

Newburger, J.W., *et al.* (1986) The treatment of Kawasaki syndrome with intravenous gamma globulin. *New England Journal of Medicine*, **315**(6), 341–347. http://www.ncbi.nlm.nih.gov/ pubmed/2426590

van der Woude, F.J., *et al.* (1985) Autoantibodies against neutrophils and monocytes: tool for diagnosis and marker of disease activity in Wegeners granulomatosis. *Lancet*, **1**(8426), 425–429. http://www.thelancet.com/journals/lancet/article/PIIS0140-6736(85)91147-X/abstract

Yazici, H., *et al.* (1990) A controlled trial of azathioprine in Behcets syndrome. *New England Journal of Medicine*, **322**(5), 281–285. http://www.ncbi.nlm.nih.gov/pubmed/2404204

Zeek, P.M. (1952) Periarteritis nodosa; a critical review. *American Journal of Clinical Pathology*, **22**(8), 777–790. http://www.ncbi.nlm.nih.gov/pubmed/14943695

Additional References

1. Basu, N., *et al.* (2010) EULAR points to consider in the development of classification and diagnostic criteria in systemic vasculitis. *Annals of the Rheumatic Diseases*, **69**, 1744–1750.

2. Fries, J.F., *et al.* (1990) The American College of Rheumatology 1990 criteria for the classification of vasculitis: summary. *Arthritis and Rheumatism*, **33**(8), 1135–1136.

3. Hunder, G.G., *et al.* (1990) The American College of Rheumatology 1990 criteria for the classification of vasculitis: introduction. *Arthritis and Rheumatism*, **33**(8), 1065–1067.

4. Jennette, J.C., *et al.* (1994) Nomenclature of systemic vasculitides: proposal of an international consensus conference. *Arthritis and Rheumatism*, **37**(2), 187–192.

5. Lapraik, C., *et al.* (2007) BSR and BHPR guidelines for the management of adults with ANCA associated vasculitis. *Rheumatology (Oxford)*, **46**(10), 1615–1616.

6. Jayne, D.R., *et al.* (2007) Randomized trial of plasma exchange or high-dosage methylprednisolone as adjunctive therapy for severe renal vasculitis. *Journal of the American Society of Nephrology*, **18**(7), 2180–2188.

7. de Groot, K., *et al.* (2005) Randomized trial of cyclophosphamide versus methotrexate for induction of remission in early systemic antineutrophil cytoplasmic antibody-associated vasculitis. *Arthritis and Rheumatism*, **52**(8), 2461–2469.

8. de Groot, K., *et al.* (2009) Pulse versus daily oral cyclophosphamide for induction of remission in antineutrophil cytoplasmic antibody-associated vasculitis: a randomized trial. *Annals of Internal Medicine*, **150**(10), 670–680.

9. Hamuryudan, V., *et al.* (1997) Azathioprine in Behcets syndrome: effects on long-term prognosis. *Arthritis and Rheumatism*, **40**(4), 769–774.

10. Newburger, J.W., *et al.* (1991) A single intravenous infusion of gamma globulin as compared with four infusions in the treatment of acute Kawasaki syndrome. *New England Journal of Medicine*, **324** (23), 1633–1639.

11. Burns, J.C., *et al.* (2008) Infliximab treatment of intravenous immunoglobulin-resistant Kawasaki disease. *Journal of Pediatrics*, **153**(6), 833–838.

12. Newburger, J.W., *et al.* (2007) Randomized trial of pulsed corticosteroid therapy for primary treatment of Kawasaki disease. *New England Journal of Medicine*, **356**(7), 663–675.

26   Polycystic Kidney Disease

Qi Qian

Division of Nephrology and Hypertension, Department of Internal Medicine,
Mayo Clinic, Rochester, Minnesota, USA

Introduction

Inherited polycystic kidney diseases (PKDs) are a large group of genetically heterogeneous disorders characterised by the development of kidney cysts leading to cystic kidney enlargement and kidney failure. Among them autosomal dominant PKD (ADPKD) and autosomal recessive PKD (ARPKD) are the major and most common forms. In the last decade impressive progress has been made in uncovering the underlying mechanisms of cystogenesis. Dysfunction of primary cilia appears to be a common feature of PKD, playing a major role in initiating a chain of downstream events leading to dedifferentiation, proliferation and apoptosis of kidney tubular epithelium and ultimately to cystic expansion of kidney tubules. A better understanding of the pathogenesis has led to identification of key therapeutic targets and design of targeted preclinical and clinical studies. For ADPKD, a number of clinical trials testing the efficacy of several drugs are being conducted and hold great promise.

Autosomal Dominant Polycystic Kidney Disease

Autosomal dominant polycystic kidney disease (ADPKD), also known as adult polycystic kidney disease (APKD), is the most common monogenic kidney disorder (1 in 400–700 live births). It involves a single gene (PKD1 or PKD2), occurs worldwide in all ethnic groups and ranks as the fourth leading cause of end-stage renal disease in adults. As its name suggests the cardinal feature of ADPKD is adult onset, progressive polycystic kidney enlargement, leading to kidney failure in more than half of the affected individuals. The true scope of ADPKD, however, is much broader. ADPKD is in fact a multisystemic disorder with progressive cyst formation in ductal organs (most prominently in kidney and liver; see Figure 26.1); cardiovascular abnormalities including mitral valve prolapse, pericardial effusion, abnormal arterial thickening, arterial dissection and aneurysms and early onset hypertension disproportional to age and kidney dysfunction; hernias of the intestine and abdominal wall and, more recently, bronchiectasis.

The basic biochemical defects which lead to the manifestations of ADPKD have been the subject of intense research. Gene type seems a major determinant of the severity of kidney disease. PKD1 mutation (85% of ADPKD cases) is associated with more severe disease than PKD2 mutation (15% of the cases). The average age of end-stage renal disease is 54.3 years for patients with PKD1 mutations compared to 74.0 years for those

Understanding Medical Research: The Studies that Shaped Medicine, First Edition. Edited by
John A. Goodfellow. © 2012 John Wiley & Sons, Ltd. Published 2012 by John Wiley & Sons, Ltd.

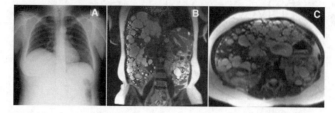

Figure 26.1 a. Chest X-ray of a 42-year-old female ADPKD patient with a serum creatinine of 1.4 mg/dL, showing an elevated right hemidiaphragm and an attenuated gastrointestinal gas pattern due to compression from cystic liver and kidneys. There was also echocardiographic evidence of right atrial compression by the enlarged liver. b. A coronal image of a noncontrast magnetic resonance imaging (MRI) of the same patient showing cystic liver and kidneys occupying almost the entire abdomen. c. A transverse view of the MRI in (B) showing enlarged cystic liver and kidneys.

with PKD2 mutations. Significant heterogeneity is seen, however, among ADPKD patients, even within the same family, in age of disease onset and rate of progression, suggesting the existence of disease modifying factors.

Currently there is no cure nor is there any medical therapy to retard the cyst growth in ADPKD. Several potential therapeutic agents shown to be effective in ameliorating cyst growth in animal models are now being tested in clinical trials.

Describing the Syndrome and Diagnosis of ADPKD
Dalgaard, Acta Medica Scandinavica Supplementum (1957)

The initial report of PKD as an inherited disease dates back as early as 1899 to Lejars (*Du gro rein polykystique de l'adulte*, Paris: Steinheil). It was Dalgaard, however, who described the autosomal dominant pattern of inheritance of ADPKD. In his landmark 1957 report, he detailed disease onset, symptoms, cause of death and autopsy findings in 350 patients. In 1987 Grantham and colleagues moved on from these clinical features to report the fine details of the cystic epithelial morphology[1]. They methodically examined 387 kidney cysts from ten ADPKD patients by scanning electron microscopy and found that the majority of the cysts were lined with a single layer of epithelium with morphological evidence of dedifferentiation and hyperplasia, consistent with insufficient terminal differentiation and active proliferation of the cyst-lining cells. They also provided evidence indicating that cyst fluids originated from active transepithelial secretion of solutes and water, rather than from sequestered glomerular filtrate. Many reports on the clinical and pathological features of ADPKD followed thereafter. Collectively, these studies form our current knowledge base of ADPKD and provide us with morphological evidence for understanding of cyst aetiology and pathogenesis.

Although cystic kidneys enlarge gradually over decades, the decline of kidney clearance typically occurs relatively rapidly in the late stage of ADPKD after the kidney parenchyma is replaced by cysts and fibrotic tissue. Thus the kidney clearance is an insensitive marker of disease progression in early stages of ADPKD. The CRISP study (The Consortium of Radiologic Imaging Studies of PKD)[2], led by Dr. Jared J. Grantham, characterised early changes in total kidney and kidney cyst volumes by magnetic resonance imaging (MRI) and the relation between the volume changes and kidney clearance. 241 patients in early stages of ADPKD (GFR>70 mL/min/BSA) were monitored yearly. During a three-year period kidney and cyst volumes were found to increase at an exponential rate, averaging a 5.27% increase in kidney volume yearly. Patients with the largest single kidney volumes (>1500 ml) had larger reductions in GFR (4.33 ml/min/year). The study concluded that kidney enlargement resulting from cyst expansion in patients with early stages ADPKD is continuous and quantifiable; moreover cystic kidney enlargement is directly related to the decline of renal function; the higher the rate of kidney enlargement, the more rapid decline in renal function.

Diagnostic modalities for ADPKD include ultrasonography, computed tomography (CT) scanning, MRI, gene-based linkage analysis and direct mutation analysis. Ultrasonography is by far the most frequently used modality because it is safe, accessible and comparatively less expensive. Pei and colleagues[3] recently conducted a comparative simulation study to assess the performance of ultrasound diagnostic criteria for both PKD1 and PKD2. Based on their study of 948 at-risk individuals from families of either PKD1 or PKD2 mutations, they proposed a new set of diagnostic criteria with a significantly improved sensitivity and specificity for all at-risk (a positive family history of ADPKD) individuals: the presence of ≥ 3 kidney cysts is sufficient for establishing the diagnosis in individuals aged 15 to 39 years; ≥ 2 cysts in each kidney is sufficient for individuals aged 40 to 59 years; and ≥ 4 cysts in each kidney is required for those aged ≥ 60 years. For evaluating potential kidney donors, in which the primary goal is to exclude ADPKD, the authors further demonstrate that the presence of < 2 kidney cysts in at-risk individuals at age > 40 has a 100% negative predictive value for ADPKD, and 0 kidney cysts at ages 30 to 39 has > 99% negative predictive value.

Accurate diagnosis and estimation of disease progression in the early stages of ADPKD are critical for the evaluation of potential treatment modalities because any treatment is futile after the kidneys have been structurally destroyed. The results from the studies by Grantham and Pei provide us with the essential tools for the diagnosis and assessment of ADPKD progression during the period when medical interventions would likely be beneficial.

Identifying the Genes and Proteins: ADPKD1 Gene and Polycystin-1
European Polycystic Kidney Disease Consortium, Cell (1994)

PKD1 gene was initially localised to the short arm of human chromosome 16 (ADPKD1) by linkage techniques in 1985[4]. It took nearly ten years before the gene was precisely mapped to chromosome 16p13.3 by the European Polycystic Kidney Disease Consortium. PKD1 is a large gene positioned within a complex duplicated area and immediately tail-to-tail with TSC2, one of the two genes responsible for the tuberous sclerosis complex. Hughes and colleagues[5] subsequently detailed the full-length PKD1 sequence that contains 46 exons spanning 52 kb of genomic DNA (MIM 601313), a 14148 bp transcript of PKD1, which encodes a protein, polycystin-1. Polycystin-1 is a 4302 amino acid glycoprotein comprised of a large, complex extracellular segment (containing a signal sequence, 2 leucine-rich repeats, a C-type lectin domain, 16 Ig-like repeats, and a sea urchin receptor for egg jelly module with a GPS cleavage site); 11 transmembrane domains; and a small cytoplasmic C-terminal tail with a coiled-coil region. Polcystin-1 has been located to primary cilia and the plasma membrane of epithelial cells and is postulated to function as a receptor of yet-to-be defined ligands. A recent study[6] shows that polycystin-1 is partially cleaved at its GPS site; a mutation created to eliminate the cleavage in mice leads to PKD, suggesting a functional significance of the cleavage.

Identifying the Genes and Proteins: ADPKD2 gene and Polycystin-2

Mochizuki et al., Science (1996)

A second gene for ADPKD was identified by positional cloning in three PKD2 families by Mochizuki and colleagues in 1996. They mapped PKD2 gene to human chromosome 4q21 and, from its full sequence (MIM 173910), uncovered polycystin-2, a membrane protein of 968 amino acids containing six transmembrane spans with intracellular amino- and carboxyl-termini. Polycystin-2 has amino acid similarity to polycystin-1, *Caenorhabditis elegan* homolog of PKD1, and transient receptor potential (Trp) channels. Polcystin-2 is highly expressed in primary cilia and the membrane of the endoplasmic reticulum and, to a much lesser degree, in the plasma membrane. Convincing evidence indicates that polycystin-2 can function as a Ca^{2+} permeable channel. It also interacts with polycystin-1 through their carboxyl termini, indicating polycystin-1 and polycystin-2 can act along a common signalling pathway.

The identification of PKD genes and proteins provides us with the fundamental knowledge to pursue a detailed understanding of the molecular pathogenesis of ADPKD.

Defining the Pathogenesis

Prior to the gene discovery, studies of ADPKD pathogenesis were focused on defining the determinants of cyst development and expansion. Using microdissection techniques, studies demonstrated that a cyst is initially a diverticulum, deriving from any tubular segment along the nephron. As the cyst enlarges it typically loses its tubular connection and becomes an isolated cyst. Further cyst expansion is promoted by concerted effects of proliferation of the cyst-lining epithelial cells, transepithelial transport of solutes and fluid, extracellular matrix remodeling and neovascularisation. These discoveries have led the researchers to focus on the signalling alterations along these pathways.

ADPKD Is a Ciliopathy
Barr et al., Nature (1999)
Pazour et al., Journal of Cell Biology (2000)

Research on the mechanisms of cystogenesis took an unexpected turn when Dr. Barr's and Pazour's groups made their seminal observations in the above papers. They found that polycystins exert a role in cilium mediated sensing, and that defects in primary cilia on which polycystins reside are associated with PKD.

The primary cilium is a nonmotile, hair-like organelle rooted in the mother centriole (the basal body) and projects out from the cell surface. Barr and colleagues showed that in *C. elegans* the homologous of PKD1 (Lov1) and PKD2 are expressed in ciliary structures of sensory neurons of the rays, hook and head. PKD1 and PKD2 are required for mating response, vulva location and chemotaxis to hermaphrodites, suggesting that polycystins are involved in transducing sensory function in cilia. Their work was paralleled by investigations by Pazour's group who found that in *Chlamydomonas* mutation of IFT88 (Tg737 in mouse and human) gene results in loss of flagella (the equivalent of primary cilia in mammalian cells). Mice harboring IFT88/Tg737 defects exhibit short cilia and die shortly after birth from PKD. Their study provided initial evidence indicating that primary cilia have important functions in kidney and that cilia defects can lead to PKD.

The discovery of ciliary polycystin expression and of cilium dysfunction affecting kidney cystogenesis has led to a general recognition that ADPKD is in fact a ciliopathy.

Cell Cycle Dysregulation
Bhunia et al., Cell (2002)
Low et al., Developmental Cell (2006)

Excessive cellular proliferation is a key pathological feature of ADPKD. In 2001 Bhunia and colleagues showed that expression of polycystin-1 activates the JAK-STAT pathway, which in turn upregulates p21(waf1) and induces cell cycle arrest in G0/G1. This process requires polycystin-2 as an essential cofactor. Mutations that disrupt the interaction of polycystin-1 and polycystin-2 prevent cell cycle arrest through this pathway. Moreover, mouse embryos lacking polycystin-1 show defective STAT1 phosphorylation and p21 (waf1) induction. These results indicate that the polycystin-1/polycystin-2 complex is able to regulate JAK/STAT pathway and mutations in either protein result in cell cycle dysregulation and hyperproliferation. Polcystin-1 has also been shown to regulate cell cycle through a direct interaction with Id2[7], a member of the helix-loop-helix (HLH) protein family that is known to regulate cell proliferation and differentiation.

The linkage between JAK-STAT pathway and primary cilia was subsequently demonstrated by Low and colleagues. They showed that polycystin-1 can undergo a proteolytic cleavage. The cleaved cytoplasmic tail is able to bind STAT6 in cilia, leading to STAT6-dependent gene expression and cell cycle progression. Cessation of tubular fluid flow increases polycystin-1 cleavage and attendant cell cycle progression. They further demonstrated that cyst-lining cells in ADPKD exhibit elevated levels of nuclear STAT6 and the polycystin-1 tail. Proteolytic cleavage of polycystin-1, a process modulated by polycystin-2 and promoted by cessation of renal tubular flow, has also been demonstrated by Chauvet and colleages[8]. These data indicate the existence of a pathway in which primary cilia and ciliary polycystins transduce mechanical (fluid flow) signals into changes of gene expression. Mutations in polycytins cause mechanical sensing defects, leading to a dysregulated gene expression.

Dysregulations of Other Signalling Pathways

Considerable evidence indicates that the activity of several major cellular signalling pathways, involving Ca^{2+}, cAMP and mammalian target of rapamycin (mTOR) are altered in cyst-lining epithelial cells of ADPKD and are related to cystogenesis.

Vassilev et al., Biochemical and Biophysical Research Communications (2001)
Nauli et al., Nature Genetics (2003)

In 2001 Vassilev and colleagues conducted exhaustive studies and unequivocally demonstrated that polycystin-2 is a Ca^{2+}-permeable channel with properties distinct from any known intracellular channels. The kinetic behavior of polycystin-2 is characterised by frequent transitions between closed and open states over a wide voltage range. Polycystin-2 channels, expressed abundantly in the endoplasmic reticulum membrane (in addition to ciliary expression), can be activated by cytosolic Ca^{2+}

elevation, but are insensitive to other major modulators known to induce intracellular Ca^{2+} release. The authors therefore assert that endoplasmic reticulum-located polycystin-2 is a novel class of Ca^{2+} release channels. They further demonstrate that mutant polycystin-2, when introduced into renal epithelial cells, causes an abnormal Ca^{2+}-stimulated intracellular Ca^{2+} release. Their observations support a possible role for a defective polycystin-2-dependent intracellular Ca^{2+} regulation in the pathogenesis of polycystic kidneys.

Their work was followed by the studies of Koulen and colleagues[9]. Using single channel experimental techniques, the authors demonstrate that polycystin-2 behaves as a Ca^{2+}-activated, high conductance endoplasmic reticulum Ca^{2+} release channel. Epithelial cells overexpressing polycystin-2 show an augmented intracellular Ca^{2+} release that is blunted with polycystin-2 mutations. Alterations in the intracellular Ca^{2+} homeostasis have also been demonstrated in $Pkd2^{+/-}$ vascular smooth muscle cells[10]. These data solidify the view of polycystin-2 being an intracellular Ca^{2+} release channel and defects of the channel may be pathogenically important.

In 2003 Nauli and co-workers carried out a series of experiments tied intracellular Ca^{2+} regulation to primary cilia. They showed that, in kidney tubular cells, ciliary polycystins jointly respond to fluid-flow by inducing an intracellular Ca^{2+} response, a response involving polycystin-2-mediated intracellular Ca^{2+} release. Cells lacking either polycystin failed to generate such a response, suggesting that polycystins contribute to renal tubular fluid-flow sensation and, through Ca^{2+} response, triggering downstream signalling cascades. Loss or dysfunction of polycystins might therefore result in ADPKD.

Polycystins can also sense mechanochemical signals in endothelial cells, osteoblasts, osteochondrocytes and smooth muscle cells. Thus, defects in the signalling mediated by ciliary polycystins seem to be a unifying mechanism underlying the multisystem nature of ADPKD.

Yamaguchi et al., Journal of Biological Chemistry (2004)

Cyclic AMP has been shown to stimulate secretion of cyst-lining epithelium and promotes cyst growth in ADPKD. In their 2004 report, Yamaguchi and colleagues demonstrated that abnormal Ca^{2+} signalling due to PKD mutations can alter the cAMP-mediated effects in renal epithelial cells. Cellular Ca^{2+} reduction induces cAMP-mediated cell proliferation, associated with elevations in B-Raf and Ras-dependent activations of B-Raf and ERK and reduction in the activity of Akt, a negative regulator of B-Raf. Their study provided further evidence of an augmented and aberrant cAMP-mediated signalling causing multiple cellular defects seen in ADPKD.

Shillingford et al., Proceedings of the National Academy of Sciences of the USA (2006)

Another change consistently found in PKD cells is the upregulation of mTOR, a serine/threonine protein kinase, known to regulate cell growth and metabolism. Shillingford and colleagues showed that the cytoplasmic tail of polycystin-1 interacts with tuberin, a protein which when mutated causes tuberous sclerosis, and through such interaction inhibits mTOR activation. PKD mutations, therefore, cause inappropriate mTOR activation. mTOR inhibition (by rapamycin) reduces renal cyst growth in two mouse PKD models and in the native kidneys of ADPKD patients with kidney transplantation. These studies were reinforced by a study[11] showing mTOR upregulation in hepatic cyst-lining epithelium and reduction in polycystic liver growth in ADPKD patients with kidney transplantation and receiving rapamycin-containing regimen. These results indicate mTOR could potentially be considered a therapeutic target for ADPKD.

Prospective Treatments

The availability of MRI techniques to accurately assess cystic kidney disease progression in a relatively short period of time has greatly facilitated clinical trial design to evaluate the effect of therapeutic agents. A number of agents targeting specific signalling pathways dysregulated in ADPKD, shown promise in PKD animal models and in pilot or retrospective human studies, have been moved to prospective clinical trials. For instance, agents targeting cAMP (vasopressin V2 receptor antagonists and somatostatin analog octreotide) and mTOR (everolimus and sirolimus) are currently being tested for patients with ADPKD. As our understanding of ADPKD pathogenesis advances, more potential therapeutic agents will be tested. It is possible that treatment for ADPKD may require a combination therapy targeting several pathways of cystogenesis.

Autosomal Recessive Polycystic Kidney Disease

Autosomal recessive polycystic kidney disease (ARPKD) is a less common disease with an incidence of 1: 20,000. It is caused by mutations in a single gene, *PKHD1*. ARPKD presents primarily *in utero* or at birth with kidney enlargement due to cystic dilatations in renal collecting ducts and biliary dysgenesis. It carries a high mortality rate. A small fraction of patients display a milder presentation with later disease manifestations characterised by hepatic portal hypertension or cholangitis and kidney failure. The kidneys at that stage are small and cystic (Figure 26.2). The lethal, infantile phenotype seems to be associated with truncating mutations in PKHD1 while the milder form correlates with missense mutations.

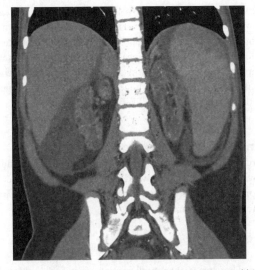

Figure 26.2 A coronal image of a contrast enhanced CT scan in an 18-year-old ARPKD patient with renal failure on maintenance dialysis, showing bilateral small, cystic kidneys and marked spleno-megaly. This patient had cirrhosis due to congenital hepatic fibrosis associated with ARPKD.

Identifying the Gene and Protein
Ward et al., Nature Genetics (2002)
The definitive identification of the *PKHD1* gene came from the work of Ward and colleagues using PCK, a rat model of PKD. The PCK rat is a recessively inherited model with features of progressive cystic kidney and liver diseases. The region on rat chromosome 9 is syntenic to the human chromosome 6 interval where *PKHD1* was initially mapped[12]. *PKHD1* spans a region of 470-kb, consists of 67 exons, and encodes a 16-kb transcript that translates to fibrocystin/polyductin, a large membrane protein with a short cytoplasmic tail and an extensive extracellular segment. A significant proportion of the extracellular segment consists of repeats of an lg-like fold of TIG/IPT domain.

Defining the Pathogenesis
As PKHD1 was discovered relatively recently, research on defining the pathogenesis of ARPKD is in its early stages. Initial work thus far has been focused on elucidating the functions of polyductin/fibrocystin and its importance in the kidney. Evidence is beginning to accumulate that the function of polyductin/fibrocystin is intimately related to primary cilia and intracellular Ca^{2+} regulation[12–15]. Polyductin/fibrocystin is expressed in multiple subcellular locations including cilia. Proteolytic cleavage can be elicited by stimulation of intracellular Ca^{2+} release and the cleavage product can potentially translocate to the nucleus. Fibrocystin also can complex with polycystin-2 to regulate Ca^{2+} responses. These studies shed light on the potential pathogenesis of ARPKD. However, the exact functions of fibrocystin/polyductin are yet to be defined.

Prospective Treatment
Therapeutic interventions for ARPKD are being tried in animal models. Several agents with expected pharmacologic effects on renal function have been shown to exert variable effects. For instance the Ca^{2+} mimetic R-568 has had no significant effect on kidney cyst growth in a rat model. However the arginine vasopressin V2 receptor antagonists (OPC-31260 and tolvaptan) and a somatostatin analog (octreotide) ameliorate the cystic growth. As our understanding of the pathogenesis of ARPKD continues to grow, more disease-relevant therapeutic targets will likely be identified.

Summary and Conclusions
Concerted research efforts have considerably advanced our understanding of PKD and continue to provide fundamental knowledge needed to select potential therapeutic targets. There is promise that effective treatment for PKD, ADPKD in particular, will be available in the foreseeable future.

Note
The papers included here represent a small fraction of research in this field. Due to space limitations, many excellent clinical and basic science research papers on PKD could not be included.

Key Outstanding Questions

1. What are the ligand(s) for polycystin-1 and fibrocystin/polyductin?
2. What are the physiological functions of polycystins and fibrocystin/polyductin?
3. What triggers cyst formation in epithelial cells bearing mutations in disease causing genes?
4. Do cysts in PKD continue to form in renal tubules throughout life?
5. Why are there phenotypic variations among ADPKD individuals from the same family with the same mutation?
6. What is the function of ciliary polycystin in connective tissues i.e., smooth muscle cells of the arterial tunica media, intestine and airway?
7. What constitute the downstream signalling pathways triggered by ciliary polycystin activation?

Key Research Centres

1. Yale School of Medicine, New Haven, United States
2. University of Kansas Medical Center, Kansas City, United States
3. Mayo Clinic College of Medicine, Rochester, United States
4. Harvard Medical School, Cambridge, United States
5. Johns Hopkins University School of Medicine, Baltimore, United States
6. Emory University School of Medicine, Atlanta, United States
7. University of Alabama at Birmingham, Birmingham, United States

References

Barr, M.M., and Sternberg, P.W. (1999) A polycystic kidney-disease gene homologue required for male mating behaviour in C. elegans. *Nature*, **401**(6751), 386–389. http://www.nature.com/nature/journal/v401/n6751/full/401386a0.html

Bhunia, A.K., *et al.* (2002) PKD1 induces p21waf1 and regulation of the cell cycle via direct activation of the JAK-STAT signaling pathway in a process requiring PKD2. *Cell*, **109**, 157–168. http://www.cell.com/retrieve/pii/S009286740200716X

Dalgaard, O.Z. (1957) Bilateral polycystic disease of the kidneys; a follow-up of two hundred and eighty-four patients and their families. *Supplement to Acta Medica Scandinavica*, **328**, 1–255.

European Polycystic Kidney Disease Consortium (1994) The polycystic kidney disease 1 gene encodes a 14 kb transcript and lies within a duplicated region on chromosome 16. *Cell*, **77**(6), 881–894. http://www.ncbi.nlm.nih.gov/pubmed/8004675

Low, S.H., *et al.* (2006) Polycystin-1, STAT6, and P100 function in a pathway that transduces ciliary mechanosensation and is activated in polycystic kidney disease. *Developmental Cell*, **10**, 57–69. http://www.cell.com/developmental-cell/retrieve/pii/S1534580705004818

Mochizuki, T., *et al.* (1996) PKD2, a gene for polycystic kidney disease that encodes an integral membrane protein. *Science*, **272**(5266), 1339–1342. http://www.sciencemag.org/content/272/5266/1339.abstract

Nauli, S.M., *et al.* (2003) Polycystins 1 and 2 mediate mechanosensation in the primary cilium of kidney cells. *Nature Genetics*, **33**, 129–137. http://www.ncbi.nlm.nih.gov/pubmed/12514735

Pazour, G.J., *et al.* (2000) Chlamydomonas IFT88 and its mouse homologue, polycystic kidney disease gene Tg737, are required for assembly of cilia and flagella. *Journal of Cellular Biology*, **151**, 709–718. http://www.ncbi.nlm.nih.gov/pmc/articles/PMC2185580/

Shillingford, J.M., *et al.* (2006) The mTOR pathway is regulated by polycystin-1, and its inhibition reverses renal cystogenesis in polycystic kidney disease. *Proceedings of the National*

Academy of Sciences of the USA, **103**(14), 5466–5471. http://www.pnas.org/content/103/14/5466.long

Vassilev, P.M., *et al.* (2001) Polycystin-2 is a novel cation channel implicated in defective intracellular Ca^{2+} homeostasis in polycystic kidney disease. *Biochemical and Biophysical Research Communications*, **282**, 341–350. http://www.sciencedirect.com/science/article/pii/S0006291X01945541

Ward, C.J., *et al.* (2002) The gene mutated in autosomal recessive polycystic kidney disease encodes a large, receptor-like protein. *Nature Genetics*, **30**, 259–269. http://www.ncbi.nlm.nih.gov/pubmed/11919560

Yamaguchi, T., *et al.* (2004) Calcium restriction allows cAMP activation of the B-Raf/ERK pathway, switching cells to a cAMP-dependent growth-stimulated phenotype. *Journal of Biological Chemistry*, **279**(39), 40419–40430. http://www.jbc.org/content/279/39/40419.long

Additional References

1. Grantham, J.J., *et al.* (1987) Cyst formation and growth in autosomal dominant polycystic kidney disease. *Kidney International*, **31**, 1145–1152.

2. Grantham, J.J., *et al.* (2006) CRISP Investigators: volume progression in polycystic kidney disease. *New England Journal of Medicine*, **354**(20), 2122–2130.

3. Pei, Y., *et al.* (2009) Unified criteria for ultrasonographic diagnosis of ADPKD. *Journal of the American Society of Nephrology*, **20**(1), 205–212.

4. Reeders, S.T., *et al.* (1985) A highly polymorphic DNA marker linked to adult polycystic kidney disease on chromosome 16. *Nature*, **317**(6037), 542–544.

5. Hughes, J., *et al.* (1995) The polycystic kidney disease 1 (PKD1) gene encodes a novel protein with multiple cell recognition domains. *Nature Genetics*, **10**(2), 151–160.

6. Yu, S., *et al.* (2007) Essential role of cleavage of polycystin-1 at G protein-coupled receptor proteolytic site for kidney tubular structure. *Proceedings of the National Academy of Sciences of the USA*, **20**(47), 18688–18693.

7. Li, X., *et al.* (2005) Polycystin-1 and polycystin-2 regulate the cell cycle through the helix-loop-helix inhibitor Id2. *Nature Cell Biology*, **7**, 1102–1112.

8. Chauvet, V., *et al.* (2004) Mechanical stimuli induce cleavage and nuclear translocation of the polycystin-1 C terminus. *Journal of Clinical Investigation*, **114**(10), 1433–1443.

9. Koulen, P., *et al.* (2002) Polycystin-2 is an intracellular calcium release channel. *Nature Cell Biology*, **4**(3), 191–197.

10. Qian, Q., *et al.* (2003) Pkd2 haploinsufficiency alters intracellular calcium regulation in vascular smooth muscle cells. *Human Molecular Genetics*, **12**(15), 1875–1880.

11. Qian, Q., *et al.* (2008) Sirolimus reduces polycystic liver volume in ADPKD patients. *Journal of the American Society of Nephrology*, **19**(3), 631–638.

12. Zerres, K., *et al.* (1994) Mapping of the gene for autosomal recessive polycystic kidney disease (ARPKD) to chromosome 6p21-cen. *Nature Genetics*, **7**(3), 429–432.

13. Hiesberger, T., *et al.* (2006) Proteolytic cleavage and nuclear translocation of fibrocystin is regulated by intracellular Ca^{2+} and activation of protein kinase. C. *Journal of Biological Chemistry*, **281**, 34357–34364.

14. Wang, S., *et al.* (2007) Fibrocystin/polyductin, found in the same protein complex with polycystin-2, regulates calcium responses in kidney epithelia. *Molecular and Cellular Biology*, **27**, 3241–3252.

15. Kaimori, J., *et al.* (2007) Polyductin undergoes notch-like processing and regulated release from primary cilia. *Human Molecular Genetics*, **16**, 942–956.

27 Glomerular Disease and the Nephrotic Syndrome

Jenny Papakrivopoulou and Robert Unwin

UCL Centre for Nephrology, Royal Free Hospital, London, UK

Introduction

A variety of systemic and primary kidney diseases can damage the filtration barrier of the kidney to cause some or all of the following clinical manifestations: proteinuria, haematuria, reduced glomerular filtration rate (GFR) and decreased sodium excretion, leading to oedema and hypertension. Proteinuria is the commonest manifestation of glomerular injury and can exist to varying degrees. Heavy proteinuria (>3.5 gr of protein/day) results in a series of metabolic disturbances that are collectively termed the 'nephrotic syndrome', and include: hypoalbuminaemia, tissue oedema, hypercholesterolaemia and hypercoagulability. Although patients may be nephrotic and have preserved renal function, progressive proteinuria can lead to permanent glomerular and tubular damage and eventual renal failure.

In this chapter we will summarise the historically important papers that have led to the concept of the nephrotic syndrome, and our current understanding of the structure and function of the glomerular filtration barrier. We will concentrate on those primary glomerular disorders that cause the nephrotic syndrome (Table 27.1), and we will discuss some of the latest discoveries about its pathogenesis. Treatment of the nephrotic syndrome will not be discussed because it remains largely empirical and nonspecifically immunosuppressive, reflecting our incomplete understanding of the underlying pathogenesis.

The Beginnings of Clinical Nephrology: Bright's Disease
Bright, Longman Green (1827)

Hippocrates was the first to make the observation that disease of the 'loins' might lead to oedema ('dropsy') that is usually accompanied by frothy urine[1]. However, the idea that diseases may have their origins in a particular organ of the body did not really come about until the 18th century, and Theodor Zwinger III (1658–1724), was the first physician to clearly attribute oedema to kidney disease[2]. The presence of protein in the urine of oedematous patients was demonstrated later by Domenico Cotugno (1735–1820)[3], although the actual link between proteinuria and oedema was made later still by William Wells (1757–1817) in 1811[2]. It wasn't until the early 19th century and the work of Richard Bright (1789–1858) that it all came together: in his book *Reports of Medical Cases* he described the association between proteinuria, oedema and kidney disease. Bright worked closely with the chemist John Bostock who described the low

Understanding Medical Research: The Studies that Shaped Medicine, First Edition. Edited by John A. Goodfellow. © 2012 John Wiley & Sons, Ltd. Published 2012 by John Wiley & Sons, Ltd.

Table 27.1 Glomerular diseases presenting as the nephrotic syndrome in adults

Disease	Aetiology	Associations
Minimal change disease	Unknown	Allergy, atopy, NSAIDs
Focal segmental glomerulosclerosis (FSGS)	Familial: podocin, TRPC6, α-actinin 4 gene mutations Sporadic: unknown	Ethnicity: African American, Infections: HIV Drugs: heroin, pamidronate
Membranous nephropathy	Autoantibody to M-type phospholipase A2 receptor	Infections: Hepatitis B, C, malaria Drugs: gold, penicillamine, NSAIDs Malignancy: breast, lung, gastrointestinal
Membranoproliferative glomerulonephritis (type I)	Unknown	Infections: Hepatitis B and C, bacterial endocarditis
Membranoproliferative glomerulonephritis (type II)	Unknown	C3 nephritic factor

Note: NSAIDs: nonsteroidal anti-inflammatory drugs; TRPC6: transient receptor potential cation 6 channel; HIV: human immunodeficiency virus.

specific gravity of urine, a reduced concentration of albumin in the blood and lipaemia in oedematous patients. Together they described in 1827 the clinical and chemical features of what we now know as the nephrotic syndrome, and they also described many of the complications of the nephrotic syndrome, such as pleural effusions and ascites. The term 'Bright's disease' was coined and became widespread by the end of the century to describe a patient with these features. However, Bright only considered chronic cases characterised by proteinuria, oedema and uraemia, and who invariably had a fatal outcome. Today we would describe such cases as examples of the nephrotic syndrome leading to chronic renal failure and hypertension. Bright did not appreciate that isolated proteinuria can persist for many years without renal damage, nor did he ever see sick children and realise the often relapsing and remitting nature of proteinuria.

By 1840 Bright and many of his colleagues had realised that his eponymous disease had different aetiologies, pathology and outcomes[4,5]. Confusion over the heterogeneity meant that even though an almost complete description of the nephrotic syndrome was evident as early as 1827, it took another century before it was a clinical entity, and another quarter of a century before this was widely accepted.

Classification of Bright's Disease
Volhard and Fahr, Springer (1914)
The 19th century saw the progress of medicine with the introduction of many new investigative tools, such as urine analysis, estimation of renal function and indirect measurements of blood pressure. The description of the anatomy of the glomerulus by William Bowman in 1842[6], along with the advent of paraffin embedding (Edwin Klebs, 1834–1913) and aniline dyes (William Perkin, 1854), allowed for more detailed

investigation of the underlying pathology of kidney disease. In 1872, the term 'glomerulonephritis' was first used by Klebs to describe the appearances of the glomeruli in post-scarlet fever acute nephritis (post-streptococcal glomerulonephritis), placing the glomerulus at the centre of the pathology of proteinuric kidney disease. In subsequent studies the description of the various renal lesions by pathologists and clinicians remained confusing and chaotic. A real breakthrough was the novel classification proposed by Volhard and Fahr in this famous monograph.

Volhard believed that the description of a disease process would only be correct if the clinical symptoms were correlated with the histological lesion and shown to be consequences of the same derangement. Their clinical and pathological text was extensively illustrated with coloured drawings of the microscopic appearances of the glomeruli, and supplemented by detailed clinical observations of patients. They divided the collective term Bright's disease into three major forms: (1) the degenerative diseases, or nephroses; (2) the inflammatory diseases, or nephritides; and (3) the arteriosclerotic diseases, or scleroses. The nephroses were subdivided further into genuine (proteinuria, oedema and normal renal function) and necrotising (proteinuria, oedema hypertension and impaired renal function). The nephritides were also divided into three stages: (1) the acute stage, (2) the chronic stage without renal impairment and (3) the end stage with renal insufficiency. All stages could be associated with proteinuria – nephritis with a nephrotic component. The last group of scleroses was subdivided into a simple benign form characterised by hypertension and sclerosis of the renal vessels, and a combination form (nephritis superimposed on sclerosis).

This classification was hugely influential and was the basis of most thinking until the introduction of the renal biopsy and the concept of the clinical nephrotic syndrome. It emphasized the difference between cases with nephritic features and those we would now call nephrotic syndrome. It wasn't until the introduction of the renal biopsy, and the application of electron microscopy, that the wide variability in histological appearances of the glomerulus in proteinuric oedematous patients was recognised, and the significance of the 'nephrotic syndrome' became fully appreciated and accepted.

The Nephrotic Syndrome
Kark et al., Annals of Internal Medicine (1958)

The term 'nephrotic syndrome' made its first appearance in an influential review by Louis Leiter in 1931[7]. Although he termed his paper 'Nephrosis', he described with great clarity the concept of 'nephrotic syndrome' and used the term on several occasions.

By the end of the 1950s, the concept of 'nephrotic syndrome' was widely accepted as the metabolic, nutritional and clinical consequence of continued massive proteinuria. The technique of percutaneous renal biopsy was first introduced and widely practised in Copenhagen[8], and perfected in its modern day form by Kark and Muehrcke[9]. The latter group published their findings in 98 renal biopsies from patients aged 15–85 in this landmark paper of 1958. They firmly established that the nephrotic syndrome has multiple underlying aetiologies which they divided into three categories: (1) primary renal disease, for example 'lipoid nephrosis' (termed minimal change disease today); (2) renal disease associated with systemic illnesses, for example SLE, amyloid and diabetes mellitus; or (3) pressure effects on the venous system draining the kidney, for example renal vein thrombosis. Today the latter category is obsolete, as we know that renal vein thrombosis is a complication rather than a cause of the nephrotic syndrome and secondary to the loss of proteins of the coagulation cascade.

Diseases intrinsic to the kidney accounted for the majority of nephrotic presentations (60%). Their histological classification incorporated the latest advances in staining techniques demonstrating the diffusely thickened basement membrane and 'spikes' of membranous nephropathy. Glomerular pathology evident on light microscopy, grouped at the time under the term glomerulonephritis, was divided into three categories: membranous, proliferative and mixed membranous and proliferative (membranoproliferative). As can be seen from Table 27.1, few modifications have occurred over the last 50 years. The introduction of immunofluorescence and the discovery of the immune-mediated nature of some glomerulonephritides have resulted in the current terminology of focal and segmental sclerosis (FSGS), which excludes the proliferative changes seen in ANCA-related vasculitis or anti-GBM disease.

'Lipoid nephrosis' was the final histological group, separate because of the lack of glomerular changes under light microscopy. This entity had been previously described by Volhard and Fahr, but had been the subject of controversy for many years. Its relapsing/remitting nature and favourable prognosis had been appreciated for years. Post-mortem examination revealed normal glomeruli, but degenerated, fat-laden tubules (hence the name) with interstitial oedema. Using the newly developed technique of electron microscopy, the authors demonstrated changes in the podocytes surrounding the glomerular capillaries, namely, fusion of 'foot processes'. Serial biopsies in one patient demonstrated the completely restored architecture of the podocytes following treatment with prednisone, newly introduced as therapy.

This histological classification forms the basis for the modern classification of primary renal diseases presenting with nephrotic syndrome. Moreover, this was the first description of a histological lesion in what is now known as minimal change disease.

Structure, Function and Pathology of the Glomerular Filtration Barrier

As early as 1924, from the technique of renal micropuncture developed by Wearn and Richards[10], it was known that macromolecules were excluded from the glomerular filtrate in Bowman's space. Elegant physiological studies in the 1940s and 1950s demonstrated that the glomerulus behaves as a sieve, restricting the passage of macromolecules with a molecular weight (MW) >70,000 Da from the glomerular ultrafiltrate[11]. With the introduction of electron microscopy (EM) in the 1950s and 1960s the mechanisms and structural basis of glomerular permeability began to be elucidated. It became clear that the structure of glomerular capillary walls was unique, in keeping with their highly specialised filtering function. The glomerular filter, beginning in the capillary wall, was shown to consist of three layers: (1) an endothelial layer with fenestrae, pore-like structures, of 50–100 nm diameter; (2) a glomerular basement membrane (GBM); and (3) an elaborate epithelial cell (podocyte) layer on the outer surface, consisting of interdigitating foot processes with slit-like pores (30–40 nm diameter) between them (Figure 27.1). Over the next 50 years the key research questions were which of these layers controlled permeability, and which one is disrupted in proteinuric kidney disease.

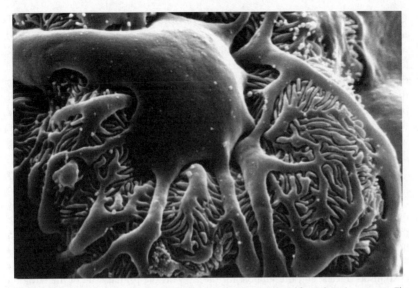

Figure 27.1 Scanning electron micrograph of normal podocyte viewed from the urinary space. The urinary side of the capillary wall is covered by the highly branched podocytes with their interdigitating foot processes. With kind permission from Springer Science and Business Media: *J. Mol. Med.*, Regulation of podocyte structure during development of nephrotic syndrome, volume 76, 1998, 172–183, Smoyer WE, Mundel P, figure 2.

Farquhar et al., Journal of Experimental Medicine (1961)

In 1961, Farquhar and her colleagues provided the first direct experimental evidence suggesting the GBM was the structure serving as the main filtration barrier. Their studies on rats, using the electron-dense tracer ferritin, were based on the assumption that a sharp drop in the concentration of the tracer should occur at the level of the structure that restricted its passage. Kidney tissue fixed at intervals of 2 minutes to 2 hours following an intravenous injection of ferritin was examined by EM. At short time intervals (2 to 15 minutes) after ferritin administration, most of the tracer was retained in the endothelial lumen, with few tracer molecules in the basement membrane, and even fewer in the epithelium. Later (1 to 2 hours) the tracer particles were still present in the lumen and within endothelial fenestrae and had accumulated on the luminal side of the basement membrane. Larger numbers of ferritin molecules were found in the epithelial cells, at the base of foot processes and in intracellular vesicles. Based on the sharp drop in ferritin observed at the level of the GBM, it was concluded that the GBM acted as the main filtration barrier. The following functional model for the glomerulus was proposed: (1) the basement membrane as the main filter; (2) the endothelium as a valve, which by the number and size of its fenestrae controls access to the filter; and (3) the epithelium as a 'monitor', which partially recovers proteins that have leaked through the filter.

Although this was an elegant theoretical model, it could only be applied to molecules the size of ferritin (480,000 Da), and the question as to whether smaller molecules were filtered in the same way remained unanswered.

Graham and Karnovsky, Journal of Experimental Medicine (1966)

In 1966 Graham and Karnovsky used horseradish peroxidase (HRP, 40,000 Da) and myeloperoxidase (MPO, 160,000–180,000 Da) as tracer molecules to investigate the location of the filtration barrier. When mice were injected with HRP, the tracer traversed the entire thickness of the glomerular capillary wall and entered the urinary space. When they used MPO, it passed rapidly through the endothelial fenestrae and across the basement membrane but was impeded at the level of the podocyte slits. They formulated the hypothesis that the GBM acts as a 'coarse' filter to exclude only very large molecules, whereas the podocyte slits, acting as a 'fine' filter, are the principal filtration barrier and determine the protein content of the glomerular ultrafiltrate.

The hypothesis of the two filtration barriers in series gained wide acceptance, as other groups obtained further evidence that the podocyte slits are the main barrier to filtration[12,13]. However, these studies were not without criticism; the main ones being that the tracers were either too small or too large when compared with albumin, and that the localisation of the histochemically detectable tracers was potentially inaccurate, because of diffusion or reabsorption of the tracer or its reaction product. In 1974 Farquhar's group published their observations using newly available electron-dense dextrans as tracers, and the support for the GBM as the primary site of the filtration barrier again strengthened. In their classic publication[14], they demonstrated that the 62,000 Da fraction of electron-dense dextran was filtered in only small amounts (similar to albumin) and that there was a sharp drop in the concentration of this tracer at the level of the GBM. Despite this progress the exact location of the barrier continued to be debated for the next 40 years.

Rodewald and Karnovsky, Journal of Cell Biology (1974)

Although early EM studies of the renal glomerulus had described a structure often seen bridging the podocyte slits it wasn't until this landmark paper by Rodewald and Karnovsky that this structure was described in detail. Using tannic acid as a new fixative, they discovered a thin, electron-dense line connecting the plasma membranes of adjacent epithelial foot processes. Sections cut tangential to the basement membrane revealed the three dimensional structure of the slit diaphragm: 'a central filament was joined to the cell membranes by regularly spaced cross bridges which appeared to alternate between the two sides of the central filament, thus giving the diaphragm a zipper-like appearance'. This arrangement gave rise to rectangular pores between the cross bridges, with a mean width of 4nm and was narrow enough to restrict passage of most serum proteins. This study was descriptive and not followed by any direct evidence for a filter function of the slit diaphragm so it remained largely ignored until the late 1990s when the molecular structure of the slit diaphragm was discovered and its importance in filtration finally understood.

Chang et al., Kidney International (1975)

Work in the 1970s and 1980s added another dimension to the complexity of glomerular permeability – charge selectivity – and shifted the focus away from the slit diaphragm. Studies by this group had already demonstrated that the clearance of uncharged molecules of a similar effective radius as albumin was much higher than albumin[15]. They postulated that some factor in addition to molecular size retarded the transglomerular passage of albumin. Since albumin is negatively charged in physiological solutions, they examined the effect of charge on glomerular permeability by using an anionic form of dextran as a tracer molecule. For any given size of sulphated dextran (1.0–5.5 nm), clearance was lower than that for neutral dextran. For molecules of ~3.6 nm, similar to the size of albumin, substitution of neutral dextran for dextran sulfate was associated with a marked reduction in clearance. They concluded: 'that the polyanionic property of albumin, together with its size, can account almost entirely for its retention within the intravascular compartment, and, thereby, for its osmotic effectiveness in regulating plasma volume', and that the observed charge selectivity was the result of electrostatic repulsion by some fixed, negatively charged component of the glomerular capillary wall.

Their conclusions were supported by morphological studies demonstrating regularly spaced, highly charged anionic sites composed of heparan sulfate proteoglycans in the outer and inner layers of the GBM[16], and a highly negatively charged coat on podocytes rich in sialic acid[17]. Two animal models of proteinuric disease had also become available (nephrotoxic serum nephritis and puromycin aminonucleoside nephrosis) and Brenner's group demonstrated loss of charge selectivity in both[18]. Farquhar's group subsequently showed that in the puromycin model, which mimics minimal change nephropathy in humans, there is loss of anionic sites from the podocytes, as well as the GBM[19].

Thus the prevailing idea in the 1980s was that the GBM was the primary site of size and charge selectivity within the filtration barrier, and that the heavy proteinuria associated with nephrotic syndrome could be explained by the loss of charge selectivity. It was postulated that in minimal change nephropathy the causative factor was a circulating cationic substance that reduced the surface negative charge to result in proteinuria.

Kestila et al., Molecular Cell (1998)

The role of the slit diaphragm remained obscure until this seminal publication. This group studied a population of children with congenital nephrotic syndrome of the Finnish type (CNE): a rare autosomal recessive disease characterised by massive proteinuria at birth and lack of a podocyte slit diaphragm. They identified the gene on chromosome 19, NPHS1, and showed it to be mutated in CNE. The gene product encoded a novel transmembrane member of the immunoglobulin superfamily, which they named 'nephrin', because of its high expression level in human embryonic renal glomeruli.

Subsequently the same group demonstrated with immunoelectron microscopy that nephrin was localised exclusively at the slit diaphragm and that its inactivation in mice causes massive proteinuria, absence of a slit diaphragm, and neonatal death[20,21]. They have also provided evidence that the extracellular domains of the nephrin molecules of two neighbouring foot processes interact in the centre of the slit to form a zipper-like structure with pores the size of albumin, or smaller, located on both sides of a central density[22]; thus elucidating the molecular basis of the structure described by Karnovsky 30 years earlier.

Following the discovery of nephrin, a multitude of new components of the slit diaphragm have been identified, some based on their structural similarity to nephrin, for example Neph1[23], others on their binding properties to nephrin, for example CD2AP[24], and others on their association with human disease, for example podocin, (autosomal recessive steroid resistant nephrotic syndrome)[25]. We now know that the slit diaphragm is a complex of several proteins and acts not only as the size barrier to protein filtration, but also as a signalling platform to regulate and maintain the shape of the podocyte foot processes through interactions with the actin cytoskeleton. This discovery has changed our understanding of the role of the slit diaphragm in filtration and placed the podocyte at the centre of the pathogenesis of proteinuric kidney disease.

Kopp et al. and Kao et al., Nature Genetics (2008)

Mutations in nephrin and podocin genes have been found to account for only a very small proportion of adult cases of nephrotic syndrome. FSGS is one of the main causes of adult nephrotic syndrome, and accounts for up to 3% of end-stage renal disease cases in the United States. It is characterised by loss of the normal foot process architecture ('effacement'), as well as areas of glomerular sclerosis/collapse. In the majority of cases the aetiology is unknown; hence the term 'idiopathic FSGS'.

In these publications, both groups undertook a genome-wide association study approach to identify susceptibility genes for idiopathic FSGS, HIV-associated FSGS and nondiabetic ESRD, based on the observation that all of these conditions are much more prevalent in African Americans. They compared populations of African Americans with European Americans, and identified variations in the nonmuscle myosin heavy chain 9 (MYH9) gene that were highly associated with the development of all three conditions in the African American population.

The heavy chain of nonmuscle myosin is expressed in podocytes and binds to actin to perform intracellular motor functions. Mutations in this gene had previously been identified in four autosomal dominant forms of macrothrombocytopaenia that are also associated with glomerular disease. Although the exact mechanism has not been elucidated yet, it is possible that accumulation of abnormal myosin disrupts the actin-myosin filaments in the podocyte foot processes, leading to foot process efface-ment and proteinuria.

These studies have underscored once again the importance of the podocyte in proteinuric kidney disease, and have identified a genetic cause for a common adult cause of the nephrotic syndrome.

Beck et al., New England Journal of Medicine (2009)

Membranous nephropathy is the commonest cause of the nephrotic syndrome in white adults over 60 years. It is an organ-specific autoimmune disease in which immune deposits of IgG and complement appear at the basal surface of podocytes. It can occur in association with a variety of conditions, for example SLE, hepatitis B and lymphoma, but in the majority of cases it is idiopathic.

The mechanism of proteinuria in membranous nephropathy was elucidated using a rat model of the disease, Heymann's nephritis, developed in the 1960s[26]. The immune deposits are formed in situ, as a result of circulating antibodies binding to megalin on podocytes. The antigen-antibody complexes then form the subepithelial deposits. Complement activation does not lead to cell lysis and death but initiates a signalling cascade resulting in loss of foot process architecture and release of oxidants and proteases that damage the underlying GBM. This causes proteinuria from loss of both the size- and charge-selective properties of the glomerular capillary wall. However, megalin is not expressed in human podocytes and for many years investigators have been searching for the antigen responsible for the human form of membranous nephropathy.

Beck and his colleagues were successful in their search as a result of a simple technical alteration. They examined serum from 37 patients with biopsy proven idiopathic membranous nephropathy and tested them for antibodies against normal human glomerular protein extracts. They used a nonreducing electrophoretic technique so that glomerular proteins remained in their native conformation. This identified auto-antibodies in 70% of patient sera against an antigen normally expressed on the podocyte cell membrane, the M-type phospholipase A2 receptor (PLA2R). This protein is a transmembrane receptor of the mannose-receptor family, but its function remains unclear. They also provided preliminary evidence for an association between the clinical features of the disease (proteinuria and nephrotic syndrome) and the presence and titre of the circulating autoantibodies.

This seminal publication was a major breakthrough in our understanding of the pathogenesis of nephrotic syndrome and it has major implications for diagnosis and treatment. Assays for anti-PLA2R autoantibody may permit the non-invasive diagnosis of membranous nephropathy, as well as provide a convenient way of monitoring the activity of the disease in response to treatment.

Summary and Conclusions

These papers summarise the slow but significant progress that has been made in our understanding of proteinuric renal disease: from its early clinical and pathological description, to its eventual basis in glomerular structure and function, and finally to the beginnings of its molecular characterisation, and the prospects for more specific forms of therapy. These papers also emphasise the importance of good clinical observation, detailed tissue histology, and later animal experimentation, which all laid the phenotypic founda-tions for the subsequent genetic and molecular advances. However, there is still much to learn about the function of the newly identified podocyte proteins, and how they might be manipulated to therapeutic effect in renal proteinuria and the nephrotic syndrome.

Key Outstanding Questions

1. Why does the slit diaphragm not clog?
2. How is the precise interdigitating pattern of the podocyte foot processes formed?
3. How are proteins assembled into the slit diaphragm?
4. What is the pathogenesis of minimal change disease?
5. Do other genes confer susceptibility to non diabetic proteinuric kidney disease?

Key Research Centres

1. UCL Centre for Nephrology, Royal Free Hospital, London, United Kingdom
2. Academic Renal Unit, University of Bristol, Bristol, United Kingdom
3. Division of Matrix Biology, Department of Medical Biochemistry and Biophysics, Karolinska Institute, Stockholm, Sweden
4. Inserm U983, Hopital Necker-Enfants Malades, Paris, France
5. Renal Division, Washington University School of Medicine, St. Louis, United States
6. Division of Nephrology, University of Washington, Seattle, United States
7. The Samuel Lunenfeld Research Institute, Mt Sinai Hospital, Toronto, Ontario, Canada

References

Beck, L.H., Jr., *et al.* (2009) M-type phospholipase A2 receptor as target antigen in idiopathic membranous nephropathy. *New England Journal of Medicine*, **361**(1), 11–21. http://www. ncbi.nlm.nih.gov/pubmed/19571279

Bright, R. (1827) *Reports of medical cases selected with a view to illustrating the symptoms and cure of diseases by a reference to morbid anatomy.* Vol. 1. Longman Green, London. http://www. christies.com/LotFinder/lot_details.aspx?intObjectID^1/$_4$1710765

Chang, R.L.S., *et al.* (1975) Permselectivity of the glomerular capillary wall: III. Restricted transport of polyanions. *Kidney International*, **8**, 212–218. http://www.nature.com/ki/ journal/v8/n4/abs/ki1975104a.html

Farquhar, M.G., *et al.* (1961) Glomerular permeability: ferritin transfer across the normal glomerular capillary wall. *Journal of Experimental Medicine*, **113**, 47–66. http://www.ncbi.nlm. nih.gov/pmc/articles/PMC2137334/

Graham, R.C., and Karnovsky, M.J. (1966) Glomerular permeability: ultrastructural cytochemical studies using peroxidases as protein tracers. *Journal of Experimental Medicine*, **124**(6), 1123–1134. http://www.ncbi.nlm.nih.gov/pmc/articles/PMC2138332/

Kao, W.H., *et al.* (Family Investigation of Nephropathy and Diabetes Research Group) (2008) MYH9 is associated with nondiabetic end-stage renal disease in African Americans. *Nature Genetics*, **40**(10), 1185–1192. http://www.ncbi.nlm.nih.gov/pubmed/18794854

Kark, R.M., *et al.* (1958) The nephrotic syndrome in adults: a common disorder with many causes. *Annals of Internal Medicine*, **49**(4), 751–774. http://www.annals.org/content/49/4/ 751.extract

Kestila, M., *et al.* (1998) Positionally cloned gene for a novel glomerular protein – nephrin – is mutated in congenital nephrotic syndrome. *Molecular Cell*, **1**, 575–582. http://www.cell.com/ molecularcell/retrieve/pii/S109727650080057X

Kopp, J.B., *et al.* (2008) MYH9 is a major-effect risk gene for focal segmental glomerulosclerosis. *Nature Genetics*, **40**(10), 1175–1184. http://www.ncbi.nlm.nih.gov/pubmed/18794856

Rodewald, R., and Karnovsky, M.J. (1974) Porous substructure of the glomerular slit diaphragm in the rat and mouse. *Journal of Cellular Biology*, **60**, 423–433. http://jcb.rupress.org/content/ 60/2/423.long

Smoyer, W.E., and Mundel, P. (1998) Regulation of podocyte structure during the development of nephrotic syndrome. *Molecular Medicine*, **76**, 172–183. http://www. inclopedia.info/regulation-of-podocytestructure-during-the-development-of-nephrotic-syndrome.html

Volhard, F., and Fahr, T.H. (1914) *Die Brightsche Nierenkrankheit, Klinik, Pathologie und Atlas.* Springer, Berlin.

Additional References

1. Chadwick, J., and Mann, W.N. (1950) *The medical works of Hippocrates.* Oxford University Press, Oxford.
2. Cameron, J.S., and Glasscock, R.J., eds. (1987) *The nephrotic syndrome.* Informa Healthcare, London.
3. Dock, W. (1922) Some early observers of albuminuria. *Annals of Medical History*, **4**, 287–290.
4. Christison, R. (1829) Observations upon the variety of dropsy which depends upon deceased kidneys. *Edinburgh Medical and Surgical Journal*, **32**, 262–291.
5. Sabatier, J.-C. (1834) Considerations and observations sur lhydropsie symptomatique dune lesion speciale des reins. *Archives generales de Medecin (Paris)*, **5**, 333–389.

6. Bowman, W. (1842) On the structure and use of the malpighian bodies of the kidney with observations on the circulation through that gland. *Philosophical Transactions of the Royal Society of London*, **132**, 57–80.

7. Leiter, L. (1931) Nephrosis. *Medicine*, **10**, 135–242.

8. Iversen, P., and Brun, C. (1952) Aspiration biopsy of the kidney. *Acta Medica Scandinavica*, **6**, 430–435.

9. Muerhcke, R.C., *et al.* (1955) Technique of percutaneous kidney biopsy in the prone position. *Journal of Urology*, **74**, 267–277.

10. Wearn, J.T., and Richards, A.N. (1924) Observations on the composition of glomerular urine, with particular reference to the problem of reabsorption in the renal tubules. *American Journal of Physiology*, **71**, 209–227.

11. Pappenheimer, J.R. (1953) Passage of molecules through capillary walls. *Physiological Reviews*, **33**, 387–423.

12. Venkatachalam, M.A., *et al.* (1970) An ultrastructural study of glomerular permeability using catalase and peroxidase as tracer proteins. *Journal of Experimental Medicine*, **132**(6), 1153–1167.

13. Oliver, C., and Essner, E. (1972) Protein transport in mouse kidney utilizing tyrosinase as an ultrastructural tracer. *Journal of Experimental Medicine*, **136**(2), 291–304.

14. Caulfield, J.P., and Farquhar, M.G. (1974) The permeability of glomerular capillaries to graded dextrans. Identification of the basement membrane as the primary filtration barrier. *Journal of Cellular Biology*, **63**(3), 883–903.

15. Chang, R.L.S., *et al.* (1975) Permselectivity of the glomerular capillary wall to macromolecules: II. Experimental studies in rats using dextran. *Biophysical Journal*, **15**, 887–906.

16. Caulfield, J.P., and Farquhar, M.G. (1976) Distribution of anionic sites in glomerular basement membranes. Their possible role in filtration and attachment. *Proceedings of the National Academy of Sciences of the USA*, **73**, 1646–1650.

17. Mohos, S.C., and Skoza, L. (1969) Glomerular sialoprotein. *Science*, **164**(887), 1519–1521.

18. Brenner, B.M., *et al.* (1978) Molecular basis of proteinuria of glomerular origin. *New England Journal of Medicine*, **298**(15), 826–833.

19. Caulfield, J.P., and Farquhar, M.G. (1978) Loss of anionic sites from the glomerular basement membrane in aminonucleoside nephrosis. *Laboratory Investigation*, **39**(5), 505–512.

20. Ruotsalainen, V., *et al.* (1999) Nephrin is specifically located at the slit diaphragm of glomerular podocytes. *Proceedings of the National Academy of Sciences of the USA*, **96**(14), 7962–7967.

21. Putaala, H., *et al.* (2001) The murine nephrin gene is specifically expressed in kidney, brain and pancreas: inactivation of the gene leads to massive proteinuria and neonatal death. *Human Molecular Genetics*, **10**(1), 1–8.

22. Wartiovaara, J., *et al.* (2004) Nephrin strands contribute to a porous slit diaphragm scaffold as revealed by electron tomography. *Journal of Clinical Investigation*, **114**(10), 1475–1483.

23. Donoviel, D.B., *et al.* (2001) Proteinuria and perinatal lethality in mice lacking NEPH1, a novel protein with homology to NEPHRIN. *Molecular Cell Biology*, **21**, 4829–4836.

24. Shih, N.Y., *et al.* (2001) CD2AP localizes to the slit diaphragm and binds to nephrin via a novel C-terminal domain. *American Journal of Pathology*, **159**, 2303–2308.

25. Boute, N., *et al.* (2000) NPHS2, encoding the glomerular protein podocin, is mutated in autosomal recessive steroid-resistant nephrotic syndrome. 2000. *Nature Genetics*, **24**, 349–354.

26. Heymann, W., *et al.* (1959) Production of nephrotic syndrome in rats by Freunds adjuvant and rat kidney suspensions. *Proceedings of the Society for Experimental Biology and Medicine*, **100**, 660–664.

28 Acquired Immunodeficiency Syndrome

Tica Pichulik and Alison Simmons

MRC Human Immunology Unit, Weatherall Institute of Molecular Medicine, University of Oxford, Oxford, UK

Introduction

HIV-1/AIDS is today recognised as a global pandemic affecting all parts of society. Among the worst affected are women and children in Sub-Saharan Africa and Asia. In 2009 the World Health Organisation published devastating statistics according to which 33.3 million people are living with HIV-1 and 1.8 million die of AIDS every year. That a further 2.6 million new infections occur every year is a stark reflection of the fact that this pandemic is far from being under control. As a result of statistics like these, HIV-1/AIDS has captured the attention of world leaders, the media and the medical and public health communities perhaps more than any other disease affecting the developing world.

Extensive scientific efforts led to the elucidation of the viral, genetic and structural organisation and the important factors that control the replication and life-cycle of HIV-1. This information facilitated the rapid development of a specific diagnostic assay for HIV-1 antibodies and, importantly, the first antiretroviral drug azidothymidine (AZT) in 1987. The scientific community has since focused on gaining further insights into the viral life-cycle, the virus-host interactions and the immune response to the virus in order to develop various treatment options and, ideally, an effective vaccine.

The Discovery of AIDS and HIV
Gottlieb et al., New England Journal of Medicine (1981)
Gallo et al., Science (1984)

In 1981, the *New York Times* reported increasing incidence of a rare lung infection, *Pneumocystis carinii* pneumonia (PCP), and an aggressive form of Kaposi's sarcoma (KS) amongst young gay men in New York and California. This condition was termed acquired immunodeficiency syndrome (AIDS) by the CDC in 1982. Only two years later, Françoise Barré-Sinoussi and Luc Montagnier published a seminal paper in Science that described the isolation of a retrovirus from lymph nodes of patients in the early phase of AIDS. In 1984 Robert Gallo and colleagues demonstrated that this retrovirus, then known as HTLV-III and now termed human immunodeficiency virus 1 (HIV-1), was the causative agent of AIDS.

The Origin and Evolution of HIV-1
Gao et al., Nature (1999)

It is now thought that HIV arose as a result of a zoonotic transmission of simian immunodeficiency virus (SIV) infecting nonhuman primates to human hunters in West Africa. Phylogenetic analyses of HIV-1 suggest that three independent cross-species transmission events gave rise to independent HIV-1 groups: major (M), nonmajor (N) and outlier (O). Groups M and N were introduced into the human population from chimpanzees through a blood borne route whereas group O may have originated from gorillas[1]. Group M is the predominant circulating HIV-1 group and can currently be divided into at least nine genetically distinct subtypes also referred to as clades, which are typically associated with certain geographical regions.

A second type of human immunodeficiency virus, HIV-2, can give rise to AIDS. HIV-2 is primarily found in West Africa and is related to SIV infecting sooty mangabey monkeys (SIVsmm)[2]. Interestingly, sooty mangabeys only rarely progress to AIDS despite high levels of viral replication and limited antiviral immune responses. Similarly, HIV-2 infection exhibits lower infectivity and virulence, and despite structural similarities to HIV-1, only rarely causes AIDS and therefore remains an interesting research area.

Advanced sequencing technologies demonstrate that HIV-1 evolves rapidly within individual patients. Diversification is driven by host immune pressures and reaches a delicate survival balance during which the virus avoids elimination without sacrificing replicative fitness induced by potentially detrimental mutations. Several intrinsic mechanisms enable rapid evolution within the host: a fast generation time with 10^{10}–10^{12} newly produced virions per day; an error-prone reverse transcriptase enzyme that lacks proofreading activity leading to the introduction of 0.2–0.3 per genome per replication cycle; and a high level of recombination with three recombination events per genome per replication cycle. This extensive viral diversity has important implications for host control of the virus as well as antiretroviral treatment and vaccine development.

Identification of Cellular Entry Receptors and Co-Receptors Required for HIV-1 Infection
Deng et al., Nature (1996)

HIV-1 infections can occur by sexual exposure, intravenous drug use, contaminated blood products or vertical transmission from mother to child during birth or through breast milk. HIV-1 infects a variety of cells comprising the innate and adaptive immune system including T cells, monocytes, macrophages, eosinophils, dendritic cells and microglial cells of the CNS.

The virus gains entry through its primary receptor CD4 which is expressed on a wide variety of immune cells. However, *in vitro* experiments demonstrated that CD4 is not sufficient to allow entry and that chemokine receptors CXCR4 and CCR5 are essential co-receptors. Further evidence was gained from the identification of a genetic variant involving a 32 base pair deletion in the CCR5 gene (CCR5-Δ32). This mutation results in a truncated C-terminus leading to down regulation of CCR5 and to a lesser extent CXCR4 expression on the cell surface. In the homozygous state it confers almost complete resistance to HIV-1 infection, and in the heterozygous state it provides partial resistance with slower disease progression[3].

The importance of CCR5 as a co-receptor for HIV-1 infection is underlined by a unique medical case[4]. An HIV-1 positive patient was treated for myeloid leukemia with chemotherapy to suppress the cancer and received a bone marrow transplant to restore the immune system. Transplant was performed from a matched donor homozygous for the CCR5-Δ32 deletion mutation. Following the transplant, undetectable levels of HIV-1 were found in the blood and neither R5 nor X4 variants could be found. After 3 years, the patient had maintained the resistance to HIV-1 and had been pronounced cured of the infection.

Co-receptor usage facilitates the interaction of the virion and the cell surface, increases the probability of fusion, and also directs the cellular tropism of HIV-1. The transmitted virus is predominantly macrophage-tropic (R5 type) as it primarily infects mucosal CCR5 expressing cells such as macrophages and memory T cells. In contrast, T cell tropic isolates (X4 type) utilise CXCR4, which is expressed on a variety of cells including naïve and resting CD4 T cells, macrophages and thymic precursors. X4 viruses usually emerge later in the course of chronic infection and are associated with disease progression[5].

The Course of HIV-1 Infection: From Transmission to the Development of AIDS

The course of HIV-1 infection can be divided into five distinct phases from the time of transmission to the development of AIDS (Figure 28.1): the initial eclipse phase which

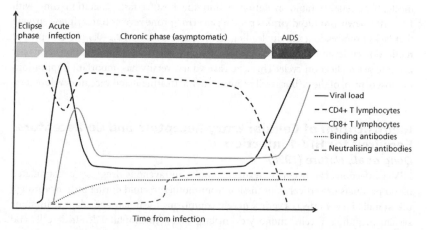

Figure 28.1 Typical time course of untreated HIV-1 infection shows a rapid increase in viraemia in the early acute phase which declines to a setpoint. This early phase of viral replication is accompanied by a rapid depletion of CD4+ lymphocytes especially in the gut-associated lymphoid tissue. The fall in viraemia coincides with the first appearance of HIV-specific CD8+ T cell responses which play an important role in temporarily controlling viral replication and rescuing CD4 counts. HIV-1 specific antibodies become detectable after the reduction in viral load; however, neutralising antibodies only begin to appear during the chronic phase of infection. The chronic phase is characterised by a stable viral load and a slow decline in CD4 counts. Continued viral replication and immune evasion finally exhausts the immune system leading to opportunistic infections and AIDS.

Source: Reproduced under the terms of *Creative Commons Attribution 3.0 License* from Martin DJ, *Immunology of HIV infection and the Host Response*, ftguonline.org.

constitutes the time between transmission and detection of viral RNA in the blood; the burst of viral replication in the acute phase; the reduction in viral load and the establishment of viral set point; the chronic phase; and the progression to AIDS.

Eclipse Phase
Zhang et al., Science (1999)

Most studies investigating the early events of HIV-1 transmission are based on *in vitro* experiments using mucosal explants and *in vivo* models of macaques infected with SIV either intravaginally or intrarectally. Sexual transmission of HIV-1 is a rare event; risk of female-to-male transmission is 0.04% per act and male-to-female transmission is 0.08% per act. However, the rate for receptive anal intercourse is much higher at 1.7% per act. The risk of transmission is increased by damage to the mucosal barrier caused by physical trauma or pre-existing genital infections, and can be reduced by male circumcision.

Single-genome studies show that about 80% of mucosally established HIV-1 infections occur by a single CCR5 tropic founder virus. Studies of the SIV vaginal challenge model indicate that HIV-1 follows a local expansion and stage dissemination model. The successful founder virus crosses the epithelia by transcytosis and infects 'resting' CD4 T cells in the underlying submucosa. Local infection is established which is supported by early innate immune responses that lead to the recruitment of additional target cells to the site of infection. Finally, the virus disseminates to the draining lymph nodes and then spreads systemically throughout the secondary lymph organs.

There is evidence that mucosal dendritic cells (DCs) play an important role in the early stages of viral dissemination to the draining lymph nodes. Mucosal DCs express high levels of the C-type lectin receptor DC-SIGN which binds to the heavily glycosylated HIV-1 envelope protein (Env). *In vitro* studies demonstrate that DC-SIGN acts as an adhesion receptor sequestering virus particles into a specialised endosomal compartment in which the virus can survive for up to three days. Furthermore, binding of HIV-1 Env to DC-SIGN triggers an intracellular signalling cascade that impairs the innate antiviral immune response and allows successful viral dissemination[6]. Following signalling through DC-SIGN, virus-bearing DCs migrate to the draining lymph nodes where they establish direct interaction with residing T cells. DC and T cell conjugates are formed to allow direct cell-to-cell transfer of sequestered virus particles from virus-bearing DCs to target cells through so-called virological synapses. This mode of transmission is more effective than infection by cell free virus as it delivers the virus directly to its entry receptor[7].

Acute Phase
Brenchley et al., Journal of Experimental Medicine (2004)
Brenchley et al., Nature Medicine (2006)

As HIV-1 reaches the draining lymph nodes, the availability of target cells increases and the virus can replicate freely leading to an exponential increase in plasma virus levels. During this acute phase, patients test positive for viral p24 antigen and anti-HIV-1 antibodies. While plasma viraemia rises, the number of CD4+ T cells rapidly decreases. Similarly to SIV infection in rhesus macaques, HIV-1 replication is particularly prominent in the gut-associated lymphoid tissue (GALT), which is predominantly populated by CCR5-expressing effector memory CD4 T cells[8]. High levels of viral replication in the GALT rapidly deplete up to 80% of CD4 T cells within the first 3 weeks of infection. T cell death is not restricted to infected cells but also affects uninfected bystander T cells.

Although the exact mechanisms causing this immunopathology are not fully understood, they are thought to be the consequence of target-cell infection and virus-induced Fas-mediated apoptosis in a unique lymphoid site. This profound depletion is associated with the destruction of the intestinal laminar propria and submucosa, allowing translocation of apoptotic microparticles and microbial products derived from commensal bacteria into the blood.

The breakdown of the integrity of the epithelial barrier of the gastrointestinal tract has been proposed as one of the main driving forces of systemic immune activation, which is characteristic for the chronic phase of HIV-1 infection in humans and SIV infection of rhesus macaques. In contrast, SIV-infected sooty mangabeys, which are a natural host for SIV infection and commonly used as a non-pathogenic primate model for HIV-infection, have minimal levels of immune activation, preserved mucosal CD4+ T cells and no evidence of microbial translocation despite chronic high levels of virus replication[9]. This indicates that immune activation plays an important role in the development of AIDS.

Establishment of Viral Set Point and the Chronic Phase
Mellors et al., Science (1996)

Following the burst of viral replication and a sharp decrease in CD4 target cells, HIV-1 replication reaches its plateau 21–28 days post infection. Thereafter it decreases to a level referred to as viral set point. The magnitude of the initial peak viraemia and set point reflect the balance between viral turnover and the immune response attempting to control the virus. The constant struggle between the host and the virus is one of the most striking features of HIV-1 infection. The set point viral load reached is predictive of the time to an AIDS defining illness and is likely to be determined by host genetic factors, the quality and quantity of the host HIV-specific immune response as well as the fitness of the transmitted founder virus.

Host Immune Mechanisms Controlling HIV-1 Infection

Identification and characterisation of both viral and host factors controlling the course of HIV-1 infection in different groups of individuals has been a powerful tool in understanding the immunopathogenesis of the virus. Most studies have focused on individuals that control the virus to low or undetectable levels for an extended period (typically over 10 years), in the absence of antiretroviral drugs. These patients are referred to as 'elite controllers' or 'long-term nonprogressors' (LTNPs). There are also cohorts of individuals that are frequently exposed to HIV-1, often through a long term relationship with an HIV infected partner, who nevertheless remain uninfected.

Cellular Restriction Factors
Mangeat et al., Nature (2003)
Stremlau et al., Nature (2004)

It has become increasingly apparent that innate immunity plays a key role in defending the host against retroviral infection. This mechanism relies on receptors that recognise pathogen-associated molecular patterns (molecular motifs common to a wide range of pathogenic organisms) as well as cellular restriction factors such as APOBEC3G, Tetherin, Trim22 and Trim5α.

Among the best-studied antiretroviral cellular host factors is APOBEC3G, a cytosine deaminase, which is selectively incorporated into progeny virions during viral assembly. Upon infection of subsequent target cells, APOBEC3G mediates the deamination of dC residues to dU on nascent proviral minus strand during reverse transcription. This results in G to A hypermutations, which in turn may render the virus defective or destabilise proviral transcripts leading to their degradation. However, in HIV-1 the viral accessory protein Vif binds to APOBEC3G in virus producing cells and targets it for proteosomal degradation. As a result Vif reduces the levels of APOBEC3G in the cell and hence the frequency of incorporation into viral particles.

The cellular restriction factor Trim5α is a ring finger protein that provides an early entry block to retroviral infection by interfering with viral uncoating and targeting the HIV-1 capsid for degradation. It plays an important role in restricting the host range of HIV-1 to humans and chimpanzees. This hypothesis is supported by *in vitro* studies demonstrating that non-human primate Trim5α can effectively block HIV-1 infection in human cell lines. In contrast the antiviral activity of human Trim5α against HIV-1 is weak and cannot control viral replication. Increasing the activity of human Trim5α may be an attractive therapeutic intervention strategy.

The Humoural Immune Response Against HIV-1
Wei et al., Nature (2003)

Antibodies are induced early during HIV-1 infection but do not protect against the acquisition of HIV-1. The lack of escape mutations from humoural response during acute infection indicates that these early antibodies are non-neutralising and have no significant effect on the dynamics of viral load or the viral set point. Why these antibodies fail to prevent HIV-1 and control viral replication during acute infection is still unknown. Neutralising antibodies are generated about 12 weeks after infection. However, there is little evidence that they actually contribute to the immune control. This is demonstrated by the fact that HIV-1 antibodies are generally incapable of neutralising the virus currently circulating within the individual from whom they were isolated.

One reason for the apparent ineffectiveness of the antibody response is that the HIV-1 Env glycoprotein has evolved several unique features to allow efficient escape from neutralising antibodies[10]. Neutralising epitopes are effectively hidden or protected by an extensive and shifting glycan shield. Antibodies against sugars are generally of low affinity and the use of self-sugars is key to the evasion strategy, as antibodies are not allowed to develop due to the risk of autoimmunity. HIV-1 Env also contains hypervariable regions which function as an effective decoy for antibody responses as it can readily mutate without the loss of viral fitness. As a consequence the great majority of HIV-1 neutralising antibodies isolated to date are only able to neutralise a few strains of HIV.

A limited number of broadly neutralising antibodies have been isolated. Compared to conventional antibodies, these isolates exhibit unique properties enabling them to overcome the challenges of Env binding. They have acquired the ability to access conserved epitopes such as the CD4 binding site, the gp41 stalk close to the membrane or a distinct glycosylation pattern.

The Importance of CD8+ Cytotoxic T Cell Response (CTLs) in Controlling Viral Replication
Fellay et al., Science (2007)

The fall in viraemia associated with transition from the acute to the chronic phase of HIV infection coincides with the first appearance of HIV CD8+ T-cells, suggesting an important role for this cell type in the control of viral replication. This is supported by data from the monkey model showing that artificial depletion of CD8+ T cells in SIV-infected rhesus macaques results in a massive burst of viraemia leading to a rapid progression to AIDS[11]. As with antibodies, the huge mutational capacity of HIV allows for the generation of viral variants that escape recognition by HIV-1 specific CTLs and, in some cases, this can lead to a loss of control and progression to AIDS[12].

An additional piece of compelling evidence for the importance of CD8+ T-cells comes from several, recent, large-scale genome-wide association studies (GWAS), which found that only polymorphisms in the human leukocyte antigen (HLA) loci can be significantly associated with control of HIV-1. This supports numerous earlier work identifying particular HLA types, most frequently HLA-B*57, with improved control of HIV-1. As the function of HLA is to present pathogen derived peptides on the cell surface of infected cells for recognition by CD8+ T-cells, this association is thought to relate to the HIV-specific CD8+ T-cells response. The reason why certain alleles are associated with a more effective HIV-specific CD8+ response is not clear but probably involves the strength and quality of peptide-specific CTL responses and the nature of the peptides presented by the molecule. Protective HLA alleles tend to present peptides from conserved regions of the viral genome, particularly the gag protein, and escape mutations in these regions are often slower to occur and associated with a fitness cost to the virus. This is demonstrated by the fact that on transmission of this virus to another individual with different HLA background such mutations disappear and the virus regains its full replicative capacity. In contrast, escape mutations in less conserved proteins such as Env, are often rapidly selected and occur with little or no impact on viral fitness.

Data from studies examining elite HIV-1 controllers suggest that CTL control of HIV-1 replication is dependent on a number of factors: (1) the recognition of a wide variety of conserved epitopes; (2) efficient degranulation, characterised by the release of perforin and granzyme B as well as increased killing of target cells; and (3) polyfunctionality, defined as the secretion of multiple cytokines including IFNg, TNFa, IL2 and MIP1b.

There are other mechanisms by which HIV escapes CTL pressure. HIV-1 down-regulates the expression of HLA class I on the surface of infected cells via its accessory protein Nef[13]. There is also compelling evidence that HIV-1 infection renders CTLs partially ineffective by causing them to remain in a pre-terminally differentiated state.

Impaired CD4+ T Cell Help
Douek et al., Nature (2002)

CD4 responses against HIV-1 are detectable in chronic infection, particularly against gag and nef, but tend to be of very low magnitude. This may in part be due to the fact that HIV-1 appears to preferentially infect and destroy HIV-1-specific CD4+ cells, probably through close contact with HIV coated DCs within lymph nodes. Moreover HIV-1 infection results in a qualitative impairment of CD4+ T cell function, which includes reduced polyfunctionality and the progressive loss of proliferative responses to HIV-1 antigen. The impairment of CD4+ T cell help during acute HIV-1 infection has important downstream effects on priming and maintenance of effective CD8$^+$ T cell responses and the generation of neutralizing antibodies. Very early administration of antiretroviral therapy during the acute phase prevents the rapid depletion of CD4$^+$ T cells and can rescue strong HIV-1-specific CD4$^+$ T cell responses.

Treatment of HIV-1 Infection by Antiretroviral Drugs
Mitsuya et al., PNAS (1985)

The first antiretroviral drug to be licensed in 1987 was AZT, a nucleotide inhibitor of the viral reverse transcriptase enzyme. The development of AZT is an example for the early attempts of structure-based drug design. In contrast to high-throughput screening of randomly elected compounds, AZT was designed with the hypothesis that a 'fraudulent base' would be able to inhibit DNA replication in cancer cells. After it failed to prove effective against cancer in mice, it was shelved until the discovery that HIV-1 is the causative agent of a human disease. The first randomised placebo controlled trials in 1985 demonstrated AZT's efficiency in extending the lives of AIDS patients leading to its immediate approval as a treatment option. However, AZT on its own turned out to be of limited use as HIV rapidly becomes resistant to this drug when used in isolation.

In recent years, additional compounds have been developed including next generation reverse transcriptase, protease inhibitors and integrase as well as fusion inhibitors that aim to block HIV-1 infection upstream of irreversible integration. Use of these drugs in a combination therapy has proven very efficient in temporarily reducing viral replication. It extends the duration and quality of life[14,15] for people living with HIV-1 as well as reduces the frequency of transmission, especially from mother to child. Importantly, their use in combination can prevent, or at least greatly slow down, the appearance of drug resistant strains.

Antiretroviral therapy is life-prolonging but unable to eradicate the virus from infected individuals due to the existence of latent viral reservoirs in quiescent CD4$^+$ T cells and macrophages. Furthermore the toxicity of treatment causes side effects and the occurrence of multidrug resistance mutations highlights the need for the discovery of new drug targets. Novel therapeutic approaches focus not only on suppressing viral replication by blocking viral entry and purging latent reservoirs, but also on new intervention strategies targeting the host immune response by inhibiting microbial translocation and thus attenuating immune activation. In addition, recent trials of a vaginal gel containing the anti-retroviral drug tenofivir suggest this maybe an effective strategy for reducing HIV-1 transmission in the absence of condom use[16,17].

HIV-1 Vaccines: Preventative versus Therapeutic

Despite effective therapeutic treatments, a highly efficacious preventive vaccine is still the greatest hope for generating long-term immunological memory and sustained protection against HIV-1 infection to end the pandemic. The current view in the field is that there is a very narrow window of opportunity between transmission and peak viraemia for a vaccine to be able to prevent the irreversible destruction of the intestinal CD4$^+$ population and clear infection before the establishment of viral reservoirs. Successful vaccine design will probably need to both elicit broadly neutralising antibodies and generate strong CD4$^+$ and CD8$^+$ T cell responses.

The unique characteristics of the virus have so far proved an insurmountable barrier to vaccine development. These include mucosal route of infection, ability to infect and kill $CD4^+$ T cells, effective strategies to evade humoural and cellular immune responses and most importantly dramatic sequence diversity. Important lessons from past vaccine trials have highlighted the problem identifying correlates of protection against HIV-1 infection indicating the nature of the immune response that a vaccine would need to induce.

Sterilizing Immunity Mediated by HIV-1-specific Antibodies
Mascola et al., Nature Medicine (2000)

Antibody-based vaccines are aimed at eliciting neutralising antibodies against the HIV-1 envelope protein to provide sterilizing immunity and block infection. Evidence that primary protection can be mediated by the humoural immune response is provided by several studies in rhesus macaques showing that passive administration of a cocktail consisting of neutralising antibodies is able to prevent SIV infection after mucosal challenge.

The design of an immunogen capable of eliciting long-lived systemic mucosal and broadly neutralising antibodies presents a major challenge. Vaccination with gp120 protein or heat-inactivated whole virus particles leads to the induction of antibodies that recognise dominant epitopes present in the hypervariable regions and are therefore either non-neutralising or ineffective against heterologous viral challenge. Alternative antigen design is focusing on using gp120 trimers or epitopes in a scaffold in order to elicit broadly neutralising antibodies.

Eliciting HIV-1-specific CTL Responses by a Therapeutic Vaccine
McMichael and Hanke, Nature Reviews Immunology (2002)

T cell-based vaccines evoke the cell-mediated immunity that may not protect against infection but could help to lower the initial burst of viraemia and viral set point thus preventing or delaying the onset of AIDS and importantly reducing transmission. In an attempt to elicit efficient CTL responses prior to infection immunogen design has focused on the study of protective HLA class I alleles and HLA-class I-restricted peptides in LTNPs. However, as LTNPs tend to share a small set of protective HLA alleles, whether these data can be used to generate effective T-cell responses in individuals lacking these protective alleles is uncertain. In addition there is evidence that HIV-1 may adapt to the CTL immune response at the population level, leading to the gradual loss of potential protective CTL responses.

Lesson Learned from Vaccine Trials
Buchbinder et al., Lancet (2008)
Rerks-Ngarm et al., New England Journal of Medicine (2009)

One of the largest HIV-1 vaccine trial carried out by Merck, the STEP trial, employed a replication incompetent human adenovirus serotype 5 (Ad5) vectored vaccine containing a clade B antigen. This vaccine induced HIV-1 specific CTL responses in phase II trials, but the large multicenter trial was prematurely terminated due to a potentially increased risk of HIV-1 acquisition in men who have sex with men. Interestingly, post-trial analyses measured strong polyfunctional CTL responses and corresponding escape mutations. Due to early termination of the trail there is not sufficient statistical power to detect significant difference between the vaccine and control groups. However, there is a suggestion that the potential increased risk of HIV-1 acquisition in the vaccine group was skewed towards individuals with pre-existing immunity against human Ad5. The hypothesis is that this might facilitate HIV-1 acquisition due to reduced T cell immunogenicity and increased activated memory CD4$^+$ cells which could serve as immediate HIV-1 targets at the mucosal sites of infection[18]. Although the impact of pre-existing Ad5 immunity remains controversial novel recombinant vaccine vectors such as chimp adenoviruses or pox viruses are being developed in order to avoid the problem of preexisting immunity.

Further confusion in the field of HIV-1 vaccine design was fueled by the most recent vaccine trial RV144 carried out in Thailand. The trial employed a combined canary-pox HIV-1 vector (ALVAC) prime with a gp120 protein (AIDSVAX) boost in an attempt to elicit both neutralising antibodies as well as CTL responses against the virus. Despite both vaccines alone lacking efficacy in previous clinical trials, the combined prime boost regime showed 31% efficacy in reducing HIV-1 infection in low-incident groups. Despite low efficacy, this trial provided the first encouraging sign that a vaccine strategy may be effective in controlling the spread of HIV-1. Unlike in the STEP trail, the RV144 vaccine regime did not induce strong CTL response or broadly neutralising antibodies in previous efficacy trials.

Taken together, these studies demonstrate that the magnitude and quality of immune responses associated with strong immunogenicity, as currently measured, may not predict the ability of a vaccine to confer effective protection against HIV-1 infection. An in-depth understanding of the immune response induced by the RV144 vaccine may help defining the immune responses responsible for the modest protection observed.

Conclusion

Since the discovery of HIV-1 as the causative agent of AIDS an impressive scientific effort has focused on elucidating the complex virus-host interaction; however, much remains to be accomplished in the fight against the virus.

Despite advances in treatment regimes and a hopeful glimmer of an effective vaccine, the HIV-1 pandemic is still growing. The complex pathogenesis of the virus and its ability to control and evade the host immune response raises the problem that highly effective treatments may need to prompt the host to induce an immune response that is better than the one elicited during natural infection. Therefore, it is difficult to foresee when a successful prophylactic treatment for HIV-1 will arrive and which form it will take: a small-molecule drug, a vaccine, a combination thereof or perhaps a totally different novel approach.

Key Outstanding Questions

1. Is it possible to develop novel treatment strategies that will break viral latency and allow eradicate of the virus?
2. Can we develop a conventional protective vaccine that will prevent infection by eliciting broadly neutralising antibodies?
3. Alternatively, can we design a T cell-based vaccine that prevents the progression to AIDS or cures the patient after infection has been established?

4. Is it possible to overcome the challenge of viral diversity and emerging drug resistance?

Key Research Centres

1. NIH Office of AIDS Research, National Institutes of Health, Bethesda, United States
2. The Ragon Institute, Massachusetts General Hospital, Charlestown, United States
3. The Centre for AIDS Interdisciplinary Research at Oxford, Oxford University, United Kingdom
4. Pasteur Institute, Paris, France
5. Center for HIV-AIDS Vaccine Immunology (CHAVI) – an international consortium of research groups

References

Brenchley, J.M., *et al.* (2004) CD4+ T cell depletion during all stages of HIV disease occurs predominantly in the gastrointestinal tract. *Journal of Experimental Medicine*, **200**(6), 749–759. http://jem.rupress.org/content/200/6/749.long

Brenchley, J.M., *et al.* (2006) Microbial translocation is a cause of systemic immune activation in chronic HIV infection. *Nature Medicine*, **12**, 1365–1371. http://www.ncbi.nlm.nih.gov/pubmed/17115046

Buchbinder, S.P., *et al.* (2008) Efficacy assessment of a cell-mediated immunity HIV-1 vaccine (the Step study), a double-blind, randomised, placebo-controlled, test-of-concept trial. *Lancet*, **372**, 1881–1893. http://www.ncbi.nlm.nih.gov/pubmed/19012954

Deng, H., *et al.* (1996) Identification of a major co-receptor for primary isolates of HIV-1. *Nature*, **381**(6584), 661–666. http://www.ncbi.nlm.nih.gov/pubmed/8649511

Douek, D.C., *et al.* (2002) HIV preferentially infects HIV-specific CD4+ T cells. *Nature*, **417** (6884), 95–98. http://www.nature.com/nature/journal/v417/n6884/full/417095a.html

Fellay, J., *et al.* (2007) A whole-genome association study of major determinants for host control of HIV-1. *Science*, **317**, 944–947. http://www.ncbi.nlm.nih.gov/pubmed/17641165

Gallo, R.C., *et al.* (1984) Frequent detection and isolation of cytopathic retroviruses (HTLV-III) from patients with AIDS and at risk for AIDS. *Science*, **224**(4648), 500–503. http://www.sciencemag.org/content/224/4648/500.abstract

Gao, F., *et al.* (1999) Origin of HIV-1 in the chimpanzee Pan troglodytes troglodytes. *Nature*, **397** (6718), 436–441. http://www.ncbi.nlm.nih.gov/pubmed/9989410

Gottlieb, M.S., *et al.* (1981) Pneumocystis carinii pneumonia and mucosal candidiasis in previously healthy homosexual men: evidence of a new acquired cellular immunodeficiency. *New England Journal of Medicine*, **305**(24), 1425–1431. http://www.ncbi.nlm.nih.gov/pubmed/6272109

Mangeat, B., *et al.* (2003) Broad antiretroviral defence by human APOBEC3G through lethal editing of nascent reverse transcripts. *Nature*, **424**(6944), 99–103. http://www.ncbi.nlm.nih.gov/pubmed/12808466

Martin, D.J. (N.d.) Immunology of HIV infection and the host response. http://www.ftguonline.org

Mascola, J.R., *et al.* (2000) Protection of macaques against vaginal transmission of a pathogenic HIV-1/SIV chimeric virus by passive infusion of neutralizing antibodies. *Nature Medicine*, **6** (2), 207–210. http://www.nature.com/doifinder/10.1038/72318

McMichael, A., and Hanke, T. (2002) The quest for an AIDS vaccine: is the CD8+ T-cell approach feasible? *Nature Reviews Immunology*, **2**(4), 283–291. http://www.nature.com/nri/journal/v2/n4/full/nri779.html

Mellors, J.W., *et al.* (1996) Prognosis in HIV-1 infection predicted by the quantity of virus in plasma. *Science*, **272**, 1167–1170. http://www.ncbi.nlm.nih.gov/pubmed/8638160

Mitsuya, H., *et al.* (1985) 30-Azido-30-deoxythymidine (BW A509U), an antiviral agent that inhibits the infectivity and cytopathic effect of human T-lymphotropic virus type III/lymphadenopathyassociated virus in vitro. PNAS, **82**(20), 7096–7100. http://www.pnas.org/content/82/20/7096.long

Rerks-Ngarm, M.D., *et al.* (2009) Vaccination with ALVAC and AIDSVAX to prevent HIV-1 infection in Thailand. *New England Journal of Medicine*, **361**, 2209–2220. http://www.ncbi.nlm.nih.gov/pubmed/19012954

Stremlau, M., *et al.* (2004) The cytoplasmic body component TRIM5alpha restricts HIV-1 infection in Old World monkeys. *Nature*, **427**, 848–853. http://www.ncbi.nlm.nih.gov/pubmed/14985764

Wei, X., *et al.* (2003) Antibody neutralization and escape by HIV-1. *Nature*, **422**, 307–312. http://www.nature.com/nature/journal/v422/n6929/full/nature01470.html

Zhang, Z., *et al.* (1999) Sexual transmission and propagation of SIV and HIV in resting and activated CD4+ T cells. *Science*, **286**(5443), 1353–1357. http://www.ncbi.nlm.nih.gov/pubmed/10558989

Additional References

1. Van Heuverswyn, F., *et al.* (2006) Human immunodeficiency viruses: SIV infection in wild gorillas. *Nature*, **444**(7116), 164.

2. Hirsch, V.M., *et al.* (1989) An African primate lentivirus (SIVsm) closely related to HIV-2. *Nature*, **339**(6223), 389–392.

3. Samson, M., *et al.* (1996) Resistance to HIV-1 infection in caucasian individuals bearing mutant alleles of the CCR-5 chemokine receptor gene. *Nature*, **382**(6593), 722–725.

4. Hütter, G., *et al.* (2009) Long-term control of HIV by CCR5 Delta32/Delta32 stem-cell transplantation. *New England Journal of Medicine*, **360**(7), 692–698.

5. Connor, R.I., *et al.* (1997) Change in coreceptor use correlates with disease progression in HIV-1-infected individuals. *Journal of Experimental Medicine*, **185**(4), 621–628.

6. Hodges, A., *et al.* (2007) Activation of the lectin DC-SIGN induces an immature dendritic cell phenotype triggering Rho-GTPase activity required for HIV-1 replication. *Nature Immunology*, **8**(6), 569–577.

7. McDonald, D., *et al.* (2003) Recruitment of HIV and its receptors to dendritic cell-T cell junctions. *Science*, **300**(5623), 1295–1297.

8. Veazey, R.S., *et al.* (1998) Gastrointestinal tract as a major site of CD4+ T cell depletion and viral replication in SIV infection. *Science*, **280**(5362), 427–431.

9. Silvestri, G., *et al.* (2003) Nonpathogenic SIV infection of sooty mangabeys is characterized by limited bystander immunopathology despite chronic high-level viremia. *Immunity*, **18**(3), 441–452.

10. Schief, W.R., *et al.* (2009) Challenges for structure-based HIV vaccine design. *Current Opinion in HIV and AIDS*, **4**(5), 431–440.

11. Schmitz, J.E., *et al.* (1999) Control of viremia in simian immunodeficiency virus infection by CD8+ lymphocytes. Science, **283**, 857–860.

12. Goulder, P.D., *et al.* (1997) Co-evolution of human immunodeficiency virus and cytotoxic T-lymphocyte responses. *Immunology Review*, **159**, 17–29.

13. Collins, K., *et al.* (1998) HIV-1 Nef protein protects infected primary human cells from killing by cytotoxic T lymphocytes. *Nature*, **391**, 397–401.

14. Hammer, S.M., *et al.* (1996) A trial comparing nucleoside monotherapy with combination therapy in HIV-infected adults with CD4 cell counts from 200 to 500 per cubic millimeter. *New England Journal of Medicine*, **335**, 1081–1090.

15. Delta Coordinating Committee (1996) Delta: a randomised double-blind controlled trial comparing combinations of zidovudine plus didanosine or zalcitabine with zidovudine alone in HIV-infected individuals. *Lancet*, **348**(9023), 283–291.

16. Abdool Karim, Q., *et al.* (2010) Effectiveness and safety of tenofovir gel, an antiretroviral microbicide, for the prevention of HIV infection in women. *Science*, **329**, 1168–1174.

17. Grant, R.M., *et al.* (2010) Preexposure chemoprophylaxis for HIV prevention in men who have sex with men. *New England Journal of Medicine*, **363**, 2587–2599.

18. Benlahrech, A., *et al.* (2009) Adenovirus vector vaccination induces expansion of memory CD4 T cells with a mucosal homing phenotype that are readily susceptible to HIV-1. *Proceedings of the National Academy of Sciences of the USA*, **106**(47), 19940–19945.

29 Transplantation

Dame Elizabeth Simpson

Division of Immunology and Inflammation, Imperial College London, London, UK

Introduction

Transplantation covers a huge range of clinical interventions. In addition to the often complex surgical procedures involved, there are immunological problems that until the last few decades prevented therapeutic transplantation of any organ or tissue that did not come from a genetically identical source. The intrinsic surgical problems and ingenuity it took to address them will not be the topic of this chapter, but rather the incremental understanding of the immunological barriers standing in the way of combining surgical and medical solutions.

Surgery and immunology were linked in the 1950s by crucial interactions between biologists and surgeons on either side of the Atlantic. For organ transplantation, the convergence of surgeon Joseph Murray in Boston with experimental immunologist Peter Medawar in London saw organ transplantation move from proof-of-principle kidney transplant from an identical twin to developments allowing use of kidneys from genetically disparate donors. For bone marrow transplantation, Donnall Thomas' pioneering studies were built round the findings that irradiation of the recipient allowed repopulation of haematopoietic lineages with donor cells. He too was influenced by the findings on induction of immunological tolerance in Medawar's laboratory.

These early studies were carried out in the 1950s when there was very little understanding of the molecules that defined donor and recipient as 'self' or 'foreign'. The American geneticist George Snell, using skin and tumour transplants in mice, was working to define the genetic loci that controlled expression of histoincompatibility determinants that provoked rejection of grafts from genetically disparate donors. He found that one particular locus, named H2, controlled the most rapid rejection, and this co-segregated with molecules identified with antibodies prepared by his London collaborator, Peter Gorer, after injecting mice of one inbred strain with cells of another.

Subsequent work uncovered complexity of this 'H2 locus'. It was found to consist of a number of closely linked, highly polymorphic genes. A comparable situation was found in humans. The gene complex controlling strong transplantation antigens in a wide range of species was named the major histocompatibility complex, MHC (HLA in humans, acronym for 'human leukocyte antigens' and named from the use of anti-leukocyte antibodies from multiparous women to identity expression of these molecules on white blood cells). However the unraveling of the human HLA complex took two decades after Snell's pioneering model work on H2 in mice, and involved a huge international collaboration of clinicians, including Jean Dausset in Paris, and scientists with interests spanning transfusion, transplantation, pregnancy and autoimmunity.

Understanding Medical Research: The Studies that Shaped Medicine, First Edition. Edited by John A. Goodfellow. © 2012 John Wiley & Sons, Ltd. Published 2012 by John Wiley & Sons, Ltd.

The involvement of MHC-encoded molecules in transplantation turned out to be key in dissecting the immune response to all nonself molecules (including viruses and other pathogens, autoantigens and some tumours) in addition to transplants from genetically dissimilar donors. Thus advances in transplantation immunology have led to fundamentally important studies of the cells and molecules controlling a wide array of physiological and pathological responses in clinical medicine.

Identification of Chromosomal Loci Encoding Major Histocompatibility Antigens in Mice and Humans
Gorer et al., Proceedings of the Royal Society B (1948)
Amos and Bach, Journal of Experimental Medicine (1968)

The choice of both of these references as the starting point in this chapter, despite the fact that their publication was 20 years apart, is logical because of the central importance of the MHC molecules for understanding immune responses directed against transplants. This 20-year period also encompasses the time when primarily antibodies were used as research tools in this area, before an understanding of how recognition by T lymphocytes, with their cell bound receptors, differed in key ways from B cells.

Identification of T and B cells as separate lymphoid lineages, with interconnected functions in mounting immune effector responses to both pathogens and transplants, allowed further developments in understanding the co-operative interactions between B and T cells. Their interaction with various types of antigen presenting cells and with elements of the innate immune system was also dependent upon these first steps. Many of the key molecular players in these interactions have now been identified. They include cell surface molecules, cytokines, chemokines and intracellular signalling cascades. While these provide us with potential therapeutic targets, their number, diversity and redundancy present an extraordinary challenge to the task.

But back to T and B cells in relation to immune responses to transplants: George Snell was medically qualified, and fascinated by the genetics of transplantation. In choosing to work at the Jackson Laboratory in Maine, United States, he had at his disposal a collection of inbred mouse strains. Their development by selective inbreeding was crucial to those working in tumour immunity, as otherwise responses to genetically encoded transplantation antigens (called 'histoincompatibility' or 'H' antigens by Snell) confused the results of tumour transplant experiments. In his studies Snell used both transplantable tumours and skin transplants exchanged between inbred mouse strains, and between various generations of mice produced by intercrossing those strains. In doing so they defined the number of H loci independently segregating in intercross and backcross mice. Because the long-term transplanted tumours he used tended to escape control by immune responses he underestimated the number of H loci, but those pioneering experiments established that there were a significant number and that they varied in strength as determined by the speed of rejection elicited. One of the strongest was H2, and it was on this antigenic system that he collaborated with Peter Gorer.

Peter Gorer was a medically qualified research scientist interested in immune responses leading to the production of agglutinating antibodies. He studied these in a limited number of inbred mouse strains, using agglutination of red blood cells (RBCs) as a readout for the presence of antibodies in the serum of mice immunised with cells from another strain. The titres of these antibodies were low, and in retrospect, knowing now that MHC molecules are barely detectable on the surface of nucleus-free mammalian RBCs, it is surprising what he was able to achieve, perhaps helped by the presence of contaminating leukocytes in his RBC preparations. However, during a sabbatical he spent in Snell's laboratory, it became clear to both researchers that the agglutination reactions Gorer measured *in vitro* were directed against the same H2 transplantation antigens that Snell defined by transplantation *in vivo*. Their 1948 paper is key, and moreover shows that the locus for H2 is closely linked to a phenotypic marker 'fused tail' to which Snell had access from the Jackson laboratory mouse mutant programme.

Twenty years after the Snell and Gorer paper, Bernard Amos and Fritz Bach reported on findings to which an international consortium of clinical research laboratories contributed. They took part in a series of workshops on HLA antigens, in which panels of sera from multiparous women were tested on panels of peripheral blood leucocytes from particular donors, using agglutination and/or cytotoxicity as the readout. Conditions under which the testing took place in different laboratories led to significant discrepancies in the results, but patterns within them could be observed by discerning eyes, including those of Dausset, Cepellini, van Rood and Paine. Eventually consensus was reached, leading to the identification of a locus, HLA, mapped to human chromosome 6. This encoded both the antigens defined by antisera, and also, and this was Bach's particular contribution, antigens triggering *in vitro* mixed lymphocyte responses (MLR) in families in which HLA loci were segregating. The notion that a separate class of lymphocytes, later called T cells, were the cells that proliferated in MLR came from a number of laboratories, including some discussed below. Subsequent research established that while T cells were the main effectors of acute and chronic allograft rejection, antibodies were responsible for hyperacute rejection.

Tolerance to Transplanted Tissue Can Be Induced Post-natally (skin grafts are rejected by 'cell mediated immunity')
Billingham et al., Philosophical Transactions of the Royal Society B (1956)
This paper is the extended account of Peter Medawar's initial *Nature* report[1] in which tolerance to skin allografts was induced following perinatal injection of tissues from the donor inbred mouse strain. This groundbreaking work demonstrated that tolerance induction was a function of the immaturity of immune system when the foreign cells were initially introduced; that is, under these circumstances the recipient came to regard the foreign cells as 'self'. Such tolerance was antigen specific, since third-party grafts were rejected, but it could be broken by injection of normal lymphocytes from mice of the recipient strain. This last point extended Medawar's previous work on skin graft rejection in rabbits[2] in which he showed that rejection was an antigen-specific immune response characterised by graft infiltrating lymphocytes.

Clinical Transplantation of Kidneys Is Feasible
Murray et al., Journal of the American Medical Association (1956)
The significance of finding that transplantation tolerance could be induced, that is, that rejection of transplants was a due to a potentially tamable immune response, was

immediately picked up by a number of Medawar's clinical colleagues, including Joseph Murray and Donall Thomas. Murray showed the technical feasibility of human kidney transplantation by transplanting a kidney from an identical twin, a life-saving venture that also illustrated the crucial importance of genetic factors. This paper discusses these and the immune barriers to transplantation in the light of Medawar's findings.

What was now needed were drugs that could be used to dampen the immune response in adulthood so that rejection could be held at bay. There was also hope that ways could be found to induce donor-specific tolerance in adult, immunologically mature recipients. Medawar's group tested cortisone and irradiation in mice and other laboratory animal species, and the limited success of these results led him to develop and antilymphocyte serum as an immunosuppressive agent aimed at removing effector cells from the circulation. The results were encouraging, and were a forerunner of using monoclonal antibodies to modulate immune responses (see 'Köhler and Milstein, *Nature* (1975)' and 'Benjamin and Waldmann, *Nature*, 1986', below). However, protocols successfully used in inbred species do not always easily transfer to the clinic. The genetic differences in outbred human populations, increasing the variables with respect both to transplantation antigens and immune responsiveness, make this particularly difficult.

Clinical Transplantation of Bone Marrow Creates Chimerism
Thomas et al., New England Journal of Medicine (1957)

Preclinical research on immunosuppressive agents in outbred animals was vigorously pursued in a number of transplant centres, and in a few basic science laboratories with the appropriate resources. In Boston azothiaprine and other chemotherapeutic agents were tested in dogs as a prelude for use in human kidney transplant patients, but the toxicity of these agents created problems, as well as their blanket immunosuppression that left recipients susceptible to infections. In New York and subsequently Seattle, Donall Thomas pioneered research on bone marrow transplantation, crucial to the treatment of patients caught in radiation accidents, and of huge potential for leukaemia patients. In this paper six detailed case reports and their associated laboratory findings on time course and levels of chimerism are presented and skilfully analysed. This provides insight into the difficulties faced in the bone marrow transplant situation where both graft-versus-host and host-versus-host immune responses take place in the presence of toxic chemotherapeutic agents. Developments now provide less damaging ways of achieving chimerism following bone marrow transplantation, with addition of donor lymphocyte infusion to harness graft-versus-leukaemia effects[3].

Following the era of clinical transplantation in the 1950s and 1960s, the subsequent discovery in the 1970s of cyclosporin[4] as a particularly effective immunosuppressive agent revolutionised organ transplantation. The fact that it has significant nephrotoxicity and also affects liver function makes it, and the other calcineurin inhibitors that followed, less than ideal. Ironically, the clinical success of using these immunosuppressive agents creates a situation in which it is more difficult to justify clinical testing of biological reagents, such as monoclonal antibodies, that might be effective in countering acute rejection and/or favouring the induction of antigen-specific tolerance.

The Thymus Controls the Ability to Reject Grafts and Humoral Responses
Miller, Proceedings of the Royal Society B (1962)

The research of Jacques Miller, another medically qualified scientist, brings us back to basic questions. He established the importance of the thymus as the source of lymphocyte populations that are responsible both for rejecting skin grafts and also for providing 'help' for antibody responses. Until the time of his studies, the function of the thymus was virtually unknown. In children undergoing heart surgery, partial removal of the thymus was common, but appeared to have no adverse effect. Miller removed the organ from neonatal mice, not to test immunological function, but to determine whether its presence was necessary for the development of thymomas following injection of an oncogenic virus. His analysis of the unexpected phenotypic finding, profound immunosuppression, is masterly, and he used all the relevant tools in the immunologist's armamentarium of that time to probe the underlying cause. His findings opened the way to the later discovery of separate T and B lymphocyte lineages and subpopulations. Taken together, Miller's work and that of others led to an understanding of T/B collaboration, that is, how helper T cells responding to one antigen can amplify responses of B cells making antibody to another antigen linked physically to the helper molecule and also to how different T subpopulations play the roles of helper and effector cells. In due course the notion of different functions and subpopulations of T cells led to the discovery of regulatory T cells, in their first incarnation called 'suppressor T cells' (see 'Gershon and Kondo, *Immunology*, 1971', discussed below).

Mutation Involving Thymus Affecting Ability to Reject Grafts
Pantelouris, Immunology (1971)

The mutation 'nude' was recognised by Pantelouris as leading to failure of the thymus to develop, as well as the hairless skin phenotype. He reported in this paper that it was associated functionally with very serious impairment of immune responses, particularly graft rejection, as well as susceptibility to premature death by infection. However, he was alert to the complexity of normal graft rejection responses, and the fact that redundancy of the immune system made it difficult to facilitate grafting of allogeneic tissues. Nevertheless, until the creation of transgenic mice with further diminished immune function (including Fcγ chain ablation), the use of mice carrying the nude mutation as recipients of allografts and even xenogenic tumours from patients was becoming widespread. Nude mice were also important in helping to define the Thy1 alloantigen as a mouse T cell marker[5], as they served as a source bereft of T cells.

Regulation of Immunity by T Cells
Gershon and Kondo, Immunology (1971)

Gershon's paper was pioneering and regarded by many immunologists at the time as heterodox. Following the idea that control of immune responses featured helper components (the helper T cells described above in 'Miller, *Proceedings of the Royal Society B*, 1962'), he explored the notion that responses could also be modulated by suppressor cells. In this paper he presented evidence of these being T cells, and named them 'suppressor T cells'. His experimental design involved complex cell transfers of different donor lymphocyte populations into irradiated recipients. The readout was an assay for serum antibodies in recipients receiving bone marrow as source of B cells, plus T helper cells from nontolerant mice, with or without the addition of T suppressor cells from tolerised mice. Recipients were immunised with sheep red cells. Because suppression was adoptively transferred from donor to recipient in this way, Gershon called it 'infectious'. It was the somewhat mischievous use of that word, as well as the complexity of the *in vivo* experimental design used to demonstrate the effect, that raised hackles.

However, by the mid-1970s a number of immunologists had been won round to the idea of suppression, and the notion of it being due to a separate lineage of T cells gained favour. The introduction of T-T hybridomas following Millstein's work on B-B hybridomas allowed the isolation of putative T suppressor hybrid clones, and the literature in this area proliferated at an astounding rate. But rather like the immune response following the acute stage of a response, this pyramid collapsed when newer molecular techniques in the early 1980s showed that the much touted suppressor hybrids did not contain rearranged antigen receptor genes, and that those encoding the critical 'IJ' molecules they were reported to secrete did not exist in the locus where they had been confidently mapped[6].

After that debacle the term 'suppressor T cells' fell into disuse, but the phenomenon of suppression did not disappear. It became clear from experiments in a number of situations that tolerance could be transferred by selected populations of T cells (see discussion following 'Köhler and Milstein, *Nature* (1975)' and 'Benjamin and Waldmann, *Nature*, 1986', below). They have been named 'regulatory T cells' or Treg, and the literature on them is now proliferating. It is also clear that in addition to the actions of Treg cells, the mechanisms of which are not yet entirely clear, other cells of the immune system, both innate and adaptive, can play a role in regulating responses. For example, B cells make antibodies that clear antigens; cytotoxic T cells kill infected target cells, reducing the antigenic load driving the response; and immature dendritic cells can give tolerogenic signals.

T Cell Responses are MHC Restricted – a Central Tenet for All T Cell Responses
Zinkemagel and Doherty, Nature (1974)

If I had to choose one paper out of the ten I have cited, I would select this one, which established the key feature of MHC restricted recognition by T cells. This is true for T cell responses to viruses, as described in this paper, but also to transplantation alloantigens, tumour antigens and autoantigens. It is true for helper, effector and regulatory T cell responses, for tolerance as well as responsiveness. It also accounts for evolution of the extraordinary polymorphism of MHC molecules, optimising the chance for responsiveness to rapidly mutating pathogens. The results presented in this paper showed that virus specific T cells could recognise MHC matched infected target cells, but not infected target cells with a nonmatching MHC from a different mouse strain. However, mice of that different strain could respond to the virus, with T cells that killed infected target cells of their own MHC type. The T cells therefore recognised both MHC and viral components.

There was much discussion over the next dozen years about how T cells could 'see' two things at once. Did they do it with one receptor specific for 'altered self' MHC, or with two receptors, one for self MHC, and the other for virus? It was not until the molecular identification of T cell receptor genes[7] in the early 1980s, followed by discovering that the viral component recognised by T cells was a very short peptide[8], and, shortly after that, the powerful structural studies of Bjorkmann[9], that it was possible to understand how T cells 'saw' their MHC molecule and the viral epitope. The peptide lay in a groove created by the folding of the two membrane-distal domains of MHC molecules. MHC polymorphism was focused on the amino acid residues lining the peptide holding groove, thus determining which peptides would fit in, and thence the topography of the MHC/peptide complex on which the TCR docked, triggering a response cascade.

The Monoclonal Antibody Revolution
Köhler and Milstein, Nature (1975)
Benjamin and Waldmann, Nature (1986)

Milstein and Kohler's paper revolutionised the making of antibodies by finding a way to immortalise single antigen-specific mouse B cells by fusing them with a mouse myeloma tumour partner and to propagate the progeny indefinitely in vitro. From cultures of such B cell hybridomas antibodies could be purified and tested for fine specificity. The immunoglobulin genes of hybridomas could also be genetically modified to improve their affinity, or to exchange murine regions of the molecule for their human counterparts, to render their use in patients less antigenic.

The ability to select a single antibody of interest from a polyclonal response against complex antigens allowed rapid advances in many applied and basic research areas that relied on the use of antibodies. These included development of antibodies defining human lymphocyte cell surface molecules. In mice alloantibodies prepared by immunisation between selected strains of inbred mice had already been developed to distinguish subpopulations of lymphocytes[10]. The array of reagents recognising different mouse lymphocyte markers was enormously extended using hybridomas, and these provided experimental tools for dissecting the cellular and molecular components of immune responses in mice.

A whole new field of endeavour was, however, opened up for probing the comparable molecules in human immune responses. This started with lymphocyte subpopulation markers, identified by immunising mice with human cells, and selecting hybrids with specificities that looked interesting. A series of international workshops provided a forum for this work, in which monoclonal antibodies with similar cellular reaction patterns were arranged in clusters, hence the term 'cluster determinants' (CD), with respect to cell surface molecules they identified. The biochemical characteristics of these could then be determined and compared with their mouse homologues. The matches were remarkable: for example, the T cell co-receptors CD4 and CD8 in humans and mice had the same structure and function, in both species marking helper T cells and cytotoxic T cells respectively; the CD3 molecule was expressed on all T cells in both species, and was composed of similar component chains. The list of human CD molecules now runs to hundreds.

Waldmann's group were the first to exploit monoclonal antibodies to T cell subpopulations in mice to modulate immune responses. Their initial paper was concerned with abrogating helper T cell help for B cell responses using depleting anti-CD4 monoclonals. They went on to use nondepleting anti-CD4 and anti-CD8 monoclonals to induce tolerance to skin allografts across multiple minor H barriers and, under some circumstances, H2 barriers. Additional alloantigens could also be tolerated on a second skin graft co-expressing them with those to which tolerance had been induced (linked suppression). The findings were made more remarkable on discovering that tolerance could be transferred into naïve recipients. Moreover, such transfers elicited the generation of more regulatory CD4 cells of recipient origin[11]; 'infectious tolerance' again, now ascribed to Treg cells.

Repertoire Selection of T Cells in the Thymus Depends on Structural Components of the T Cell Receptor and Self MHC Molecules
von Boehmer and Kisielow, Science (1990)

T cells develop in the thymus from precursors of bone marrow origin. Differentiation involves a rearrangement of their alpha and beta T cell receptor genes, similar to the rearrangement of immunoglobulin genes in B cells. The rearrangement maximises diversity by being random. Undesirable responses to self-components are mostly removed by deletion in the thymus. When that breaks down, as it does in AIRE gene mutants, overwhelming autoimmunity occurs[12]. Some self-reactive T cells escape from the thymus to the periphery, where they can be held in check by Treg cells. When these are absent, as in Foxp3 mutants[13], again severe autoimmune disease occurs. However, cross-reactivity of T cells for self components following response to extrinsic antigens can trigger autoimmune diseases such as multiple sclerosis[14].

While deletion by negative selection is clearly important to prevent autoimmunity, the presence of an effective T cell repertoire is key for responses involving T cells. In the absence of T cells with appropriate antigen-specific receptors a response cannot be elicited. This occurs during the development of some tumours[15]. While the notion of negative selection was clear, that of positive selection remained vague until von Boehmer and Kisielow demonstrated both types of thymic selection using their T cell receptor (TCR) transgenic mouse strain specific for an endogenous self component, HY, a minor histocompatibility antigen expressed only in males. Negative selection was examined by comparing males with females. The TCR itself was restricted by the H2^b MHC allele, H2D^b, so that negative selection of T cells carrying the TCR transgene only took place in males with this MHC allele. The novelty of this paper is the clear demonstration that positive selection is also MHC restricted; H2^b female mice carrying the TCR transgene showed the characteristic thymic pattern of T cell maturation, with selection into the appropriate CD8 compartment, while H2^d mice did not. They hypothesised similar being true for selection of CD4 cells, and that TCR rearrangements with very low affinity for self-MHC fail to be selected, dying in the thymus. These are important concepts both for addressing fundamental questions about repertoire selection and to explore therapeutic approaches for controlling immune responses in transplantation, autoimmunity and cancer.

Key Outstanding Questions

1. Can antigen-specific transplantation tolerance in the clinical setting be reliably achieved?

2. Can functional tolerance be induced without compromising protective immune responses to pathogens, possibly by combining biologicals (monoclonal antibodies) and selected chemotherapies?
3. Will manipulation of Tregs provide another therapeutic avenue in the search for transplant-specific tolerance?
4. Can donor-specific haematopoietic stem cell transplantation (HSCT) be developed free of graft-versus-host disease (GVHD) risk, to establish chimerism, and hence tolerance, prior to organ transplantation?
5. Will the current worldwide NIH-funded project to identify biomarkers of tolerance in the rare transplant patients who retain grafts following cessation of immunosuppression yield clues as to how tolerance can be achieved in other settings?

Key Research Centres

1. Dr Jeff Bluestone, UCSF Diabetes Center and Immune Tolerance Network, University of California, San Francisco, United States
2. Prof Hermann Waldmann, Sir William Dunn School of Pathology, University of Oxford, Oxford, United Kingdom
3. Dr Lawrence Turka, Renal-Electrolyte and Hypertension, University of Pennsylvania, Philadelphia, United States
4. Prof Robert Lechler, King's Health Partners Academic Health Sciences Centre, King's College, London, United Kingdom
5. Dr Megan Sykes, Transplantation Biology Research Center, Massachusetts General Hospital, Boston, United States

Research on transplantation is marked by a significant number of Nobel prize winners. Those cited in this chapter are Medawar, Snell, Dausset, Murray, Thomas, Doherty and Zinkemagel, Milstein and Kohler. Basic scientists and clinical scientists have both played key roles in the progress in understanding the complexity of immune responses elicited by transplants, and have extended this to related pathologies.

Acknowledgements

I would like to thank Francesco Dazzi (Imperial College, London) and Julian Dyson (Imperial College, London) for their critical reading of the manuscript.

References

Amos, D.B., and Bach, F.H. (1968) Phenotypic expressions of the major histocompatibility locus in man (HL-A), leukocyte antigens and mixed leukocyte culture reactivity. *Journal of Experimental Medicine*, **128**, 623637. http://www.ncbi.nlm.nih.gov/pmc/articles/PMC2138544/

Benjamin, R.J., and Waldmann, H. (1986) Induction of tolerance by monoclonal antibody therapy. *Nature*, **320**, 449451. http://www.nature.com/nature/journal/v320/n6061/abs/320449a0.html

Billingham, R.E., *et al.* (1956) Quantitative studies on tissue transplantation immunity. III actively acquired tolerance. *Philosophical Transactions of the Royal Society B: Biological Sciences*, **239**, 357414. http://rspb.royalsocietypublishing.org/content/143/910/58.abstract

Gershon, R.K., and Kondo, K. (1971) Infectious immunological tolerance. *Immunology*, **21**, 903 914. http://www.ncbi.nlm.nih.gov/pmc/articles/PMC1408252/

Gorer, P.A., *et al.* (1948) Studies on the genetic and antigenic basis of tumour transplantation: linkage between a histocompatibility gene and fused in mice. *Proceedings of the Royal Society B: Biological Sciences*, **135**, 499505. http://rspb.royalsocietypublishing.org/content/135/881/499. abstract

Köhler, G., and Milstein, C. (1975) Continuous cultures of fused cells secreting antibody of predefined specificity. *Nature*, **256**, 495497. http://www.nature.com/nature/journal/v256/n5517/abs/256495a0.html

Miller, J.F.A.P. (1962) Effect of neonatal thymectomy on the immunological responsiveness of the mouse. *Proceedings of the Royal Society B: Biological Sciences*, **156**, 415428. http://rspb.royalsocietypublishing.org/content/156/964/415.abstract

Murray, J.E., *et al.* (1956) Successful homotransplantation of the human kidney between identical twins. *Journal of the American Medical Association*, **160**, 277282. http://jama.ama-assn.org/content/160/4/277.abstract

Pantelouris, E.M. (1971) Observations on the immunobiology of nude mice. *Immunology*, **20**, 247252. http://www.ncbi.nlm.nih.gov/pmc/articles/PMC1455799/

Thomas, E.D., *et al.* (1957) Intravenous infusion of bone marrow in patients receiving radiation and chemotherapy. *New England Journal of Medicine*, **257**, 491496. http://www.ncbi.nlm.nih.gov/pubmed/13464965

von Boehmer, H., and Kisielow, P. (1990) Self-nonself discrimination by T cells. *Science*, **248**, 13691373. http://www.sciencemag.org/content/248/4961/1369.abstract

Zinkemagel, R.M., and Doherty, P.C. (1974) Restriction of in vitro mediated cytotoxicity in lymphocytic choriomeningitis within a syngeneic or semi-allogeneic system. *Nature*, **248**, 701 702. http://www.nature.com/nature/journal/v248/n5450/abs/248701a0.html

Additional References

1. Billingham, R.E., *et al.* (1953) Actively acquired tolerance of foreign cells. *Nature*, **172**, 603 606.

2. Medawar, P.B. (1944) The behaviour and fate of skin autografts in rabbits: a report to the War Wounds Committee of the Medical Research Council. *Journal of Anatomy*, **78**, 176199.

3. Dazzi, F., *et al.* (2000) Durability of responses following donor lymphocyte infusions for patients who relapse after allogeneic stem cell transplantation for chronic myeloid leukemia. *Blood*, **96**(8), 27122716.

4. Borel, J.F., *et al.* (1977) Effects of the new anti-lymphocyte peptide cyclosporin A in animals. *Immunology*, **32**(6), 10171025.

5. Reif, A.E., and Allen, J.M. (1966) Mouse thymic iso-antigens. *Nature*, **209**, 521523.

6. Kronenberg, M., *et al.* (1983) RNA transcripts for I-J polypeptides are apparently not encoded between the I-A and I-E subregions of the murine major histocompatibility complex. *Proceedings of the National Academy of Sciences of the USA*, **80**, 57045708.

7. Hedrick, S.M., *et al.* (1984) Isolation of cDNA clones encoding T cell-specific membrane-associated proteins. *Nature*, **308**, 149153.

8. Townsend, A.R., *et al.* (1985) Cytotoxic T cells recognize fragments of the influenza nucleoprotein. *Cell*, **42**, 457467.

9. Bjorkman, P.J., *et al.* (1987) Structure of the human class I histocompatibility antigen, HLA-A2. *Nature*, **329**, 506518.

10. Cantor, H., and Boyse, E.A. (1975) Functional subclasses of T lymphocytes bearing different Ly antigens. *Journal of Experimental Medicine*, **141**, 13901399.

11. Qin, S., *et al.* (1993) Infectious transplantation tolerance. *Science*, **259**, 974977.

12. Björses, P., *et al.* (2000) Mutations in the AIRE gene: effects on subcellular location and transactivation function of the autoimmune polyendocrinopathy-candidiasis-ectodermal dystrophy protein. *American Journal of Human Genetics*, **66**, 378392.

13. Fontenot, J.D., *et al.* (2003) Foxp3 programs the development and function of CD4±CD25± regulatory T cells. *Nature Immunology*, **4**, 330336.

14. Lang, H.L., *et al.* (2002) A functional and structural basis for TCR cross-reactivity in multiple sclerosis. *Nature Immunology*, **3**(10), 940943.

15. DeglInnocenti, E., *et al.* (2005) Peripheral T cell tolerance occurs early during spontaneous prostate cancer development and can be rescued by dendritic cell immunization. *European Journal of Immunology*, **35**, 6675.

30　Autoimmunity

Jonathan C.W. Edwards and Geraldine Cambridge

Centre for Rheumatology, Division of Medicine, University College London,
London, UK

Introduction

Autoimmunity is a historical term centred on the concept of inappropriate adaptive immune responses to self: loss of self-tolerance. In clinical practice it has often been used loosely to cover inflammatory disease not explained by environmental agents. However, inflammatory disorders, such as ankylosing spondylitis, may show no evidence of immune response to self, and some autoimmune disorders, like myasthenia gravis, are not inflammatory. Moreover spontaneous autoimmunity in man must be distinguished from experimentally induced loss of self-tolerance in animals, which often has little to do with human disease. Thus the scope of any discussion of 'autoimmunity' needs to be made clear. This chapter will focus on disease based on *spontaneous loss of adaptive self-tolerance in humans.*

In retrospect the evolution of ideas about autoimmunity in the 20th century was slow. For the first 50 years the concept was largely disregarded despite early evidence of auto-antibodies. When, around midcentury, infectious disease physicians became 'immunologists', they transposed ideas about rheumatic fever, invoking cross-reactivity between pathogens and host, to autoimmune states like rheumatoid arthritis. This paradigm may have delayed progress since the validity of 'molecular mimicry' remains doubtful even in rheumatic fever and certainly in chronic autoimmune disease (perhaps the only established example is in post-infective polyneuropathy[1]). In addition, following the demonstration that antibody responses depend on permissive signals from T cells, there emerged an assumption that autoimmune disease is, like a normal immune response, 'T cell driven'. However, this paradigm has also been problematic since it is hard to find either evidence or explanation for acquisition of T cell autoreactivity in adult life.

Autoimmune responses increasingly look to be not so much standard adaptive responses to forbidden antigens but rather primarily dysregulated responses specific to a restricted number of self-antigens. The bulk of evidence relates to dysregulation of B cell behaviour. Evidence for disordered selection of T cells is more difficult to find.

The ten papers discussed below have been chosen because they illustrate key points in the development of ideas relating to autoimmunity. Understanding of autoimmunity remains in a state of flux, but the advent of highly specific biological therapeutic agents promises to provide a powerful means for probing pathogenic mechanisms in a way that can directly benefit patients.

Understanding Medical Research: The Studies that Shaped Medicine, First Edition. Edited by
John A. Goodfellow. © 2012 John Wiley & Sons, Ltd. Published 2012 by John Wiley & Sons, Ltd.

Is 'Horror Autotoxicus' Possible?
Donath and Landsteiner, Zeitschrift für Klinische Medizin (1904)

Paul Ehrlich famously decreed that reaction to self, or 'horror autotoxicus' was impossible; he was to be proved wrong. The centenary has recently been marked of the description by Donath and Landsteiner of self-reactive antibodies in patients with certain types of haemolytic anaemia. This is where the concept of autoimmunity starts[2]. The haemolytic anaemias have subsequently turned out to be complex and heterogeneous, and auto-antibodies do not always play a role. Antibodies to polymorphic antigens in patients receiving donated blood have always been a bigger practical issue. Nevertheless the demonstration that a human immune system could produce antibodies to self was of great historic importance, even if its validity was questioned widely until other examples were identified. Moreover the auto-antibodies of haemolytic anaemia and cryoglobulinaemia provide a good example of the aberrant nature of auto-antibody dynamics that has become a common theme in other conditions. Auto-antibodies carrying a heavy chain framework determinant recognised by the 9G4 monoclonal antibody have an inherent capacity to bind self red cells[3]. 9G4 B cells are found in normal people but do not produce antibody. There is something innately unusual about regulation of 9G4 B cells that fails in a number of autoimmune disorders.

Is Collagen Vascular Disease a Systemic Reaction to Dying Self?
Hargreaves, Mayo Clinical Proceedings (1949)

Serious interest in autoimmunity developed with the discovery of serum factors, subsequently proved to be auto-antibodies, in what had been called 'collagen vascular diseases': notably rheumatoid arthritis and systemic lupus erythematosus (SLE). The term collagen vascular disease was based on an idea of a common pathological lesion known as fibrinoid necrosis of collagen, exhibiting various patterns of cell death, fibrin deposition and collagen degradation. Pathological changes can affect many organ systems, often with involvement of blood vessel walls: hence 'vascular' in the name.

In 1940 Waaler[4] had shown that sera from patients with rheumatoid arthritis would agglutinate sheep red cells coated with IgG (see Chapter 23 on rheumatoid arthritis). Interest grew in the potential role of serum factors in widespread tissue pathology. In SLE the 'fibrinoid' tends to bind haematoxylin, indicating release of DNA into tissue matrix from dead cells ('haematoxyphil bodies'). In 1948 Hargreaves described the 'L.E. cell' phenomenon, in which phagocytosed nuclear debris was seen within granulocytes in agitated blood from SLE patients. A year later Hargreaves showed that the phenomenon could be reproduced by adding serum from SLE patients to cells from bone marrow. Subsequently, the serum factors responsible for this were found to be auto-antibodies to nuclear material.

Two aspects of Hargreaves's study are noteworthy. Recognition of the potential role of immune complexes in disease had already evolved from reactions to horse serum used to treat tetanus and Hargreaves's studies led on to the view that complexes formed by auto-antibodies could produce multisystem disease. The factors responsible for the targeting of specific organs like renal glomeruli or synovium were not understood but seemed likely to be related more to vascular physiology and tissue reactivity than to specific tissue antigens – hence 'non-organ-specific autoimmunity'. The study was also significant in that it suggested that SLE might relate to interference between the immune response to foreign agents and the body's innate, normally 'silent' mechanisms for disposal of its own nuclear debris. The idea was born, and remains alive today, that autoimmunity may often represent a 'misalliance' between adaptive and innate immune mechanisms that leads to dysregulation of tolerance mechanisms.

Might Auto-antibodies Cause Organ-Specific Disease?
Roitt et al., Biochemistry Journal (1958)

The familiar clinical concept of autoimmunity became established in the late 1950s with the demonstration of organ-specific auto-antibodies in conditions such as thyroiditis, pernicious anaemia and chronic hepatitis. Doniach and others developed immunoflu-orescent techniques to show that sera from patients with a range of clinical disorders would bind intracellular components in tissue sections. In many cases the antibody reactivities made sense in terms of potential pathogenic role. Antibodies to thyroid tissue were associated with thyroid dysfunction, antibodies to parietal cells with failure of absorption of vitamin B12 etc. However, other specificities were puzzling. Antibodies to a mitochondrial component are associated with primary biliary cirrhosis and antibodies to what proved to be topoisomerase-1 with scleroderma. The pathogenic significance of these antibodies remains controversial.

Although several auto-antibody reactivities were documented most were found to be to one of a small number of antigens: perhaps 50 gene products out of a potential of ~40,000. (Auto-antibodies to a wider range of antigens have now been described but they account for a tiny fraction of cases.) Moreover, these seemed to be universal and unaffected by time or geography; there are no autoimmune epidemics. A number of organ-specific auto-antibody targets are endocrine glands and targets in non-organ-specific disease include several molecules involved in innate immune signalling, such as IgG Fc, C1q and DNA. The suggestion arose that there might be something about B cell tolerance to these antigens that is inherently unstable, independent of environment.

Can Instability of B Cell Tolerance Be Modeled in Animals?
Helyer and Howie, Nature (1963)

The idea that B cell tolerance to certain self-components, like DNA, is inherently unstable, was confirmed in this study by the discovery that strains of inbred mice can develop spontaneous autoimmunity reminiscent of human SLE. Not only did disease in early strains resemble SLE but also, subsequently, a wide of range genetic alterations was found to mimic a stereotyped range of syndromes: chiefly SLE or endocrine disease. With the advent of genetic manipulation SLE-like syndromes have been found in association with deletion or over-expression of a number of B cell activation threshold factors, including complement components, immunoglobulin Fc receptors, cytokines such as interleukin 10 and the B cell trophic factor BAFF. Similar genetic abnormalities (e.g. C1q deficiency) have been identified in a small proportion of human SLE cases[5].

These spontaneous autoimmune states in animals based on alterations in thresholds in innate signalling should be contrasted with experiments in which autoreactivity is induced by large doses of mycobacterial adjuvant material, or by direct genetic manipulation of T or B cell receptor repertoires. Such models may demonstrate that it is feasible to generate an auto-antibody response to almost any self-antigen but probably do not shed light on the regulatory errors that lead to auto-antibody production in man.

Are B Cell Dynamics as Important as Reactivity?
Zetterval and Link, Clinical and Experimental Immunology (1970)

Although the central concept in autoimmunity is a loss of tolerance to self, in one clinical syndrome the evidence for adaptive immune disturbance comes chiefly from disordered B cell dynamics rather than specific autoreactivity. In multiple sclerosis (MS) evidence for disturbed adaptive immunity first came from raised immunoglobulin levels in CSF as described in this study. CSF protein levels are raised in many inflammatory states but in MS there is a specific increase in immunoglobulin. Moreover, the immunoglobulin differs from that in serum in being oligoclonal indicating that it is synthesised ectopically within central nervous system. It seems likely that these immunoglobulins are auto-reactive since the selective entry into, or survival within, the CSF space of the respective B cells is likely to depend on B cell surface immunoglobulin specificity. However, it is still unclear what antigenic specificities distinguish these immunoglobulins from others.

In recent years evidence of dysregulated antibody production, rather than just production of antibody to a 'wrong' antigen, has been found in a range of autoimmune disorders. In Sjögren's syndrome generalised hypergammaglobulinaemia is a prominent feature[6], and high levels of one or more immunoglobulin isotype are common in SLE and rheumatoid arthritis. Responses to autoantigens frequently show skewing of Ig class distribution, diverging from the normal progression from IgM to IgG and IgA isotypes. The reasons for this remain largely unknown but the implication is that the relative instability of B cell self-tolerance relates to regulatory signals that have different significance for B cells committed to different immunoglobulin isotypes. This is in keeping with the finding that normal people frequently have low affinity auto-anti-bodies, usually of IgM class. The protection against loss of self-tolerance appears often to be at the level of class switching and/or affinity maturation.

How Can Autoreactive B Cells Get T Cell Help?
Roosnek and Lanzavecchia, Journal of Experimental Medicine (1991)

The concept of autoimmunity predates T cell biology. During the 1980s it became accepted that in a normal adaptive immune response antibody production by B cells was dependent on a permissive signal from T cells known as 'help'. The new paradigm was that adaptive immune responses are 'T cell driven'. However, this concept soon presented paradoxes in autoimmunity. Some autoantigens, like DNA, should not be recognised by T cells. For others, such as IgG Fc, repeated studies failed to find greater T cell responses to the B cell antigen in patients compared to controls. Even at present the evidence for the existence of autoreactive T cells in autoimmune disease patients, not present in normal people, is very limited. T cells reactive with insulin peptides do appear to behave differently in patients with type I diabetes as compared to healthy controls but the consistency and significance of these differences remain uncertain[7]. In most other situations where T cell responses to B cell autoantigens have been studied the results are inconclusive. The demonstration of increased T cell reactivity to specific antigens is technically complex and this may be a factor. T cell proliferation in experimental systems is threshold dependent to the extent that reactivity to self can be readily demonstrated in normal T cell populations. This makes interpretation difficult. Nevertheless, in contrast to the routine diagnostic use of auto-antibody tests, no diagnostic test involving T cell autoreactivity exists.

This inconsistency led to investigation of ways in which auto-antibody responses might occur without loss of T cell tolerance to the B cell autoantigen. The occurrence of auto-antibodies to IgG Fc (rheumatoid factors) in normal people following infection or blood transfusion suggested a possible explanation that Roosnek and Lanzavecchia were able to demonstrate *in vitro*. If B cells recognising IgG (rheumatoid factor B cells) come into contact with immune complexes containing IgG bound to foreign antigen X then X can be endocytosed and peptide fragments presented to anti-X T cells. The rheumatoid factor B cell then receives 'bystander' help, as if it were an anti-X B cell.

A similar 'piggy-back' mechanism had been mooted for the expansion of anti-DNA B cells in SLE, involving the endocytosis of DNA attached to nucleic acid binding proteins that could be presented to T cells recognising the protein rather than DNA. The involvement of such a mechanism has been studied in detail by Datta[8] and others, in both human SLE and lupus-like disease in mice. T cell responses to nucleic acid binding proteins do appear to be involved in anti-DNA antibody production, but whether or not there is genuine loss of T cell tolerance in human disease remains less clear. The concept of aberrant signalling in loss of B cell tolerance to self has further expanded in the last two decades. Marshak Rothstein and colleagues[9] have suggested that the ability of DNA to bind to Toll-like receptor-9 and for certain nucleoproteins to bind Toll-like receptor 7 might alter the threshold for loss of tolerance by providing an extra pro-survival signal for autoreactive B cells in SLE.

The concept of aberrant interaction with antigen has the additional implication that there may be no meaningful sense in which either B cells or T cells 'drive' the process. One important possibility is that certain auto-antibody species, as a result of engaging their antigen, can generate signals that by altering thresholds can convert anergic T cells to autoreactive T cells. These autoreactive T cells may then be able to provide help for further auto-antibody production. This scenario can also be seen as being initiated on the T cell side by chance encounter with environmental adjuvant signals.

Does B Cell/T Cell Antigen Discordance Occur *In Vivo*?
Dieterich et al., Nature Medicine (1997)

Coeliac disease holds an anomalous position in the field of autoimmunity. It appears to be a response to foreign antigen, yet a response 'turned against host'. Relatively recently it became clear that auto-antibodies are present in the disease despite the targeting of T cells to the foreign wheat protein gliadin. In 1997 Dieterich and colleagues showed that the auto-antibodies are directed to tissue transglutaminase, demonstrating definitively that disease can involve B and T cell responses to different antigens. Although the precise mechanism is not established, it seems likely that the loss of B cell tolerance in the presence of a T cell response to a foreign antigen occurs through a 'piggy-back' mechanism involving the two different antigens. This does not prove that all autoimmune disorders involve antigenic discordance, but it adds weight to the idea that this is a common explanation for unstable tolerance to certain self-antigens.

What Roles Do Innate Thresholds Play?
Hugot et al., Nature (2001)

Evidence for aberrant interactions between T and B cells (and between B cells and antigen) suggests that each of a number of autoimmune diseases may represent a different weak link in the regulatory 'software' that controls antibody production. In several cases these weak links appear to involve molecules with innate immune functions that make them behave in an aberrant way as antigens. A further demonstration of the interplay between innate and adaptive mechanisms has come from the demonstration of a genetic predisposition to Crohn's disease linked with an intracellular component of innate immune responsiveness known as the inflammasome. The inflammasome regulates cytokine and other responses to a wide range of nonspecific noxious stimuli. Allelic variants of NOD-2 confer susceptibility to Crohn's disease. The simple interpretation of this is that Crohn's disease is not truly an autoimmune disorder, but rather a state of oversensitivity of the innate immune response. Nevertheless a proportion of patients with Crohn's disease have antibodies which recognise a complex carbohydrate antigen present both on the yeast *Saccharomyces cerevisiae* and on host cell surface receptors including the concanavalin A receptor on T cells: a further possible twist to the relationship between adaptive and innate responses in autoimmunity[10]. It also illustrates the point that self-antigens are not necessarily exclusive to self. DNA, complex carbohydrate groups and post-translational modifications of proteins such as citrullination are all examples of antigens recognised in autoimmune disorders that are in a sense neither self nor nonself.

Are There Genetic Effects on T Cell Tolerance?
Finnish-German APECED Consortium, Nature Genetics (1997)

In the preceding discussion it was mentioned that evidence for loss of T cell tolerance to self is hard to find in autoimmunity, despite widespread evidence of loss of B cell tolerance. There may, however, be an exception to this in the context of a rare syndrome known as APECED, in which multiple endocrine autoimmunity is associated with a defect in thymic availability of self-antigens because of an abnormality in the AIRE gene. T cells recognising self should normally be deleted after contact with antigen in the thymus but if availability of self-antigen in the thymus is defective this may be expected to fail to occur.

What Does Therapeutic Depletion of B or T Cells Tell Us?
Herold et al., New England Journal of Medicine (2002)

Until recently therapeutic agents for autoimmune disease were largely limited to corticosteroids and cytostatic agents borrowed from oncology with a nonspecific immunosuppressive capacity. Beneficial effects of such agents are hard to interpret in detailed pathophysiological terms. The advent of biological agents has changed this dramatically, providing an opportunity to test theoretical frameworks in a therapeutic way. We can now ask which cells and which mediators are essential to disease.

Definitive evidence of benefit from biologic agents has so far come chiefly in rheumatoid arthritis with blockade of TNF, IL-6 and costimulation (using CTLA4-Ig) and B cell depletion with rituximab as discussed in the chapter on rheumatoid arthritis[11-13]. In broader terms B cell depletion appears to produce benefit in a wide range of auto-antibody-associated disease, but not, as might be expected in conditions without auto-antibodies[13].

Table 30.1 Evidence for loss of self-tolerance in human autoimmune disease

Syndrome	Antigens Implicated in Loss of Self-Tolerance	
	B Cell Antigens	T Cells Antigens
Rheumatoid arthritis	IgG Fc	NK: Possibly any foreign antigen in immune complex
	Peptidyl-Citrulline	NK: Possibly any citrullinated protein (foreign or host)
SLE	DNA	NK: possibly any DNA
	Nucleoprotein (Ro, Sm)	NK: evidence hard to obtain
	C1q	NK: possibly any foreign antigen in immune complex
Scleroderma	Toposiomerase-1	NK: evidence for Topo-1 is negative
Myasthenia gravis	Acetylcholine receptor, muscle-specific Kinase	NK: limited evidence for AChR responses
Grave's disease	Thyroid peroxidase	NK
Coeliac disease	Tissue transglutaminase	Gliadin
Multiple sclerosis	NK, possibly oligoclonal bands	NK
Sarcoidosis	Complex carbohydrates, possibly peanut agglutinin receptor	NK
Crohn's disease	Mannan complex on *Saccharomyces*	NK

Note: NK = not known.

   Attempts to deplete T cells in autoimmune disease predated B cell depletion by at least ten years. However, in rheumatoid arthritis, where trials were most extensive, efficacy was consistency lacking. At the time this was a major disappointment although now it might seem relatively unsurprising. Nevertheless, the need to be aware of the heterogeneity and complexity of autoimmune dynamics was emphasised when it became clear that in type I diabetes mellitus T cell targeting with anti-CD3 could produce significant benefit[11]. Again, this appears to be telling us that endocrine autoimmune disease may be much more critically dependent on changes in T cell reactivity than in other forms of autoimmunity. The complex interactions between B and T cells mean that interpretation still needs to be cautious but as more biological agents become available, it may not be too long before truly rational, disease tailored, remission inducing therapy becomes routine in a wide range of these disorders.

Conclusions

The detailed theoretical framework for autoimmunity remains in flux. Nevertheless, certain central concepts stand out[13]. The core evidence for spontaneous human autoimmunity remains the presence of auto-antibodies, indicating loss of B cell tolerance. Association with MHC Class II and other evidence supports the idea that loss of B cell tolerance involves interaction with T cells but evidence for loss of T cell tolerance remains scarce. See Table 30.1. In conditions such as coeliac disease and rheumatoid arthritis there are good reasons to think it is not involved. Circumstantial evidence for loss of T cell tolerance is strongest in autoimmune disorders targeting endocrine glands, such as type I diabetes, and the dysregulated dynamics in these disorders may be fundamentally different from those of non-organ-specific autoimmune states.

Evidence both from epidemiology in man and genetic studies in mice strongly suggests that B cell tolerance to a small number of self-antigens is unstable. Once spontaneous autoimmunity has developed it is usually permanent, suggesting a vicious cycle develops. Although a shift from tolerance to autoimmunity might be triggered by an environmental insult epidemiology argues against this, being more consistent with one or more stochastic events within the adaptive response itself in line with the random nature of the genesis of B and T cell receptor diversity. We all make B cells recognising self-antigens every day and in almost every case negative regulatory mechanisms prevail. However, if autoreactive B cell clones with antibodies capable of binding self-antigen and engaging innate immune signalling systems in aberrant ways are generated in a favourable local environment then negative regulation may be outweighed by positive proliferation signals.

Key Outstanding Questions

The central remaining question for each autoimmune disease is the nature of the acquired event or events that transform a healthy, if genetically predisposed, individual into a long-term disease sufferer. We would like to understand the basis of 'disease memory'. It is still unclear how much this is purely dependent on the loss of B cell tolerance we observe or some as yet unconfirmed change in T cell reactivity. Discriminating between the two is not easy. Type 1 diabetes and, subsequently, other autoimmune diseases such as rheumatoid arthritis, have been found to be associated with a variant of the PTPN22 gene, the product of which was first recognised as a threshold in T cell receptor signalling, which might implicate errors of T cell tolerance. More recently the gene product has also been implicated in B cell receptor signalling and specifically B cell receptor editing; another candidate event for the transition to loss of tolerance. A continuing attraction of this field of research is that there are still key questions to address – tough ones, but almost certainly soluble ones!

References

Dieterich, W., *et al.* (1997) Identification of tissue transglutaminase as the autoantigen of celiac disease. *Nature Medicine*, **3**, 797–801. http://www.nature.com/nm/journal/v3/n7/abs/nm0797-797.html

Donath, J., and Landsteiner, K. (1904) Ueber paroysmale hemoglobinurie. *Zeitschrift fr Klinische Medizin*, **58**, 173–189. http://www.nap.edu/html/biomems/klandsteiner.pdf

Finnish-German APECED Consortium (1997) An autoimmune disease, APECED, caused by mutations in a novel gene featuring two PHD-type zinc-finger domains. *Nature Genetics*, **17** (4), 399–403. http://www.nature.com/ng/journal/v17/n4/abs/ng1297-399.html

Hargreaves, M.M. (1949) Production in vitro of the L.E. cell phenomenon; use of normal bone marrow elements and blood plasma from patients with acute disseminated lupus erythematosus. *Mayo Clinical Proceedings*, **24**(9), 234–237. http://www.ncbi.nlm.nih.gov/pubmed/18119558

Helyer, B.J., and Howie, J.B. (1963) Renal disease associated with positive lupus erythematosus tests in a cross-bred strain of mice. *Nature (London)*, **197**, 197. http://www.nature.com/nature/journal/v197/n4863/abs/197197a0.html

Herold, K.C., *et al.* (2002) Anti-CD3 monoclonal antibody in new-onset type 1 diabetes mellitus. *New England Journal of Medicine*, **346**(22), 1692–1698. http://www.ncbi.nlm.nih.gov/pubmed/12037148

Hugot, J.P., *et al.* (2001) Association of NOD2 leucine rich repeat variants with susceptibility to Crohn's disease. *Nature*, **411**, 599–603. http://www.nature.com/nature/journal/v411/n6837/full/411599a0.html

Roitt, I.M., *et al.* (1958) The nature of the thyroid auto-antibodies present in patients with Hashimoto's thyroiditis (lymphadenoid goitre). *Biochemical Journal*, **69**(2), 248–256. http://www.ncbi.nlm.nih.gov/pmc/articles/PMC1196545/

Roosnek, E., and Lanzavecchia, A. (1991) Efficient and selective presentation of antigen-antibody complexes by rheumatoid factor B cells. *Journal of Experimental Medicine*, **173**, 487–489. http://www.ncbi.nlm.nih.gov/pmc/articles/PMC2118796/

Zetterval, O., and Link, H. (1970) Electrophoretic distribution of kappa and lambda immunoglobulin light chain determinants in serum and cerebrospinal fluid in multiple sclerosis. *Clinical & Experimental Immunology*, **7**(3), 365–372. http://www.ncbi.nlm.nih.gov/pmc/articles/PMC1712736/

Additional References

1. Willison, H.J., and Plomp, J.J. (2008) Anti-ganglioside antibodies and the presynaptic motor nerve terminal. *Annals of the New York Academy of Science*, **1132**, 114–123.

2. Zouali, M. (2005) *Molecular autoimmunity*. Springer, New York.

3. Schutte, M.E., *et al.* (1993) VH4.21-encoded natural auto-antibodies with anti-i specificity mirror those associated with cold hemagglutinin disease. *Journal of Immunology*, **151**(11), 6569–6576.

4. Waaler, E. (1940) On occurrence of factor in human serum activating specific agglutination of sheep blood corpuscles. *Acta Pathologica Microbiologica Scandinavica*, **17**, 172–175.

5. Kirschfink, M, *et al.* (1993) Complete functional C1q deficiency associated with systemic lupus erythematosus. *Clinical & Experimental Immunology*, **94**, 267–272.

6. Bunim, J.J. (1965) The frequent occurrence of hypergammaglobulinemia and multiple tissue antibodies in Sj—gren's syndrome. *Annals of the New York Academy of Science*, **124**(2), 852–859.

7. Wilson, D.B. (2005) Immunology: insulin auto-antigenicity in type 1 diabetes. *Nature*, **438** (7067), E5.

8. Datta, S.K. (2003) Major peptide autoepitopes for nucleosome-centered T and B cell interaction in human and murine lupus. *Annals of the New York Academy of Science*, **987**, 79–90.

9. Laum C.M., *et al.* (2005) RNA-associated autoantigens activate B cells by combined B cell antigen receptor/Toll-like receptor 7 engagement. *Journal of Experimental Medicine*, **202**(9), 1171–1177.

10. Main, J., *et al.* (1988) Antibody to Saccharomyces cerevisiae (bakers' yeast) in Crohn's disease. *British Medical Journal*, **297**(6656), 1105–1106.

11. Elliott, M.J., *et al.* (1994) Randomised double-blind comparison of chimeric monoclonal antibody to tumour necrosis factor alpha (cA2) versus placebo in rheumatoid arthritis. *Lancet*, **344**(8930), 1105–1110.

12. Maini, R.N., *et al.* (2006) Double-blind randomized controlled clinical trial of the interleukin-6 receptor antagonist, tocilizumab, in European patients with rheumatoid arthritis who had an incomplete response to methotrexate. *Arthritis and Rheumatism*, **54**(9), 2817–2829.

13. Edwards, J.C., and Cambridge, G. (2006) B-cell targeting in rheumatoid arthritis and other autoimmune diseases. *Nature Reviews Immunology*, **6**(5), 394–403.

31 The Biochemistry of Depression

Philip J. Cowen

Department of Psychiatry, University of Oxford, Oxford, UK

Introduction

Clinical depression (major depression) is a common condition with a substantial morbidity and significant mortality. About 14% of the global burden of disease has been attributed to neuropsychiatric disorders and recurrent depression is the largest single contributor to this burden. The personal and social antecedents of depression have been well characterised; however, the neurochemical basis of the illness is still poorly understood and this has inhibited the development of better medical treatments. Although current antidepressant medications may be safer than their predecessors they work on the same general pharmacological principles and are no more efficacious.

There have been some longstanding clues to what might be the nature of the biochemical changes in depression. For example, certain medical conditions such as hypothyroidism and hyperparathyroidism are associated with high rates of depressive symptomatology and more recently similar effects have been seen during treatment with interferons. However, the main driver of research in this area has been the pharmacological effects of antidepressant drugs. It has been argued, for example, that the prominent effects of these agents on monoamines suggest that disturbances in monoamine function might be important in the pathophysiology of clinical depression. Logically of course this is not *necessarily* the case; however, hypotheses based on the action of useful treatments do have heuristic value in situations where knowledge is limited.

A Laboratory Test for Depression?
Carroll et al., Archives of General Psychiatry (1981)

The fact that many depressed patients hyperscrete cortisol had been known since the 1960s. This paper by Carroll and colleagues represented a bold attempt to put depression on the same footing as general medical conditions by developing a specific laboratory test for the condition. The test involved administration of 1 mg dexamethasone in the evening followed by a 4 p.m. blood sample for cortisol the next day. Failure to suppress cortisol was highly predictive of melancholic depression; a subtype of depression associated with prominent biological features, including psychomotor retardation, early morning waking, weight loss and diminished sense of pleasure.

Carroll and colleagues argued that the dexamethasone suppression test (DST) could be used as a laboratory diagnosis of melancholic depression. This could be clinically useful because patients with melancholic depression are more likely to respond to

Understanding Medical Research: The Studies that Shaped Medicine, First Edition. Edited by
John A. Goodfellow. © 2012 John Wiley & Sons, Ltd. Published 2012 by John Wiley & Sons, Ltd.

somatic treatments such as antidepressant medications and less likely to be helped by psychotherapy. Further it appeared that normalisation of the DST in depressed patients was associated with clinical recovery.

Subsequent research has led to a qualification of these claims. In particular, failure to suppress cortisol to dexamethasone is not a specific test for depression because it is also seen in patients with Alzheimer's disease and anorexia nervosa. However, there is no doubt that patients with depression hypersecrete cortisol compared to controls, and this could be of pathophysiological importance bearing in mind the increased rate of depression seen in patients with Cushing's disease. The abnormalities of mood seen in Cushing's disease resolve when cortisol levels are decreased; raising the possibility that drugs which lower cortisol levels or block the action of cortisol at glucocorticoid receptors might have clinical antidepressant properties. Thus far the latter hypothesis has not yielded clearly positive results during clinical trials. In fact there is evidence that depression is associated with subsensitivity of glucocorticoid receptors which results in impaired feedback control of the hypothalamo-pituitary-adrenal (HPA) axis. One action of conventional antidepressant treatment is to increase the availability of glucocorticoid receptors. From this viewpoint it is not clear that the use of agents that block glucocorticoid receptors is necessarily the correct strategy to treat depressed patients.

Overall the hope that the DST would provide a useful laboratory test for the diagnosis of depression and effective subsequent guidance of appropriate treatment has not been borne out. However, depressed patients clearly have abnormalities in HPA axis function and the use of the DST spawned a large research effort which has probably not yet reached full fruition.

Hypersecretion of Cortisol as a State-Independent Marker of Depression
Vreeburg et al., Archives of General Psychiatry (2009)

Much of the work investigating the role of cortisol in the pathophysiology of depression was based on the view that increased cortisol secretion was a state marker of illness which remitted as the depression resolved or was successfully treated. This does appear to be the case for certain aspects of cortisol hypersecretion in depression. Technical advances in the measurement of cortisol enabled free cortisol to be measured in saliva samples. This permitted more extensive investigations of cortisol secretion in large epidemiological cohorts.

The salivary cortisol response to waking is a reliable increase in cortisol that occurs in healthy individuals in the 30 minutes or so that elapse after waking. This increase is a response to the release of endogenous corticotrophin releasing hormone (CRH). It has good within-subject reliability and a significant heritability. This paper by Vreeburg and colleagues measured waking salivary cortisol in about 1500 participants. They foud that patients with current depression had increased waking cortisol, but intriguingly so did patients who have been depressed but who are clinically recovered.

This finding suggests that the increase in waking salivary cortisol seen in depressed patients may be independent of current clinical state and appears to represent a trait marker, so that even when patients are recovered from illness they continue to hypersecrete cortisol. It leaves open the question as to whether the increase in waking cortisol is a longstanding vulnerability marker or instead be a consequence of depression or treatment. However, smaller scale investigations have revealed that people at increased risk of depression through familial loading also hypersecrete waking cortisol even when they have never experienced clinical illness.

Taken together these findings suggest that abnormalities in HPA axis function are present in people at risk of depression and continue to manifest themselves during depression and after recovery. Some aspects of cortisol hypersecretion may therefore function as a vulnerability factor; increasing the risk that an individual will experience depression when exposed to adverse life events. It is also possible that continued hypersecretion of cortisol over the life span could explain the increased risk of certain general medical abnormalities found in depressed patients including for example cardiovascular disease and diabetes.

The origin of the increase in waking salivary cortisol in depression and those at risk of depression isn't clear. It seems likely that childhood adversity can affect the development of the HPA axis, but it is also possible that genetic inheritance might be a factor. For example, some studies have reported that carriers of the short allele of the serotonin transporter gene secrete more cortisol in response to waking.

Noradrenaline Dysfunction in Depressed Patients
Checkley et al., British Journal of Psychiatry (1981)

The chance discovery that tricyclic antidepressants (TCA) were therapeutically useful in depressed patients is the cornerstone of the monoamine theory. Experimental work in animals revealed that TCAs enhance the function of noradrenaline and serotonin by preventing the reuptake of these neurotransmitters into the presynaptic nerve ending. From this it was hypothesised that the biochemical causation of depression might be linked to a functional deficiency of noradrenaline (the catecholamine theory) or serotonin (the indoleamine hypothesis).

This paper by Checkley and colleagues adopts a novel approach to investigating this question by using the so-called neuroendocrine challenge methodology. The use of this approach rests on the fact that monoamine pathways innervate the hypothalamus where they provoke the release of hormone releasing factors such as growth hormone releasing hormone (GHRH) and prolactin releasing factor (PRF). Therefore if monoamine pathways are stimulated with a selective drug the size of the hormone response provides an indication of the functional activity of the relevant neurotransmitter, at least in the hypothalamus. It is important in these studies to make sure that patients are free of antidepressant medication because these drugs themselves of course will alter mono-amine function.

The work by Checkley and colleagues provides a classic demonstration of the use of a neuroendocrine challenge paradigm in patients with endogenous (melancholic) depression. They show that the growth hormone response to the selective α_2-adrenoceptor agonist clonidine is blunted in such patients, consistent with a functional subsensitivity of the postsynaptic α_2-adrenoceptors which regulate the secretion of growth hormone. Interestingly, there was no difference between patients and controls in the ability of clonidine to produce sedation and hypotension. Because the latter effects of clonidine are also mediated by post-synaptic α_2-adrenoceptors it suggests that the in α_2-adrenoceptor functional deficit in depressed patients may be restricted to certain brain regions.

Follow-up studies by Checkley and his colleagues suggested that the growth hormone response to clonidine remained impaired when patients had recovered clinically and withdrawn from antidepressant treatment. This is consistent with a trait abnormality in noradrenaline function which persists after clinical remission from illness.

Role for Noradrenaline in Depressive Relapse
Berman et al., Archives of General Psychiatry (1999)

The finding by Checkley and colleagues of a persistent abnormality in noradrenaline function in recovered depressed patients raised the possibility that noradrenaline could play a role in depressive relapse. Berman and colleagues used alpha methyl paratyrosine (AMPT) to block noradrenaline synthesis in the human brain. AMPT inhibits the activity of tyrosine hydroxylase and this prevents the conversion of the amino acid tyrosine to L-dopa. It is important to note that AMPT thereby decreases dopamine synthesis as well as that of noradrenaline.

In healthy volunteers AMPT does not result in clinical depression. In recovered depressed patients withdrawn from antidepressant treatment AMPT causes a striking transient clinical relapse. This suggests that patients with recurrent depression have a specific psychological vulnerability to depletion of noradrenaline and dopamine. Whether this is present before or develops during the course of recurrent depression is not clear. Dietary manipulations which specifically diminish dopamine neurotransmission do not cause relapse in recovered depressed patients, suggesting that AMPT mediates relapse through noradrenaline or perhaps noradrenaline and dopamine working together.

Serotonin and Depression: A Possible Link with Suicide
Asberg et al., Science (1976)

As noted previously, antidepressant drugs also potentiate the activity of serotonin in the central nervous system. Methods for detecting serotonin abnormalities in depressed patients have gradually improved such that modern investigations are able to image serotonin receptors directly in the human brain using ligand imaging in conjunction with positron emission tomography (PET).

This paper by Asberg and colleagues played a pioneering role in investigations of serotonin function by identifying lower levels of the serotonin metabolite, 5-hydroxindoleacteic acid (5-HIAA), in the cerebrospinal fluid (CSF) of unmedicated depressed patients. Interestingly their findings indicated a bimodal distribution of 5-HIAA in the depressed population suggesting distinct biochemical subtypes (i.e. that low serotonin availability might characterise only a subgroup of depressed patients). Suicide attempts and completed suicide were more common amongst people with low 5-HIAA and within this group levels of the serotonin metabolite correlated inversely with the severity of depression.

Generally, the finding of a bimodal distribution of 5-HIAA in the CSF of depressed patients has not been widely replicated. However, there is evidence that low 5-HIAA is associated with both suicidal behaviour and impulsive aggression towards others across psychiatric diagnoses; also affecting, for example, people with personality disorders. This has led to suggestions that the aspect of serotonin function that is captured by a measure of low CSF 5-HIAA is probably related to a trait measure of personality involving low impulse control.

Low Serotonin Function in Depression Detected by Neuroendocrine Challenge
Heninger et al., Archives of General Psychiatry (1984)

As we saw in the study by Checkley, neuroendocrine challenge tests provide a feasible and relatively non-invasive method of assessing neurotransmitter function in the hypothalamus. This paper by Heninger and colleagues represents one of the first applications of this technique to the measurements of serotonin function in depression. The authors used the amino acid precursor of serotonin, tryptophan, as a means of increasing brain serotonin function. When intravenous tryptophan is administered to healthy volunteers there is an increase in plasma prolactin because serotonin pathways play an excitatory role in prolactin release.

In unmedicated depressed patients, administration of tryptophan produced a much lower prolactin response than that seen in controls. This suggests that depression is associated with diminished serotonin neurotransmission, at least in the hypothalamus. The finding that depressed patients have lowered prolactin release has been widely replicated. Because prolactin release to other challenges appears normal in depression (for example to dopamine receptor blockade), this suggests that depression is characterised by impairment in presynaptic serotonin neurotransmission. This could reflect a deficiency in serotonin synthesis or in its release from the nerve terminal. Serotonin mediated prolactin release in recovered depressed patients has not been much studied. However, the evidence to date suggests that impaired prolactin release to serotonin challenge persists after clinical recovery and therefore may represent a trait marker of illness.

PET Imaging of the 5-HT1A Receptor in Depression
Drevets et al., Biological Psychiatry (1999)

The development of WAY100635 as a selective serotonin$_{1A}$ (5-HT$_{1A}$) receptor antagonist was followed by positron labelling and application as a means of measuring binding 5-HT$_{1A}$ receptor availability in the living human brain. The 5-HT$_{1A}$ receptor is a serotonin receptor subtype that plays a key role in both the regulation of serotonin release and the effects of serotonin at postsynaptic sites in the limbic system and cerebral cortex. 5-HT$_{1A}$ receptors regulate serotonin release by acting as autoreceptors on serotonin cell bodies in the brain stem raphe nuclei: the origin of the ascending serotonin neural projection. Activation of 5-HT$_{1A}$ receptors decreases serotonin cell body firing and diminishes serotonin release in terminal fields.

This paper by Drevets and colleagues was the first report of 5-HT$_{1A}$ receptor binding in unmedicated depressed patients. They found widespread reductions in 5-HT$_{1A}$ receptor availability in both the serotonin cell bodies in brain stem and in postsynaptic cortical locations. This finding confirms that unmedicated depressed patients have abnormalities in serotonin mechanisms in key brain regions. It is not, however, straightforward to align the PET findings with the functional deficiency of serotonin release suggested by neuroendocrine studies. This is because decreased availability of 5-HT$_{1A}$ autoreceptors should result in disinhibition of serotonin cell bodies and an increase in serotonin release from nerve terminals. The lowering of 5-HT$_{1A}$ receptor binding might be an adaptive response that occurs as a consequence of the low activity of serotonin neurons.

The finding of low 5-HT$_{1A}$ binding in depressed patients has been generally replicated although there are exceptions which need to be resolved. Again, while the data are not completely clear, current evidence suggests that abnormalities in 5-HT$_{1A}$ receptor binding in depression are still present in patients who have recovered and been withdrawn from treatment. Once again it appears as though this abnormality might be state independent and reflect a vulnerability marker rather than a mechanism involved directly in mediating abnormal mood. It is also important to note that diminished 5-HT$_{1A}$ receptor binding measured by PET and WAY 100635 has also been reported in patients with other psychiatric disorders, for example panic disorder and chronic fatigue syndrome. However, this might be explained on the basis that the latter two conditions have a high lifetime comorbidity with depression.

Tryptophan Depletion Provokes Relapse in Recovered Depressed Patients
Smith et al., Lancet (1997)

The studies above provide reasonable evidence that patients with depression manifest a range of abnormalities in serotonin activity. It is not clear in what way these abnormalities might relate to the depressive condition or its clinical course given their persistence after clinical recovery and withdrawal of medication.

One way to address this question is to lower serotonin neurotransmission and assess the psychological effects in both healthy controls and people at risk of depressive illness. This is essentially an analogous approach to that seen earlier in the study of Berman using AMPT. The amino acid precursor of serotonin, tryptophan, can be depleted in the plasma and brain by administration of an amino acid mixture which lacks tryptophan (an essential amino acid). This technique is called 'tryptophan depletion'. Serotonin synthesis is dependent on tryptophan availability; therefore lowering plasma and brain tryptophan decreases brain serotonin levels.

In healthy subjects without significant risk factors for depression tryptophan depletion causes some impairment in learning and memory but does not produce a clinical lowering of mood. However, in patients suffering from recurrent depression, but who are well and withdrawn from antidepressant treatment, tryptophan depletion causes an acute, transient return of clinical depressive symptomatology. In people at high familial risk of depression who have not suffered clinical illness, tryptophan depletion causes only a subclinical lowering of mood.

These findings suggest that high familial risk of depression is associated with a mild affective vulnerability to low brain serotonin levels, but this is greatly exaggerated by recurrent depressive episodes. This is consistent with clinical data which indicate that the risk of suffering depression becomes greater as patients experience a growing number of episodes and that one mechanism possibly underpinning this effect is a growing psychological sensitivity to low brain serotonin function.

An Interaction between a Serotonin Genetic Mechanism and Environmental Stress
Caspi et al., Science (2003)

Ongoing stresses and adverse life events play an important role in triggering depression. It is therefore important to formulate how particular biochemical mechanisms could interact with environmental stress to produce clinical illness in individuals. The serotonin transporter is a protein receptor that plays a critical role in the re-uptake of serotonin from the synaptic cleft and drugs that inhibit the transporter, such as selective serotonin reuptake inhibitors (SSRIs), are widely used in the management of clinical depression.

The gene for the serotonin transporter has a number of allelic variants and one in the promoter region is thought to influence tissue expression. In essence this means that our carriers of the short form of the variant gene (s) would be expected to express fewer serotonin re-uptake sites than carriers of the long form (l).

The above paper by Caspi and colleagues was seminal in showing a gene-environment interaction such that individuals who carried the s allele of the transporter gene polymorphism were more likely to become depressed when exposed to stressful life events than carriers of the l allele. This is an important conceptual advance because it shows how individual genetic variation in specific serotonin mechanisms might lead individuals to show increased psychological reaction to environment adversity. It has long been recognised that there is great individual variation in susceptibility to the depressogenic effects of adverse life events, and this study shows a potential serotonergic mechanism which might account for some of this variation.

Again it is a little difficult to link decreased expression of serotonin transporter sites with increased vulnerability to depression because lower serotonin transporter availability would be expected to increase synaptic serotonin levels, which is of course what antidepressant medications like SSRIs actually do. However, it is quite possible that the effects of the s allele to increase vulnerability could be expressed in other ways, for example through effects on neurodevelopment and the activity of the neural circuitry that underpins emotional processing. It must be acknowledged that replication of the effect reported by Caspi has not been entirely consistent and a meta-analysis suggested that interaction between serotonin transporter gene variation, life stress and environment might be unreliable. However, the meta-analysis itself has been strongly criticised. Nonetheless, this approach provides a useful model of the way one might try to integrate biological and social factors to provide a fuller understanding of the pathophysiology of depression.

Beyond Monoamines: A Role for GABA and Glutamate in Depression
Sanacora et al., Archives of General Psychiatry (2004)

Many of the papers described above provide good evidence that abnormalities of serotonin and noradrenaline mechanisms are present in depressed patients both during illness and after recovery. However, it seems unlikely that decreases in noradrenaline and serotonin activity are either necessary or sufficient to cause depressive illness because neither tryptophan depletion nor AMPT cause depression in healthy individuals. In addition, while the currently available antidepressant treatments are highly effective at increasing monoamine neurotransmission, their efficacy in the treatment of depression is often modest and new approaches are clearly needed.

γ-aminobutyric acid (GABA) and glutamate are key neurotransmitters in the brain, subserving inhibitory and excitatory neurotransmission respectively. Their investigation has recently been made more feasible by developments in proton magnetic resonance spectroscopy (MRS), and this study by Sanacora and colleagues in a large sample of unmedicated depressed patients employs MRS to show clear reductions in cortical GABA and increases in glutamate.

This opens several new lines of research into the biochemistry of depression. The decrease in cortical GABA has been confirmed in other studies but the changes in glutamate appear more variable and dependent on the brain region examined. However, the finding has led to an increase in research on the possible antidepressant effects of glutamate and GABA-modifying drugs. In this respect it is of great interest that placebo controlled trials have shown rapid antidepressant effects of the NMDA receptor antagonist ketamine in patients with treatment resistant depression. The speed of response suggests that glutamatergic manipulations may provide a novel approach to antidepressant development.

Conclusion

Better methodologies have allowed the demonstration of some reliable biochemical abnormalities in patients with depression, particularly in noradrenaline and serotonin neurotransmission. In addition, many depressed patients hypersecrete cortisol. The fact that depletion of serotonin and noradrenaline can cause depressive relapse in recovered patients shows the potential importance of these monoamines in triggering clinical symptomatology in those at high risk through previous episodes of illness. It should be noted, however, that in all the neurobiological studies to date there is much overlap in neurochemical measures between depressed patients and controls. This means that the abnormalities described in this article cannot yet be used as reliable diagnostic markers of illness.

Several difficulties need to be resolved. For example, we do not know how the abnormalities in monoamines and cortisol relate to the expression and experience of the depressed state. The fact that many of the described abnormalities persist after clinical recovery suggests that there may be more involved in vulnerability to depression rather than the pathological mood state itself. Finally, it seems unlikely that further development of monoamine therapies will lead to substantially better treatments than those currently available so pharmacological manipulations involving other neurochemical mechanisms, for example GABA and glutamate, need to be explored.

Key Questions Remaining

1. How do the biochemical abnormalities found in depressed patients link to the production of clinical symptomatology in terms of relevant neural circuitry?
2. Can we develop integrated models to explain the key role of psychosocial stress on the risk of depression by understanding how stress influences brain neurochemistry?
3. Can we identify which abnormalities in recovered depressed patients are consequences of illness and its treatment and which predate the development of depression? Such abnormalities might be useful predictors of those at risk of depression and might also be targeted in primary prevention strategies.
4. Can we develop neurochemical tests which will identify those patients who will respond to particular pharmacological manipulations?
5. How does manipulation of monoamines with antidepressant drugs influence the neuropsychological mechanisms involved in the regulation and experience of emotion?

References

Asberg, M., *et al.* (1975) 'Serotonin depression' – a biochemical subgroup within the affective disorders. *Science*, **191**, 478–480. http://www.sciencemag.org/content/191/4226/478.2.Abstract

Berman, R.M., *et al.* (1999) Transient depressive relapse induced by catecholamine depletion. *Archives of General Psychiatry*, **56**, 395–403. http://archpsyc.ama-assn.org/cgi/content/full/56/5/395

Carroll, B.J., *et al.* (1981) A specific laboratory test for the diagnosis of melancholia. *Archives of General Psychiatry*, **38**, 15–22. http://archpsyc.ama-assn.org/cgi/content/abstract/38/1/15

Caspi, A., *et al.* (2003) Influence of life stress on depression: moderation by polymorphism in the 5-HTT gene. *Science*, **5631**, 386–389. http://www.ncbi.nlm.nih.gov/pubmed/12869766

Checkley, S.A., *et al.* (1981) Growth hormone and other responses to clonidine in patients with endogenous depression. *British Journal of Psychiatry*, **138**, 51–55. http://bjp.rcpsych.org/cgi/content/abstract/138/1/51

Drevets, W.C., *et al.* (1999) PET imaging of serotonin 1A receptor binding in depression. *Biological Psychiatry*, **46**, 1375–1387. http://www.biologicalpsychiatryjournal.com/article/S0006-3223(99)00189-4/Abstract

Heninger, G.R., *et al.* (1984) Serotonergic function in depression. *Archives of General Psychiatry*, **41**, 398–402. http://archpsyc.ama-assn.org/cgi/content/abstract/41/4/398

Sanacora, G., *et al.* (2004) Subtype-specific alterations of g-aminobutyric acid and glutamate in patients with major depressive disorder. *Archives of General Psychiatry*, **61**, 705–713. http://archpsyc.ama-assn.org/cgi/content/full/61/7/705

Smith, K.A., *et al.* (1997) Relapse of depression after rapid depletion of tryptophan. *Lancet*, **349**, 915–919. http://www.ncbi.nlm.nih.gov/pubmed/9093253

Vreeburg, S.A., *et al.* (2009) Major depressive disorder and hypothalmic-pituitary-adrenal axis activity. *Archives of General Psychiatry*, **66**, 617–626. http://archpsyc.ama-assn.org/cgi/content/full/66/6/617

Additional References

1. Caspi, A., *et al.* (2010) Genetic sensitivity to the environment: the case of the serotonin transporter gene and its implications for studying complex diseases and traits. *American Journal of Psychiatry*. doi 10.1176/appi.ajp.2010.09101452

2. Cowen, P.J. (2008) Serotonin and depression: pathophysiological mechanism or marketing myth? *Trends in Pharmaceutical Science*, **29**, 433–436.

3. Cowen, P.J. (2010) Not fade away: the HPA axis and depression. *Psychological Medicine*, **40**, 1–4.

4. Currier, D., and Mann, J.J. (2008) Stress, genes and the biology of suicidal behaviour. *Psychiatric Clinics of North America*, **341**, 247–269.

5. Harmer, C.J., *et al.* (2009) Why do antidepressants take so long to work? A cognitive neuropsychological model of antidepressant drug action. *British Journal of Psychiatry*, **195**, 102–108.

6. Kraft, J.B., *et al.* (2006) Analysis of association between the serotonin transporter and antidepressant response in a large clinical sample. *Biological Psychiatry*, **61**, 734–747.

7. Price, J.L., and Drevets, W.C. (2009) Neurocircuitry of mood disorders. *Neuropsychopharmacology*, **35**, 192–216.

8. Prince, M., *et al.* (2007) No health without mental health. *Lancet*, **370**, 859–877.

9. Ruhe, H.G., *et al.* (2007) is indirectly related to norepinephrine and dopamine levels in humans: a meta-analysis of monoamine depletion studies. *Molecular Psychiatry*, **12**, 331–359.

10. Sanacora, K.J., *et al.* (2002) Glutamate and GABA systems as targets for novel antidepressant and mood stabilizing treatments. *Molecular Psychiatry*, **7**(Suppl. 1), S71–S80.

32　Schizophrenia and the Dopamine Hypothesis

Mandy Johnstone and Dame Eve C. Johnstone

Centre for Clinical Brain Sciences, University Department of Psychiatry, University of Edinburgh, Edinburgh, UK

Introduction

Schizophrenia is a chronic, severe and disabling mental disorder affecting around 1 in every 100 people. It has a slight preponderance in men, and the mean age of onset in men is about 23 and in women about 27 or 28 with a second peak of incidence of about 40–45 years of age. In general the frequency is similar throughout the world but it is probably commoner in some minority ethnic groups and in urban areas.

Schizophrenia is characterised by positive symptoms (i.e. those that most people don't normally experience), negative symptoms (or deficits) and also cognitive impairment. Positive symptoms include delusions, auditory hallucinations and thought disorder and are typical manifestations of psychosis. Negative symptoms are thought of as the loss of normal traits or abilities and include flattening or blunted affect and emotion, poverty of speech, a lack of volitional drive, loss of feelings, social withdrawal and decreased spontaneous movement.

What Is the Dopamine Hypothesis?

The dopamine hypothesis of schizophrenia or psychosis is the theory that argues that the unusual behaviour and experiences associated with schizophrenia (or extended to psychosis in general) can be fully or largely explained by changes in dopamine function in the brain. At its most basic, the dopamine hypothesis postulates that an excess of dopamine subcortically is associated with the positive symptoms whereas the negative and cognitive symptoms of schizophrenia are believed to arise from a deficit of dopamine in the cortex.

The pharmacological treatment of schizophrenia began with the discovery of drugs that alleviated the symptoms of psychosis. For centuries the root of the plant *Rauwolfia serpentine* had been used to treat psychosis, the active substance of which was found to be the alkaloid reserpine in 1952. Most of the effective drug treatments in psychiatry were introduced at about the same time between 1945 and 1955. Essentially they were all introduced into psychiatry in a serendipitous basis and antipsychotics are a good example of this. In 1951 Paul Charpentier synthesised the first antipsychotic drug, the phenothiazine chlorpromazine, which was introduced into clinical practice in 1952 by Delay and Deniker. The finding that this class of compounds was effective in reducing positive symptoms of psychosis drove drug development, and this observation was

Understanding Medical Research: The Studies that Shaped Medicine, First Edition. Edited by John A. Goodfellow. © 2012 John Wiley & Sons, Ltd. Published 2012 by John Wiley & Sons, Ltd.

subsequently extended to other antipsychotic drug classes including butyrophenones such as haloperidol. This link was further strengthened by experiments in the 1970s which suggested that the binding affinity of antipsychotics for dopamine D_2-receptors seemed to be important. More recent advances in neuroscience have enhanced our knowledge of neurotransmission, allowing the refining of hypotheses regarding drug action and the pharmacological mechanism of schizophrenia and providing a theoretical basis for the development of new pharmacological agents.

A further source of hypotheses regarding the pharmacological basis of schizophrenia developed from the elucidation of the basis of drugs that induce psychotic symptoms. Although the drug-induced psychoses do not exactly mimic the entire picture of schizophrenia, they do produce individual symptoms that are clinically similar. Compounds that induce psychosis include lysergic acid diethylamide (LSD), L-dihydroxyphenylalanine (L-DOPA), cocaine, amphetamine and phencyclidine (PCP). In discussion of the dopamine hypothesis and schizophrenia, we will initially focus on the literature relating to psychosis induced by drugs that increase dopaminergic activity and then turn to discuss the antipsychotic mechanism of neuroleptics.

Amphetamine-Induced Psychosis
Connell, Maudsley Monographs (1958)

In this the fifth of the *Maudsley Monographs*, Dr. Connell begins by reviewing the literature of cases of mental symptoms accompanying overdose of amphetamines which was a valuable and substantial piece of work at that time, being published only 3 years after the introduction of the drug. He described 42 patients as having developed schizophrenia-like psychoses while taking amphetamines and reached a general conclusion whilst also imparting a well-meaning warning relating to the social dangers associated with amphetamine intoxication. He stated:

> *Psychosis associated with amphetamine usage is much more frequent than would be expected from reports in the literature. . . . The clinical picture is primarily a paranoid psychosis with ideas of reference, delusions of persecution, auditory and visual hallucinations in a setting of clear consciousness. . . . The mental picture may be indistinguishable from acute or chronic paranoid schizophrenia.*

In addition to the principal psychotic symptoms mentioned, Connell noted that disorientation was unusual. Furthermore, although the presentation was very similar to an acute paranoid schizophrenic state, it differed in its duration usually clearing within a week (three quarters usually recovered within a week, and almost all of the remaining cases cleared within a month). Dr Connell went on to discuss the biochemical tests available for testing for the presence of amphetamine, dexamphetamine and methylamphetamine.

A far larger series of 500 cases of patients who developed psychiatric complications following methamphetamine use was later studied in Japan by Tatetsu[1]. As many as 92% showed some form of mostly mild psychiatric complications, but 19% developed a schizophrenia-like psychosis. Tatetsu, like Connell, described a rapid clinical improvement in most after the drug was withdrawn but unfortunately, unlike Connell's study, many did not make a full recovery. Following the publication of these two series of cases of amphetamine psychosis, many more cases of drug-induced schizophrenia-like psychoses have been reported in the literature. Other stimulant drugs associated with the development of psychotic symptoms resembling those of schizophrenia include cocaine, phenmetrazine, methylphenidate (Ritalin) and ephedrine.

Experimental Studies of Amphetamine
Griffith et al., Amphetamine and Related Compounds (1970)

Interesting questions were raised from the studies describing amphetamine-induced psychosis. Does everyone who takes amphetamines develop psychotic symptoms, or do they occur only in those predisposed to schizophrenia? Or is it that those individuals predisposed to schizophrenia are more likely to take amphetamines or other illicit drugs? One way to answer these questions would be to give amphetamines to healthy volunteers in controlled conditions. These types of experiments would be difficult to get ethical approval for nowadays but were performed 40 years ago by Griffith and colleagues. They gave 10 mg of amphetamine hourly to four volunteers who cumulatively had about 50 mg of the drug daily. All four became paranoid and developed delusions of reference after taking the drug for between 1 and 5 days. Angrist and Gershon[2] gave four individuals higher total doses over a period of up to 75 hours. Two of the four developed clear-cut psychotic symptoms including paranoid delusions and olfactory and auditory hallucinations. The other two volunteers described partial symptoms. Collectively these studies demonstrate that if sufficient amphetamine is taken, then psychotic symptoms will develop. It is believed that the amphetamine taken is acting as a dopamine agonist, over-stimulating dopamine receptors and causing the synapse to be flooded with this neurotransmitter, the functional excess of which causes people to experience delusions and hallucinations. The behavioural consequences of acute and chronic amphetamine treatment were further studied by Kokkinidis and Anisman[3]. They hypothesised that amphetamine-induced psychosis and the symptomatology associated with schizophrenia are related to alterations in both norephinephrine and dopamine activity, although animal studies have shown that the amphetamine-induced psychosis predominately relates to dopamine rather than norephinephrine.

Discovery of Antipsychotic Drugs
Delay and Deniker, Congres de Médicins Aliénistes et Neurologistes de France (1952)

Precisely how certain drugs such as amphetamine induce psychotic states remains unknown; however, it has become clear that stimulation of the dopamine system produces psychotic symptoms similar to schizophrenia. The serendipitous discovery of compounds that successfully treat schizophrenic symptoms by blocking dopamine receptors in the brain (i.e. dopamine antagonists) has significantly progressed our understanding of the role dopamine plays. In 1952 Delay and Deniker introduced the first antipsychotic, chlorpromazine, into psychiatric practice. This discovery marked a seminal advance in the field, providing a new class of drugs to relieve the fundamental symptoms of schizophrenia. For psychiatrists working in the front line, its introduction transformed disturbed wards.

Chlorpromazine was first synthesized in December 1951 by Paul Charpentier in the French pharmaceutical company Rhône-Poulenc Laboratories of Specia in Paris, and released for use as a possible potentiator of general anaesthesia in May 1952. Three parent analogues of chlorpromazine were developed; one of these, promethazine, was extensively used because of its good antihistamine activity; and another, dietnazine, was subsequently used in Parkinson's disease. The French army surgeon Henri Laborit was interested in post-operative shock, and began initially using promethazine, finding that it relaxed and calmed his patients before going on to also test chlorpromazine. Chlorpromazine produced a state of 'artificial hibernation', where the patient remained conscious but showed a marked indifference to their surroundings and became hypothermic. Laborit was the first to suggest that these properties might make it of use to his psychiatric colleagues[4]; however, it was not until Delay and Deniker began a systematic study of the effects of chlorpromazine on 38 patients suffering from mania and acute psychosis that the extraordinary usefulness of the drug became evident. Their early findings with chlorpromazine at Saint-Anne's Hospital showed that a daily dose of 75 mg was sufficient for controlling behaviour, and they presented these findings at the centennial meeting of the Société Médico-Psychologique on 25 May 1952. During the 6 months that followed, a further six publications from them firmly set the stage for the introduction of chlorpromazine into psychiatric practice: it became available on prescription in France in 1952. Laborit, Deniker and Lehmann were awarded the prestigious Albert Lasker Award in 1957 for their work on chlorpromazine.

In 1957 Paul Janssen discovered a propriophenone with morphine-like qualities that he set to structurally modify to enhance its potency. He produced a butyrophenone which when injected into mice produced behavioural changes symptomatic of both morphine and chlorpromazine. The mice initially showed morphine-like excitement before becoming progressively calm, sedated and perhaps catatonic[5]. Further modifications were made in order to remove the morphine-like qualities and increase the antipsychotic effects. This produced a compound (R1625) which was many more times more active than chlorpromazine as well as longer lasting and devoid of anti-adrenergic effects. It was by far the most powerful antipsychotic at the time, and in clinical trials was shown to be effective in controlling paranoia, delusions, hallucinations and manic symptoms and was called Haloperidol[5]. Interestingly, the first clinical trial results published[6] commented on the significant and clinically relevant side effects of Haloperidol: 'Its neuroleptic properties are powerful: the typical patient shows a marked parkinsonism with akinesia, hypertonia, asthenia-aboulia, emotional inhibition of great therapeutic interest'.

Dopamine and Parkinson's Disease
Hornykiewicz, British Medicine Bulletin (1973)

Antipsychotic medication also produced extra-pyramidal side effects including movement disorders, stiffness and slowness resembling those associated with Parkinson's disease. Hornykiewicz established that dopamine concentrations are significantly reduced in the corpus callosum and other areas of post-mortem brain from patients affected with Parkinson's disease. It was postulated that impaired dopaminergic transmission is the primary cause of the symptoms, secondary to degeneration of the nigro-striatal and other dopaminergic pathways. Therefore the symptoms of Parkinson's disease seemed to be due to a failure of the dopamine system. The extra-pyramidal side effects of antipsychotics drugs were thus considered further evidence of their anti-dopaminergic action. In this context, it is also interesting to note that L-DOPA, a dopamine precursor, can induce a paranoid psychosis, presumably by bringing about a hyperdopaminergic state.

Dopamine Blockade and the Efficacy of Antipsychotic Drugs

Carlsson and Lindqvist, Acta Pharmacologica Toxicologica (1963)

This paper is often quoted as the origin of the dopamine hypothesis and describes, for the first time, the enhancement of dopamine and noradrenaline metabolism brought about by the effects of chlorpromazine and haloperidol on the brain. It showed that the antipsychotics stimulated the turnover of catecholamines in mice. They postulated that the drugs blocked catecholamine receptors bringing about a compensatory increase of tyrosine hydroxylase activity. Carlsson and collaborators had earlier found that reserpine, the active substance in extracts of *Rauwolfia serpentine*, appeared to owe its effects on behaviour to the depletion of monoamines. This hypothesis was particularly attractive as delivery of L-DOPA reversed the behavioural effects of reserpine, whereas delivery of a precursor (5-hydroxytryptophan) of the neurotransmitter serotonin did not. The fact that after such treatment there was no increase in adrenaline or nor-adrenaline, but there was an increase in the precursor dopamine, suggested reserpine was acting as an agonist in the brain. Carlsson developed techniques for quantifying the amount of dopamine in brain tissues. His work, showing the reversal of the movement disorder in mice by L-DOPA, paved the way for the use of L-DOPA in patients with Parkinson's disease. Carlsson and Lindqvist, together with others[7], showed that both chlorpromazine and haloperidol accelerated the turnover of dopamine and noradrenaline. This accelerated turnover was not accompanied by any changes in steady-state levels, and since it was known that they antagonised the behavioural effects of L-DOPA, it was proposed that these drugs block the post-synaptic monoamine receptors and thereby alter a negative feedback mechanism which controls synthesis, release and metabolism of monoamines.

Avrid Carlsson published many papers over the years investigating the role of dopamine in the brain and whilst working for Astra AB derived the first marketed selective serotonin reuptake inhibitor. For his contribution to the advancement of knowledge in physiology and medicine, together with Paul Greengard and Eric Kandel, he was awarded the Nobel Prize in 2000.

Seeman et al., Nature (1976)

The relevance of dopaminergic mechanisms to the action of the typical neuroleptic drugs was supported by the finding that there is a strong correlation between the clinical potency of these drugs and their ability to block dopamine D_2 receptors in *in vitro* assays (see Figure 32.1). This study set out to determine whether all antipsychotic drugs, regardless of their chemical structure, would block the binding of haloperidol. This was done by testing binding of ^3H-haloperidol and ^3H-dopamine on calf and rat caudate homogenates. The results in Figure 32.1 show that there is a good correlation between the

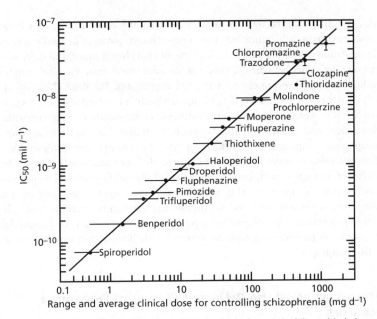

Figure 32.1 The clinical efficacy of antipsychotic drugs depends on their ability to block dopamine receptors. This graph shows the relationship between the IC_{50} values for the different antipsychotic drugs shown in blocking the binding of [³H] Haloperidol to rat striatal fractions. The abscissa indicates the average values and ranges of doses used in controlling symptoms of schizophrenia. Reprinted by permission from Macmillan Publishers Ltd: Seeman *et al.*, *Nature* (1976).

antipsychotic potencies and the IC_{50} values (the concentrations of the antipsychotic drugs which reduce the stereospecific component of ³H-haloperidol binding by 50%) for blocking the neuroleptic receptor. The assay can therefore be used to screen potentially useful antipsychotic drugs. The antipsychotic drugs also block the binding of ³H-dopamine and the IC_{50} values for this effect correlates qualitatively with the clinical antipsychotic potencies.

Johnstone et al., Lancet (1978)

Thus far most of the evidence supporting the dopamine hypothesis had been conducted in animal systems. This 1978 paper was one of the first studies testing the dopamine hypothesis as it related to human patients with acute schizophrenia. In a double-blind trial in which 45 patients with acute schizophrenia participated the cis (or alpha)-isomer of flupenthixol (which blocks the dopamine receptor) was found to be significantly more effective than both the trans (or beta)-flupenthixol (which does not block the receptor) and placebo. Before treatment started, and then weekly, the mental states of the patients were rated. The 45 patients with acute untreated schizophrenic symptoms were randomly and blindly allocated to one of three groups-one with α-flupenthixol, one with β-flupenthixol, and one with placebo. In all three groups there was a significant tendency for the patients in all three groups to improve. Even the patients in the placebo group improved, and in the first 2 weeks there was no difference at all between the patients in the three groups, but in the third and fourth weeks, the difference between α-flupenthixol and the other two groups became obvious and statistically significant. The nonspecific symptoms of depression, anxiety and retardation were never particularly severe, did not change much, and there was no significant difference between the effects of the three treatments. 'Positive' symptoms of schizophrenia were present to a marked degree, and the drug effect could be confined to the 'positive' symptoms and appeared only in the third and fourth weeks of the trial. It was as great in patients with evidence of deterioration as in patients without deterioration, and was less in patients who had affective disturbance in addition to schizophrenia symptoms. It is in the most typically schizophrenic patients that the differential effect is most obvious between the different treatments. On the basis therefore of findings from this study, we can conclude that flupenthixol is an effective 'antischizophrenic' agent and this activity can be confined to the α-isomer. These findings are consistent with the hypothesis that dopamine-receptor blockade is the only requirement for antipsychotic activity and suggests that the antipsychotic effect occurs in patients with typically schizophrenic illnesses but may be limited to positive symptoms.

Determination of the Different Classes of Dopamine Receptors
Kebabian and Greengard, Science (1971)
Kebabian et al., Proceedings of the National Academy of Sciences of the USA (1972)

Quantitative methods for measuring catecholamine activity in the striatum developed in the 1960s, and these same homogenates and membranes of striatal tissues were used to study dopaminergic receptors. Having established that the action of dopamine in the sympathetic ganglia was to elevate adenylate cyclase, Kebabian and Greengard took homogenates of the caudate nucleus of the striatum and showed that they also have adenosine $3':5'$-cyclic monophosphate (cAMP) elevated by dopamine. These stimulatory effects were inhibited by low concentrations of either chlorpromazine or haloperidol and dopamine acts to elevate cAMP. Kebabian and his colleagues first noticed in their caudate nucleus homogenates that the effects of neuroleptics on the dopamine-enhanced increase in adenylate cyclase could be divided into two classes according to their receptor–effector coupling and were designated D_1 and D_2. Subsequent studies showed that the D_1 receptors responded to dopaminergic agonists and antagonists, whereas D_2-receptors responded to phenothiazines (e.g. chlorpromazine), butyrophenones (e.g. haloperidol) and the substituted benzamides (e.g. sulpride). In the late 1980s advances in molecular biology led to the cloning of five different dopamine receptors, with additional gene variants of these five receptor subtypes being identified. Initially using an adrenergic receptor gene as a hybridization probe, related genes (including a cDNA for the D_2-receptor) were isolated and called RGB-2. Sequencing showed it to belong to the G-protein-coupled receptor family. Following this initial cloning effort, the 1990s led to the discovery of three new receptor types: D_3, D_4 and D_5. These five dopamine receptor subtypes fall into one of the two receptor classes originally defined by Kebabian and his colleagues[8]. These are referred to as D_1-like class while D_3 and D_4 receptors are similar to the dopamine D_2-like class.

Atypical Antipsychotics
Kane et al., Archives of General Psychiatry (1988)

In 1988 John Kane published a multicentre double-blind clinical trial comparing the so-called atypical antipsychotic clozapine with chlorpromazine. The efficacy of antipsychotic drugs has been extensively studied in numerous double-blind placebo-controlled trials, and despite the magnitude of the medication effect for most, as much as 10–20% of patients derive little benefit from so-called typical neuroleptic drug therapies. Furthermore, data from maintenance trials show that even amongst those patients that initially respond to an antipsychotic, 20–30% may relapse during the first year or two of maintenance drug treatment. Clozapine is a relatively weak D_2-blocker with wide ranging pharmacological effects. There is much interest in determining the mechanism of action to explain clozapine's effects in treatment-resistant patients. This has focused on developing drugs that block D_2-receptors and also block serotonin receptors (i.e. so-called atypical antipsychotics). Initially introduced many years before, clozapine had been withdrawn from use in many parts of the world in 1976 due to granulocytopenia developing in 16 patients in Finland in 1975, with 13 developing agranulocytosis and 8 dying as a result of overwhelming secondary infection. Some countries continued to allow its use for carefully selected treatment-resistant patients but have to comply with intensive precautionary monitoring of white blood cell and differential counts. The superiority of clozapine in this clinical trial was impressive in both its rigorous manner in which patients were defined and selected and because of the superiority consistently shown across a range of items on the brief psychiatric rating scale as well as the clinical global impression scale findings. Given its superiority in treating individual suffering from treatment-resistant schizophrenia, there is a need to explore the exact mechanism by which clozapine exerts its clinical effects.

A clinically efficacious antipsychotic that appeared to operate outside of the dopaminergic system was something of an anomaly and raised questions about the relevance of the dopaminergic theory.

A Revised Dopamine Theory of Schizophrenia
Kapur and Remington, American Journal of Psychiatry (1996) and Biological Psychiatry (2001)

Kapur and Remington have proposed that the antipsychotic action of clozapine and other atypical drugs does not involve serotonin or other neurotransmitter systems but only the dopamine system and D_2-receptors in particular. They proposed that the effects of these drugs are from a fast on-off of the dopamine D_2-receptor, meaning that the faster the dissociation, the fewer motor side effects that the patient will experience. This provides a revival of the dopamine hypothesis and provides a promising alternative for future drug development.

Imaging Dopamine Receptors
Laruelle, Quarterly Journal of Nuclear Medicine (1998)

Modern imaging techniques provide much promise for the future elucidation of the dopamine hypothesis. Dopamine receptor expression and action can be assessed while patients are alive using positron emission tomography, a scanning technique that uses a radiolabelled substance to produce three-dimensional images showing chemical activity in brain tissues. We are still at an early stage of applying this technology to studying schizophrenia with conflicting pioneering studies. Some have shown evidence of an excess of D_2-receptors in schizophrenia, whereas others have shown no difference between patients and controls.

Summary and Conclusions

In summary, the evidence that stimulant drugs increase levels of dopamine in the brain and induce symptoms resembling psychosis, and that patients treated with dopamine enhancing drugs, such as amphetamines, can develop psychotic symptoms resembling those of schizophrenia provides evidence for the dopamine hypothesis. Furthermore, the serendipitous discovery of antipsychotic drugs, whose binding affinity to dopamine receptors (particularly D_2) appears to correlate closely with therapeutic potency, further strengthens dopamine's role. Similarly, recent advances in schizophrenia genetics have suggested that there may be specific modifications in genes involved in dopamine function in people with schizophrenia, and further elucidation of the underlying genetic and molecular pathways will hopefully provide a rationale basis for future drug discovery.

Key Outstanding Questions

1. How do antidopaminergic drugs bring about a clinical effect over a period of weeks when their molecular actions occur in minutes?
2. Glutamate is also implicated in the pathogenesis of schizophrenia. Phenylcyclidine and ketamine both block glutamate receptors and are known to cause psychosis similar to schizophrenia. How does this tie in with the dopaminergic theory?
3. There have been multiple aetiological theories proposed for psychosis and schizophrenia over the past several years including exciting discoveries of gene mutations and structural and functional anatomical anomalies. How do these correlate with the dopamine hypothesis?

Key Research Centres

1. Professor Eve Johnstone and Professor Stephen Lawrie, Psychiatric Neuroimaging Research Group, Division of Psychiatry, University of Edinburgh, Edinburgh, United Kingdom
2. Professor Marc Laruelle, Chair in Biological Psychiatry, Division of Neurosciences & Mental Health, Imperial College London, United Kingdom
3. Professor Shitij Kapur, Professor of Schizophrenia, Institute of Psychiatry & Head of Schizophrenia, Imaging & Therapeutics, Kings College London, United Kingdom
4. Professor John Kane, Director, Psychiatric Research, Long Island Jewish-Hillside Medical Center, Glen Oaks, and Department of Psychiatry, College of Physicians & Surgeons, Columbia University, New York, United States

References

Carlsson, A., and Lindqvist, M. (1963) Effect of chlorpromazine and haloperidol on formation of 3-methoxy-tyramine and normetanephrine in mouse brain. *Acta Pharmacologica Toxicologica*, **20**, 140–144. http://www.ncbi.nlm.nih.gov/pmc/articles/PMC2655089/

Connell, P.H. (1958) *Amphetamine psychosis*. Maudsley Monographs. http://onlinelibrary.wiley.com/doi/10.1111/j.1360-0443.1990.tb00619.x/abstract

Delay, J., and Deniker, P. (1952) Le traitement des psychoses par une méthode neuroleptique dérivée de l'hibernothérapie. In: *Congres de Médicins Aliénistes et Neurologistes de France*, ed. P. Cossa. Maisson Editeurs Libraires de L'Académie de Médicine, Paris, 497–502.

Griffith, J.D., *et al.* (1970) Experimental psychosis induced by the administration of d-amphetamine. In: *Amphetamine and related compounds*, ed. E. Costa and S. Garattini. Raven Press, New York, 897–904.

Hornykiewicz, O. (1973) Dopamine in the basal ganglia: its role and thereapeutic implications (including the clinical use of L-DOPA). *British Medical Bulletin*, **29**, 172–178. http://bmb.oxfordjournals.org/content/29/2/172.long

Johnstone, E.C., *et al.* (1978) Mechanism of the antipsychotic effect in the treatment of acute schizophrenia. *Lancet*, 848–851. http://www.thelancet.com/journals/lancet/article/PIIS0140-6736%2878%2990193-9/Abstract

Kane, J., *et al.* (1988) Clozapine for the treatment-resistant schizophrenic: a double-blind comparison with chlorpromazine. *Archives of General Psychiatry*, **45**, 789–796. http://archpsyc.amaassn.org/cgi/content/abstract/45/9/789

Kapur, S., and Remington, G. (1996) Serotonin-dopamine interaction and its relevance to schizophrenia. *American Journal of Psychiatry*, **153**, 466–476. http://ajp.psychiatryonline.org/cgi/content/abstract/153/4/466

Kapur, S., and Remington, G. (2001) Dopamine D(2) receptors and their role in atypical antipsychotic action: still necessary and may even be sufficient. *Biological Psychiatry*, **50**, 873–883 http://www.biologicalpsychiatryjournal.com/article/S0006-3223%2801%2901251-3/abstract

Kebabian, J.W., and Greengard, P. (1971) Dopamine-sensitive adenyl cyclase: possible role in synaptic transmission. *Science*, **174**, 1346–1349. http://www.sciencemag.org/content/174/4016/1346.abstract

Kebabian, J.W., *et al.* (1972) Dopamine-sensitive adenylate cyclase in caudate nucleus of rat, and its similarity to the 'dopamine receptor'. *Proceedings of the National Academy of Sciences of the USA*, **69**, 2145–2149. http://www.ncbi.nlm.nih.gov/pmc/articles/PMC426888/

Laruelle, M. (1998) Imaging dopamine transmission in schizophrenia. A review and meta-analysis. *Quarterly Journal of Nuclear Medicine*, **42**, 211–221. http://www.minervamedica.it/en/journals/nuclear–med-molecular-imaging/article.php?cod¥R39Y1998N03A0211

Seeman, P., *et al.* (1976) Antipsychotic drug doses and neuroleptic/dopamine receptors. *Nature*, **261**, 717–719. http://www.nature.com/nature/journal/v261/n5562/abs/261717a0.html

Additional References

1. Tatetsu, S. (1972) Metamphetamine psychosis. In: *Current concepts of amphetamine abuse*, ed. E.H. Elinwood. NIMH, Rockville, MD.

2. Angrist, B.M., and Gershon, S. (1970) The phenomenology of experimentally induced amphetamine psychosis: preliminary observations. *Biological Psychiatry*, **2**, 95–107.

3. Kokkinidis, L., and Anisman, H. (1981) Amphetamine psychosis and schizophrenia – a dual model. *Neuroscience and Behavior Review*, **5**(4), 449–461.

4. Laborit, H., *et al.* (1952) Un nouveau stabilisateur végétatif (LE4560 RP). *Presse Médecin*, **60**, 206–208.

5. Jansen, P. (1970) The butyrophenone story. In: *Discoveries in biological psychiatry*, ed. F.J. Ayd and B. Blackwell. Lippincott, Philadelphia.

6. Divrey, P., *et al.* (1959) Étude et expérimentation cliniques du R 1625 ou haloperidol, nouveau neuroleptique et 'neurodystleptique'. *Acta Neurologica Psychologica (Belg)*, **59**, 337–367.

7. Anden, N.E., *et al.* (1964) Effects of chlorpromazine and haloperidol and reserpine on the levels of phenolic acids in rabbit corpus striatum. *Life Science*, **3**, 149–158.

8. Kebabian, J.W., and Calne, D.B. (1979) Multiple receptors for dopamine. *Nature*, **277**,

33 Alzheimer's Disease

Gordon Wilcock[1] and Alistair Burns[2]

[1]Dementia Clinical Research Group, Experimental Medicine Division, University of Oxford, Oxford, UK
[2]Department of Old Age Psychiatry, School of Medicine, University of Manchester, Manchester, UK

Introduction

It is now well known that Alzheimer's disease (AD) is the most common cause of dementia, irrespective of the age of the person affected. However, until 40 years ago this condition was associated only with early-onset disease (i.e. in those aged 65 years or younger). Dementia in older people was thought by many to be a part of ageing, or due to 'arteriosclerosis', or both.

This chapter charts the development of the conceptual changes in our knowledge of AD, including those that have paved the way for the development of therapeutic strategies.

Our choice of studies reflects some of the key developments in dementia over the past 30 years: the pathological basis of Alzheimer's disease, the treatments based on those brain changes, the rich panoply of symptomatology of the expression of dementia and the ways the condition is diagnosed. The ten chosen either are landmark papers or represent developments in important conceptual fields. They are necessarily a personal choice, and although we have also pointed the reader in the direction of others when discussing the chosen ten, there are many omissions that some will feel important.

Alzheimer's Original Description of the Disease
Alzheimer, Allg. Z. Psychiat. Psych. Gerichtl. Med. (1907; English reprint, 1995)

Alois Alzheimer first described the disease that is named after him at a meeting of the South West German Psychiatrists in Tübingen in 1906, a year before his findings were published. Although the pathological description is attributed to Alzheimer, he worked very closely with Emil Kraepelin who named the condition after Alzheimer in his psychiatric textbook which was published in 1910. The original paper briefly describes his findings. He followed this with a more lengthy description of such cases in 1911, with the emphasis suggesting that senile dementia could also occur in people who were young.

Alzheimer's first case was actually that of a 51-year-old woman. Her first symptom was not memory loss but rather paranoid jealousy of her husband, which was soon followed by a relatively rapid loss of memory, and she became disorientated in her home, hid things and also had other paranoid delusions. After being committed to an institution

Understanding Medical Research: The Studies that Shaped Medicine, First Edition. Edited by John A. Goodfellow. © 2012 John Wiley & Sons, Ltd. Published 2012 by John Wiley & Sons, Ltd.

she became completely disoriented in time and space, was unable to understand things people said to her and also failed to recognise who people were. Her memory was seriously impaired, and she had difficulty reading and writing, and also developed dyspraxia. Eventually she became bedridden and developed the consequences of this. He described increasing 'imbecility' as the disease progressed until her death $4^1/_2$ years after onset.

The autopsy showed generalised atrophic changes with some 'arteriosclerotic changes in the larger vascular tissues'. He described the now well-known neurofibrillary tangle pathology and also what he called 'minute miliary foci caused by the deposition of a special substance in the cortex'. This refers to the amyloid plaque deposition. He also describes glial changes and some abnormalities of the blood vessels.

Interestingly this patient is different to the majority of people that we see these days with dementia caused by Alzheimer's disease. She was very much younger and some of the initial symptoms are not those that are usually associated with the condition in older people (e.g. the very marked behavioural changes and paranoid delusions that were the first symptoms).

For many years Alzheimer's name was associated only with cases of presenile dementia. It wasn't until the work of Tomlinson and others[1] that it became generally accepted that the pathology of Alzheimer's disease was the most common finding in the brains of older people who became demented, and it is this latter group that make up the majority of Alzheimer's disease cases. It therefore took more than 70 years for the importance of Alzheimer's original findings to be realised, and to act as a foundation for the explosion of research into Alzheimer's disease and the dementias that we have all been aware of over the last 30 years.

Loss of Subcortical Neurones from the Basal Nucleus of Meynert
Whitehouse et al., Annals of Neurology (1981)

It was known that there was a variable reduction in the number of cortical neurones in Alzheimer's patients and also of cholinergic markers. Whitehouse's work related this to a loss of subcortical projection neurones synapsing with neocortical neurones.

The literature at that time indicated that the main source of extrinsic cholinergic input to the neocortex was the basal nucleus of Meynert which projected diffusely to neocortical structures. It is part of a continuous band of cells that includes the diagonal band of Broca and the septal nuclei, and together they are responsible for cholinergic projections to many relevant structures including the hippocampus and cortex. Animal research had shown that destruction of this nucleus resulted in a selective reduction in cholinergic presynaptic neocortical markers. Whitehouse and his co-workers were the first to follow this up in AD and examined the basal forebrain in a 75-year-old Caucasian male with a diagnosis of Alzheimer's disease, comparing their findings with a control case. The difference between the two was striking with a 90% loss of large cholinergic neurones from the basal nucleus in their index case. In addition, they reported AD-type neurofibrillary tangles in cells in this nucleus. Their work was subsequently verified in numerous studies on larger numbers of subjects and is widely accepted as evidence of malfunction of a system, possibly starting with subcortical pathology, rather than just malfunction of a cortical neurotransmitter.

These findings supported the cholinergic hypothesis and the possible role of the cholinergic system as a target for therapeutic strategies. It was subsequently demonstrated that the cholinergic neurones in the basal nucleus were influenced by neurotrophic factors such as nerve growth factor (NGF). This in turn led to another therapeutic strategy, albeit in its early stages, involving the possibility of supporting the neurones in the basal nucleus using neurotrophic substances, such as recombinant human NGF. Delivering NGF itself to the brain is complicated because it would have to cross the blood–brain barrier and if given orally would also need to survive degradation in the gastrointestinal tract. Until now, proof of concept studies of this have used neurosurgical procedures; either implanting catheters that deliver NGF directly to the basal nucleus or implanting fibroblasts that have been genetically modified to produce it.

Preliminary evidence from animal research and these early trials with a small number of AD patients are stimulating further development of this approach and a search for molecules with NGF like activity that could be administered by less invasive routes. Thus Whitehouse's work has not only underpinned the cholinergic hypothesis and the resulting symptomatic pharmacological developments, but also suggested a more fundamental disease modifying strategy.

The Relationship between the Pathology of Alzheimer's Disease and the Clinical Syndrome
Wilcock and Esiri, Journal of Neurological Science (1982)

A series of comprehensive studies in Newcastle, United Kingdom in the 1960s[1,2] showed that there was a correlation between the number of amyloid plaques (derived from a standardised count in 12 areas of the cerebral cortex) and the severity of dementia as assessed on a clinical rating scale. While the number of tangles had been noted, and it was observed that they were increased in number in people with dementia compared to normal controls, they were not studied in detail and not specifically related to the clinical symptomatology.

Gordon Wilcock and Margaret Esiri examined 59 patients who had been admitted to hospitals in Oxford and who had come to them post mortem, a partnership which emphasizes the utility of a true and meaningful collaboration between clinicians and neuropathologists. Clinically, 14 of the patients were free of dementia, 35 had Alzheimer's disease and 10 had a mixture of cerebrovascular disease and Alzheimer's disease. The group, importantly, had been assessed in the 3-month period before death and allocated a score according to the stage of dementia as well as two specific neuropsychological tests. In people with a clinical diagnosis of Alzheimer's disease, a highly significant correlation was present between the severity of dementia and the number of tangles in the cerebral cortex, but a less statistically significant and somewhat inconsistent correlation was found between the clinical syndrome of dementia and the number of amyloid plaques. The temporal lobe and hippocampus were the areas most severely affected.

The tension between complementary neuropathological views of dementia has been around for some time with supporters of amyloid as the fundamental feature of Alzheimer's disease and those arguing that tangles are at least as important. Interestingly, a third hypothesis has arisen more recently suggesting that synaptic loss is the primary clinical pathological correlate of significance in dementia. Current treatments based on deficits in the acetylcholine system in the brain could be related to either and represent a downstream effect of the main core pathological process.

The conclusion of the Wilcock and Esiri paper is that tangle counts provide a more reliable measure of the presence of and severity of dementia due to Alzheimer's disease, but that this is lessened when there is significant cerebrovascular disease. Recent studies such as the Nun Study[3] have shown that the pathological underpinning of the syndrome of dementia is a complex one, with significant plaques and tangles being found in people without the clinical syndrome of dementia. Furthermore vascular disease has an additive value on underlying Alzheimer's pathology, increasing the likelihood of dementia. Wilcock and Esiri's early paper was a refreshing and insightful contribution to the clinco-pathological debate which has raged for some years. This will continue, fuelled by the recent lack of success of anti-amyloid agents on the symptoms of people with dementia.

Standardising Diagnostic Criteria for Research Studies
McKhann et al., Neurology (1984)

There was a pressing need in the early 1980s for a set of clinical diagnostic criteria which predicted the presence of Alzheimer's disease pathology. The National Institute of Neurological and Communicative Disorders and Stroke and the Alzheimer's Disease and Related Disorders Association (NINCDS/ADRDA) established a group looking at the need to refine the extant diagnostic criteria. Twenty percent or more of people with a clinical diagnosis of Alzheimer's disease were found post mortem to have other conditions, and it was argued that if the results of clinical trials were to be interpreted in a meaningful way, then having accurate diagnostic criteria available was important. The procedure which was followed is an exemplar of how such diagnostic criteria should be developed: subgroups addressed individual topics such as medical history, clinical examination, neuropsychological testing and laboratory assessments, and then the report was discussed and debated in plenary session. It was important that the criteria were consistent with those clinical sets of criteria which were available in the US *Diagnostic and Statistical Manual* and the European *International Classification in Diseases.*

What followed must be one of the most quoted papers in the literature in dementia. The criteria were neatly divided into three. Firstly were those for 'probable' Alzheimer's disease which included 'supportive criteria' (such as gradual onset and gradual progression), and others that would make the diagnosis unlikely (e.g. evidence of cerebrovascular disease). Secondly were criteria for 'possible' Alzheimer's disease (meaning there was no doubt that dementia existed; the debate referred to the extent of the contribution of a second systemic or brain disorder which might give rise to similar symptoms). Thirdly were criteria for 'definite' AD (requiring both clinical and histopathological evidence). There was also a section describing the clinical information needed to carry out a research programme.

The NINCDS–ADRDA criteria have been the mainstay of the diagnosis of Alzheimer's disease for research studies for 25 years. Their success can be partly attributed to their role in setting down research and diagnostic criteria which were easy to follow and based in clinical practice. They did not suggest any assessments or tests that were not generally available in practice or which were not undertaken routinely for investigation of people with dementia. They quickly became the gold standard as their strength was a very high specificity for the diagnosis of Alzheimer's disease, in other words, one could be very sure that if someone satisfied the criteria they had Alzheimer's disease. However, there would be people with Alzheimer's disease who did not meet the criteria, exactly what is needed for research studies as opposed to clinical practice.

Revising the NINCDS–ADRDA Criteria
Dubois et al., Lancet Neurology (2007)

The 1984 criteria stood the test of time until 2007 when an authoritative revision was published. There was a sense that the NINCDS-ADRDA criteria had fallen behind the huge growth in scientific knowledge of Alzheimer's disease over the preceding 25 years. In particular, more accurate and sophisticated imaging techniques had become available and were being validated, including structural MRI, and also functional and molecular imaging using positron emission tomography. Biochemical analysis of cerebrospinal fluid was similarly yielding increasingly positive results.

In addition, the concept of Alzheimer's disease was being broadened to encompass the recognised prodromata of dementia, for example possible pre-dementia AD, such as mild cognitive impairment (MCI). Research diagnostic criteria for other disorders causing dementia were also recently developed such as those for vascular dementia[4,5] and dementia with Lewy bodies[6]. Since 1984 knowledge of the neuropsychological findings in Alzheimer's disease had also moved on, for example the diagnostic relevance of episodic memory as a core clinical feature of the amnesia.

Dubois and colleagues proposed that the majority of the criteria continued to be firmly based in the common experience of clinical practice but emphasised that there should now be at least one or more abnormal biomarkers present such as structural MRI, molecular imaging or cerebrospinal fluid analysis of the levels of amyloid peptides (the core of the senile plaque) or tau (a protein associated with neurofibrillary tangles).

Some related concepts were introduced and defined in the suggested revision. These included (1) MCI, where there are subjective complaints of memory problems or other cognitive symptoms and objective evidence of deficits in either, but with generally preserved activities of daily living in people who do not meet the diagnostic criteria for dementia; (2) amnestic MCI (the same but more specific and focusing only on amnesia); (3) preclinical Alzheimer's disease (the long asymptomatic period between the first brain lesions and the first appearance of symptoms); (4) prodromal Alzheimer's disease (the symptomatic predementia phase of Alzheimer's disease); and (5) Alzheimer's disease dementia itself (i.e. that which we all recognise when Alzheimer's disease becomes symptomatic).

A designation of possible Alzheimer's disease was not included because it was felt that the new diagnostic criteria would be sufficiently specific for this not to be needed. The criteria for definite Alzheimer's disease included the presence of the clinical criteria plus the histological changes of Alzheimer's disease in the brain or genetic evidence of a mutation on chromosome 1, 14 or 21. The core clinical criteria were the same. It may well be another 20 years or so before these diagnostic criteria are updated again depending on how well they stand up to evaluation.

The Symptoms of Alzheimer's Disease
Burns et al., British Journal of Psychiatry (1990)

The presentation of dementia can be described in three areas; a neuropsychological component (essentially loss of memory and problems with language), an activities of daily living domain (where these are impaired in the early stages of dementia, so-called instrumental activities of daily living, or in the later stage where things like washing and dressing are impaired, designated basic activities of daily living) and behavioural and psychological symptoms. The last category consists of a variety of psychiatric symptoms (such as depression, delusions and misidentifications and hallucinations) and behavioural disturbances (such as agitation, aggression and wandering). Alzheimer's first description included a vivid vignette of behavioural disturbance, but for many years it was considered that it was the neuropsychological component which was the only defining feature of the syndrome of dementia. The other components were considered secondary, in fact almost epiphenomena, and therefore of less importance. However, there began a realisation in the 1980s that these other features were very prominent and, in terms of distress for patients and carers, were often much more important than loss of memory.

In a series of four interlinked papers, Burns and colleagues described these phenomena in a sample of 178 patients with Alzheimer's disease. This was a simple descriptive study without an elaborate methodology. The main finding was that symptoms were much more common than had previously been thought. For example; 1 in 5 had had persecutory delusions since the onset of the illness; about 1 in 10 had experienced either visual or auditory hallucinations; nearly two thirds of the group had at least one symptom of depression; and a quarter satisfied diagnostic criteria for depression. Finally, aggression and wandering were present in 1 in 5; urinary incontinence in half; and binge eating, hyperorality and sexual disinhibition in a little under 10%.

While no standard instrument was available to assess these features (one, the Mousepad[7], was developed later), this series of the four papers underscored the importance of these symptoms in people with dementia and suggested, probably for the first time, that they were not merely epiphenomena.

Cholinesterase Inhibitors as Treatment for AD
Summers et al., New England Journal of Medicine (1986)
Kaduszkiewicz et al., British Medical Journal (2005)

There was considerable research activity in the 1990s to evaluate cholinesterase inhibitors. The first was Tacrine which was originally developed as an antidelirium agent to be given intravenously in people in emergency rooms in the United States. This led to the first trial which suggested it might be beneficial in people with Alzheimer's disease. Tacrine had serious liver side effects and tolerability problems, and so the development of the next three cholinesterase inhibitors was awaited with interest: Donepezil (Aricept), Rivastigmine (Exelon) and Galantamine (Reminyl). These were introduced and accepted by the National Institute for Health and Clinical Excellence (NICE)[8] as being suitable for prescription on the National Health Service in the United Kingdom for people with mild to moderate Alzheimer's disease. Although now accepted as effective, their benefits are modest and their introduction was associated with a degree of controversy.

NICE, while approving them originally in 2001, routinely re-reviewed them in 2005, and their initial response on this occasion was that none should be available on the National Health Service because of a lack of cost-effectiveness. This led to a fierce public campaign by the medical profession, the Alzheimer's Society and the pharmaceutical industry, resulting in a revised decision (i.e. that they could be prescribed in people with moderate, but not mild, Alzheimer's disease). Whereas the general view was that the medications were modestly to moderately effective, there remained a lot of scepticism, from NICE and others, as to their exact role.

The systematic review from Kaduszkiewicz and colleagues was published at a crucial time in 2005: it aimed to assess the scientific evidence justifying the prescription of these agents, and the authors found 22 trials which met the inclusion criteria. The majority of studies showed positive results in terms of cognition (the Alzheimer's Disease Assessment Scale being the most commonly used instrument) with differences of between 1.5 and 5.9 points in favour of the drugs. Benefits were reported from the Clinicians Interview Based Impression of Change scale. This is a global scale indicating whether the patient has improved, stayed the same, or deteriorated since the beginning of treatment. The scales were introduced to reflect the totality of symptoms of dementia described above. Significant methodological problems were found in the studies, such as multiple testing without correction for multiplicity of outcome measures or exclusion of patients after randomisation. The overall conclusion was that because of the flawed methods and small clinical benefits, the scientific basis for the recommendation of the cholinesterase drugs in people with Alzheimer's disease was questionable. Although other systematic reviews have been undertaken and, generally speaking, the benefits of the medications are not in doubt[9-11], the paper was important because it set down in a dispassionate way many of the methodological flaws occurring in trials of medication for patients with Alzheimer's disease and called into question the received wisdom that they should be fully prescribed.

The Possible Central Role of 'Amyloid'
Goate et al., Nature (1991)
Goate's paper stimulated a great explosion of interest in attempts to modify the underlying pathology of Alzheimer's disease in the hope of developing a treatment, or even a 'cure'. This was the first objective evidence that an abnormality in the amyloid precursor protein (APP) was associated with AD. This work, led by John Hardy, explored the relationship between mutations in the APP gene and Alzheimer's disease based upon the knowledge that some families with early-onset AD showed a linkage to chromosome 21 markers. The APP gene was known to be situated on chromosome 21, and the concept was further supported by the finding of Alzheimer-type pathology in the brains of people with Down's syndrome (trisomy 21).

Goate and colleagues reported, in a specific family kindred with early-onset AD, linkage to a point mutation in the APP gene which resulted in an amino-acid substitution (Val Ile) close to the carboxy terminus of the β-amyloid peptide. They found a second unrelated family with the same variant suggesting that in some cases Alzheimer's disease was probably caused by a mutation in the APP gene. This led to increasing interest in the possible genetic background to familial cases, mainly in younger families, with the expectation that such knowledge would unravel pathological processes that may also be happening in the brain in older people, even though there was not the same genetic linkage.

Subsequent research led to the concept of the 'amyloid cascade hypothesis' placing the development of amyloid in the brain at the beginning of a long cascade of events contributing to the development of Alzheimer's disease. Equally importantly, it paved the way for animal models in which the pathology was reproduced in transgenic mice. Although often described as animal models of Alzheimer's disease, one has to remember that in fact these are mostly models of amyloid production and have little other AD pathology in their brain. Nevertheless they acted as a useful workbench for developing anti-amyloid strategies that were then transferable to the clinical arena for evaluation.

The amyloid cascade hypothesis tended to divert interest away from the role of neurofibrillary tangles and other potential pathology. Tangles represent a disruption of normal cytoskeleton and internal transport systems secondary to the hyper-phosphorylation of the protein called tau. Since neuronal death is the final cause of the development of dementia in AD, the tangles could be conceived as of equal importance as a possible final common pathway. However, their intracellular location made attempts to explore their therapeutic potential more difficult, but this is now being addressed.

Risk Factor Genes for Alzheimer's Disease: APOE 4
Saunders et al., Neurology (1993)

Apolipoproteins are proteins that bind to lipids. One of these, apolipoprotein E (APOE), involved the first susceptibility polymorphism for Alzheimer's disease. There are three APOE alleles (2, 3 and 4) universally distributed in the population, and APOE 4 was the first risk factor gene identified for late-onset Alzheimer's disease. This potential linkage was explored because of the high rate of specific binding of amyloid beta peptide and APOE protein noted in AD. Initially the hypothesis was tested in late onset familial cases, but Saunders and colleagues extended their studies to several series of sporadic Alzheimer's disease patients and found that the APOE 4 allele was also significantly associated with sporadic AD. The other alleles are associated with a lesser risk, and it is possible that 2 may be 'protective'.

In a separate study, Corder and coworkers[12] showed that the risk of developing Alzheimer's disease increased fourfold, from 20% to 90%, with an increase in the number of APOE 4 alleles, and that the age of onset decreased from 84 to 68 years. Their work has subsequently been confirmed many times and it has become quite clear that the APOE 4 gene dose is a significant risk factor.

The existence of a susceptibility gene for the clinical expression of AD type dementia led to the search for others. A significant number of other risk factor genes have been identified, but none with such a strong association as APOE 4. It is important to remember, however, that not all people who develop Alzheimer's disease possess an APOE 4 allele and that many people who possess this allele do not develop dementia. It therefore must interact with other factors, rather than being simply causal.

Time to Reconsider the Amyloid Cascade Hypothesis? Amyloid Removal from the Brain Does Not Benefit AD Sufferers
Holmes et al., Lancet (2008)

Animal studies showed that innoculating transgenic mice with Aβ peptide resulted in an antibody response to the peptide that cleared the amyloid out of the brain. Based on this finding, a phase 1 clinical trial was established in Alzheimer's disease sufferers using a synthetic Aβ peptide with an adjuvant. This failed to show convincing clinical benefit even in those who responded by producing an adequate antibody level. Most importantly a small number of subjects from this trial came to autopsy, and it was confirmed that their brains contained significantly less amyloid than those of control subjects, similar to the findings in the transgenic mouse model. Showing that clearance of amyloid was associated with little benefit to the patients is disappointing, and one of the most important findings in this area. This picture could be interpreted as indicating that the anti-amyloid strategies are misconceived, or alternatively that the clinical trial methodology is not yet adequate or that treatment is being administered too late in the disease.

Further evaluation of the immunotherapeutic approach is underway, and recently a phase 2 trial using a synthetic monoclonal antibody against amyloid was reported. The overall results were also disappointing, but there was a suggestion that subjects who did not carry an APOE 4 allele were more likely to respond. This differential response requires further evaluation.

The central role of the amyloid cascade hypothesis as a target for treatment is therefore now being reconsidered but not as yet abandoned. It is possible that other approaches, such as modulation or prevention of amyloid deposition, may be therapeutically beneficial in Alzheimer's disease. A number of what initially seemed to be promising therapeutic strategies have similarly been unsuccessful when translated into the clinical environment. These have included attempts with a compound called tramiprosate to prevent amyloid beta peptide from aggregating into the fibrils, thus possibly preventing plaque deposition, and strategies to reduce amyloid beta peptide production. These use drugs that reduce amyloid beta peptide formation by the abnormal cleavage of the amyloid precursor protein molecule that occurs in AD. This is controlled by three enzyme systems known as the alpha-secretase, beta-secretase and gamma-secretase pathways.

Alpha-secretase cleavage is part of the normal processing of APP, but beta- and gamma-secretase cleavage results in the formation of the 42 amino acid Aβ peptide: the foundation of β-amyloid production. Inhibitors of gamma-secretase and modulators of this enzyme system have been developed. One example is Tarenflurbil which initially seemed to be promising at a Phase 2 clinical trial level but was disappointing when evaluated in a definitive Phase 3 trial programme[13]. Similar strategies, e.g. beta-secretase inhibitors, are still under development and evaluation.

Key Outstanding Questions

1. Will anti-amyloid strategies prove to be effective therapies?
2. Is prevention/reduction of neurofibrillary tangle formation feasible and effective?
3. Can we achieve earlier, pre-symptomatic, diagnosis of dementia? Is there a biomarker to aid this?
4. Are there any lifestyle modifications that will delay or prevent dementia?

Key Research Centres

There are too many major research centres contributing to Alzheimer's disease research, and it would be invidious to 'pick out' a few. We have therefore listed four major internet links that will provide a wealth of information and also links to current research.

Alzheimer's Research Forum, an international online research database that updates weekly: http://www.alzforum.org

Alzheimer's Research Trust: http://www.alzheimers-research.org.uk

DeNDRoN – the UK Dementias and Neurodegenerative Diseases Research Network: http://www.dendron.org.uk

UK Alzheimer's Society: http://alzheimers.org.uk

References

Alzheimer, A. (1907) Uber einen eigenartige Erkrankung der Hirnrinde. *Allg. Z. für Psychiat. Psych. Gerichtl. Med.*, **64**, 146–148. (For translation, see Stelzmann, R.A., *et al.* (1995) An English translation of Alzheimer's 1907 paper, 'Uber einen eigenartige Erkrankung der Hirnrinde' *Clinical Anatomy*, **8**, 329–431. http://onlinelibrary.wiley.com/doi/10.1002/ca.980080612/abstract)

Burns, A., *et al.* (1990) Psychiatric phenomena in Alzheimer's disease. I–IV: disorders of thought content, perception, mood, behaviour. *British Journal of Psychiatry*, **157**, 72–94. http://bjp.rcpsych.org/cgi/content/abstract/157/1/72

Dubois, B., *et al.* (2007) Research criteria for the diagnosis of Alzheimer's disease: revising the NINCDS–ADRDA criteria. *Lancet Neurology*, **6**(8), 734–746. http://www.ncbi.nlm.nih.gov/pubmed/17616482

Goate, A., *et al.* (1991) Segregation of a missense mutation in the amyloid precursor protein gene with familial Alzheimer's disease. *Nature*, **349**, 704–706. http://www.ncbi.nlm.nih.gov/pubmed/1671712

Holmes, C., *et al.* (2008) Long-term effects of $A\beta_{42}$ immunisation in Alzheimer's disease: follow-up of a randomised, placebo-controlled phase 1 trial. *Lancet*, **372**, 216–223. http://www.ncbi.nlm.nih.gov/pubmed/18640458

Kaduszkiewicz, H., *et al.* (2005) Cholinesterase inhibitors for patients with Alzheimer's disease: systematic review of randomised clinical trials. *British Medical Journal*, **331**, 321–327. http://www.ncbi.nlm.nih.gov/pubmed/16081444

McKhann, G., *et al.* (1984) Clinical diagnosis of Alzheimer's disease: report of the NINCDS–ADRDA Work Group under the auspices of Department of Health and Human Services Task Force on Alzheimer's Disease. *Neurology*, **34**(7), 939–944. http://www.neurology.org/content/34/7/939.abstract

Saunders, A.M., *et al.* (1993) Association of apolipoprotein E allele epsilon 4 with late-onset familial and sporadic Alzheimer's disease. *Neurology*, **43**, 1467–1472. http://www.neurology.org/content/43/8/1467.abstract

Summers, W.K., *et al.* (1986) Oral tetrahydroaminoacridine in long-term treatment of senile dementia, Alzheimer type. *New England Journal of Medicine*, **20**(315), 1241–1245. http://www.ncbi.nlm.nih.gov/pubmed/2430180

Whitehouse, P.J., *et al.* (1981) Alzheimer disease: evidence for selective loss of cholinergic neurons in the nucleus basalis. *Annals of Neurology*, **10**, 122–1226. http://onlinelibrary.wiley.com/doi/10.1002/ana.410100203/abstract

Wilcock, G.K., and Esiri, M.M. (1982) Plaques, tangles and dementia: a quantitative study. *Journal of the Neurological Sciences*, **56**, 343–356. http://www.sciencedirect.com/science/article/pii/0022510X82901551

Additional References

1. Tomlinson, B.E., *et al.* (1970) Observations on the brains of demented old people. *Journal of the Neurological Sciences*, **11**, 205–242.
2. Roth, M., *et al.* (1966) Correlation between scores for dementia and counts of 'senile plaques' in cerebral grey matter of elderly subjects. *Nature*, **209**(5018), 109–110.
3. Riley, K.P., *et al.* (2005) Early life linguistic ability, late life cognitive function, and neuropathology: findings from the Nun Study. *Neurobiology and Aging*, **3**(26), 341–347.
4. Chui, H.C., *et al.* (2000) Clinical criteria for the diagnosis of vascular dementia: a multicenter study of comparability and interrater reliability. *Archives of Neurology*, **57**, 191–196.
5. Román, G.C. (2003) Vascular dementia: distinguishing characteristics, treatment, and prevention. *Journal of the American Geriatric Society*, **51**(Suppl. 5), S296–S304.
6. McKeith, I.G. (2006) Consensus guidelines for the clinical and pathologic diagnosis of dementia with Lewy bodies (DLB), report of the Consortium on DLB International Workshop. *Journal of Alzheimer's Disease*, **9**(Suppl. 3), 417–423.
7. Allen, N.H., *et al.* (1996) Manchester and Oxford Universities Scale for the Psychopathological Assessment of Dementia (MOUSEPAD). *British Journal of Psychiatry*, **3**(169), 293–307.
8. National Institute for Health and Clinical Excellence (2005) *NICE appraisal consultation document: Donepezil, Rivastigmine, Galantamine and Memantine for the treatment of Alzheimer's disease.* NICE, London.
9. Birks, J. (2006) Cholinesterase inhibitors for Alzheimer's disease. *Cochrane Database Systematic Review*, January 25(1).
10. Birks, J., and Harvey, R.J. (2006) Donepezil for dementia due to Alzheimer's disease. *Cochrane Database Systematic Review*, January 25(1).
11. Loy, C., and Schneider, L. (2006) Galantamine for Alzheimer's disease and mild cognitive impairment. *Cochrane Database Systematic Review*, January 25(1).
12. Corder, E.H., *et al.* (1993) Gene dose of apolipoprotein E type 4 allele and the risk of Alzheimer's disease in late onset families. *Science*, **261**, 921–923.
13. Green, R.C., *et al.* for the Tarenflurbil Phase 3 Study Group. (2009) Effect of tarenflurbil on cognitive decline and activities of daily living in patients with mild Alzheimer's disease: a randomized controlled trial. *Journal of the American Medical Association*, **302**, 2557–2564.

Index

Understanding Medical Research: The Studies that Shaped Medicine, First Edition. Edited by
John A. Goodfellow. © 2012 John Wiley & Sons, Ltd. Published 2012 by John Wiley & Sons, Ltd.